Rehabilitation Medicine

THE MANAGEMENT OF PHYSICAL DISABILITIES

Second Edition

. . . that which is everybody's business is nobody's business

Izaak Walton
Compleat Angler

By the same author:
REHABILITATION OF THE SEVERELY DISABLED
Vol. 1—Evaluation of a Disabled Living Unit
Vol. 2—Management

Rehabilitation Medicine

THE MANAGEMENT OF PHYSICAL DISABILITIES
Second Edition

Edited by
P. J. R. NICHOLS
MA, DM (Oxon.), FRCP, DPhysMed (Lond.)
Director of Mary Marlborough Lodge, Disabled Living Research Unit (DHSS Demonstration Centre for Rehabilitation), Nuffield Orthopaedic Centre, Headington, Oxford, Director of the Oxford Rehabilitation Research Unit (DHSS), Nuffield Department of Orthopaedic Surgery, University of Oxford.

BUTTERWORTHS
LONDON · BOSTON
Sydney · Wellington · Durban · Toronto

First published 1976
Second edition 1980
Reprinted 1981

ISBN 0 407 00175 1

© Butterworth & Co (Publishers) Ltd 1980

British Library Cataloguing in Publication Data

Rehabilitation medicine. – 2nd ed.
  1. Physically handicapped – Rehabilitation
  I. Nicholls, Philip John Russell
  615'.8   RM930   80–4289

  ISBN 0-407-00175-1

Typeset by Scribe Design, Gillingham, Kent
Printed in England by Redwood Burn Ltd.
Trowbridge and Esher

Preface to the Second Edition

In this edition there are new chapters on head injury, spinal paralysis, the sexual problems of physically disabled people, the psychological aspects of physical disabilities, and research in rehabilitation.

The original text has been revised and updated, although some chapters required much less than others.

I am very grateful to my original collaborator, Dr Ann Hamilton, for help in the revision and for her chapter on sexual problems. I am also indebted to my friends and colleagues who have contributed chapters and those who have helped with their comments and criticisms, and in reading and revising manuscripts.

I particularly wish to thank Mrs N. Wright and Mrs E. Payne for all their hard work in typing and checking references.

P. J. R. N.

Preface to the First Edition

During the past few years, general interest in rehabilitation has been awakened and as a subject it has been seen to be one of the growing points of medicine. It is difficult to define as a subject in itself, as it is an integral part of much of clinical medicine and most of rehabilitation is applied commonsense and an understanding of people who have become ill or disabled. All clinicians should be concerned with the rehabilitation of their patients, but there are many who will not have had the opportunity as students, nor in their post-graduate years, to develop an understanding of the wider aspects of patient care called 'rehabilitation'. This book is an attempt to describe the 'rehabilitation approach' to common clinical problems and to describe the contribution of the physiotherapist and occupational therapist to the management of these patients.

Perhaps an apposite title would be *The Management of the Moderately Disabled*, indicating its place as a companion volume to *Rehabilitation of the Severely Disabled*.

The secret of rehabilitation is the giving of the right help at the right time. The help needed may be simple advice or reassurance, or it may be intensive physiotherapy, or it may be the supply of a complex appliance and training in its use, or it may be vocational guidance and retraining.

This book is written for all those who have an interest in their patients beyond the immediate problems of diagnosis and therapeutics. It is hoped that general practitioners in particular will find it of interest and value for they must often be the co-ordinators of the health and care services, and many patients needing rehabilitation are never referred to hospital.

Above all, we hope that this book will convince its reader of the need for integration between hospital and community services if rehabilitation is going to become a reality for those who need it.

In order to avoid a lot of repetition, we have used rheumatoid arthritis as a model to describe the 'totality' of the rehabilitation approach. In the chapter on rheumatoid arthritis we have described in considerable detail the procedures and advice relating to domestic arrangement and activities of daily living. A similar amount of detail would have been appropriate in other chapters but would have involved unnecessary repetition. Readers are therefore asked to refer back to the chapter on rheumatoid arthritis when considering other disabilities, for the details of advice are appropriate whatever the physical disability.

P. J. R. N.
E. A. H.

Acknowledgements

We would like to express our sincere gratitude to all who have helped by sharing their knowledge and experiences of rehabilitation with us. Our views and attitudes are continually changing under the influence of our colleagues through the patients they refer to us, by consultations, by case conferences and by private discussions. In this sense we owe a considerable debt of gratitude to all the medical staff of the Nuffield Orthopaedic Centre and the Nuffield Department of Orthopaedic Surgery, and in particular Dr A. G. Mowat.

We are also indebted to Dr D.J. Lane and Dr W.S. Hamilton of the Chest Clinic, Churchill Hospital for help with the chapter on chronic bronchitis.

Dr E. Williams read the manuscript and contributed many helpful suggestions which have been incorporated.

We would like to pay tribute to Mrs C. Newman, Mrs E. Payne and Mrs N. Wright who undertook the typing.

Contributors

E. A. HAMILTON
MA, BM, BCh, MRCP, DPhysMed,
Mary Marlborough Lodge, Nuffield Orthopaedic Centre, Headington, Oxford
Assistant Medical Officer, Oxford Artificial Limb and Appliance Centre, Nuffield
Orthopaedic Centre, Headington, Oxford.
Rivermead Rehabilitation Centre, Oxford.

B. L. HAZLEMAN
MB, MRCP,
Consultant Rheumatologist, Addenbrookes Hospital, Cambridge

P. R. MARTIN
BSc, DipPsych, DPhil,
Research Clinical Psychologist, Oxford Rehabilitation Research Unit, Nuffield
Department of Orthopaedic Surgery, University of Oxford.

M. J. ROSE
FRCS,
Clinical Lecturer, Oxford Rehabilitation Research Unit, Nuffield Department of
Orthopaedic Surgery, University of Oxford

J. R. SILVER
MB, BS, MRCP(Ed),
Consultant in Spinal Injuries, National Spinal Injuries Centre, Stoke Mandeville
Hospital, Aylesbury, Buckinghamshire

C. B. WYNN PARRY
MBE, MA, DM, FRCP, FRCS,
Consultant in Rheumatology and Director of Rehabilitation, Royal National
Orthopaedic Hospital, Stanmore, Middlesex

Contents

1 Organization of Rehabilitation Services

INTRODUCTION

In the early years of this century, the spa towns were centres for much of the physical treatment used in the management of patients. They specialized for the most part in the treatment of 'rheumatism' and other medical disorders of the locomotor system. In addition to hydrotherapy (or balneotherapy) the physical treatments employed included electrotherapy (heat, light and electrical stimulation), movements, manipulation and massage. In 1931, the Section of Balneology and Climatology of the Royal Society of Medicine fused with the Section of Electrotherapeutics and formed the Section of Physical Medicine, and the speciality of 'Physical Medicine' was created.

The majority of patients for whom physical treatment is prescribed are those suffering from 'rheumatic conditions' which are subject to natural remissions and exacerbations. The response to treatment will depend on the patient's motivation as well as the personality of the therapist.

Thus, the scientific evaluation of physical therapy is very difficult, and much physical therapy remains empirical in nature and unproven in value.

Partly because of the inexactness of diagnosis and treatment, and partly because physical therapy is only a part of the total management of patients, the term 'physical medicine' has fallen into disrepute. 'Rheumatology' has emerged as a clinical specialty with close links to General (Internal) Medicine. _Rehabilitation_ is an appropriate term to embrace the many physical, social and organizational aspects of the after-care of most patients who require more than acute, short-term definitive care.

REHABILITATION

Principles
Although the term 'rehabilitation' has taken on many different meanings, in its widest sense it 'signifies the whole process of restoring a disabled person to a condition in which he is able, as early as possible, to resume a normal life'.*

*From Report of the Committee of Enquiry on the Rehabilitation, Training and Resettlement of Disabled Persons (1956), par. 5. Chaired by the Rt. Hon. Lord Piercy, Cmd. 987. London; HMSO.

There can therefore be no doubt that it is the concern of all clinicians but with a differing emphasis in different specialties.

There is a relative lack of interest among the medical professions in the problems of convalescence. Publications on the subject are scanty, little research has been undertaken, and little attention has been devoted to the medical aspects of recovery. The main interests of clinicians often lie only in diagnosis and acute definitive treatment. The doctor's role in the convalescent period is often considered of minimal importance, and the patient's attitude during the period is traditionally passive.

Rehabilitation is 'creative convalescence', and as such, represents that active contribution made by medical, paramedical staff and patient to the restoration of health during the recovery phase which follows the intensive definitive treatment.

The rehabilitation principles laid down by Robert Jones in his 'curative workshops' during the First World War were not widely taken up during the 20 years of peace, but in the Second World War, specialists of various clinical disciplines in the armed forces and emergency medical services combined to establish the modern approach of full-time intensive orthopaedic rehabilitation and converted 'convalescence' into 'rehabilitation'. The pattern was developed by grouping patients with similar disabilities, narrowing the remedial aims of each group, increasing the number of groups or classes and grading their activity to enable patients to make a graduated progression through the classes as functional improvement occurred. Each class had an activity programme based on a few simple, remedial exercises, e.g. 'quadriceps setting exercises' or 'walking exercises' or 'shoulder mobilizing exercises' or 'spinal extension exercises'. Management was augmented by specific physiotherapy, occupational therapy, and hydrotherapy where necessary.

Most patients admitted to hospital require little in the way of complex rehabilitation, *providing the supervising clinician clearly communicates to the patient, relatives and family doctor, the expected progress of the disease and the outcome of treatment.* The will to recover, which is inherent in most patients, is intensified where confidence in those who give medical care is shown to be justified by good treatment and manifest understanding of their problems.

Some patients, however, do benefit considerably from periods of intensive rehabilitation and a more closely supervised convalescence. Such patients need admission to a centre which is structurally and functionally orientated towards recovery; where a purposive atmosphere instils confidence; and where the individual skills of a rehabilitation team are integrated and co-ordinated to assist each patient to achieve maximal functional efficiency. Within the category of patients needing these special rehabilitation facilities are those with multiple injuries; those with complex lesions — such as crush injuries of the hands or injuries of the head or spine; and those requiring a high standard of physical fitness before return to work is possible.

The intensive full-time regime, and the later integration of retraining for work with the initial rehabilitative exercise programme are of the utmost benefit.

The majority of patients with illnesses and injuries which have had efficient primary definitive treatment can be rehabilitated within the organization of the District General Hospital as in-patients, as out-patients on a Day Hospital basis, or as residents in a hostel. With adequate rehabilitation, the incidence of prolonged morbidity can be significantly reduced, and the duration of disability can be shortened, provided patients start their planned rehabilitation soon after the onset of disability.

There is considerable evidence that delay in *making* decisions and delay in *communicating* decisions can increase morbidity and delay return to work.

The advantage of organized rehabilitation lies in its ability to combine an integrated medical and functional assessment with the co-ordination of the activities of the many agencies (medical, social, educational and industrial) concerned with a patient's return to work. There is a particular advantage to be gained by combining the medical and industrial sections into a single rehabilitation unit, so enabling the patient's rehabilitation to progress smoothly without unnecessary delays.

Probably one in three patients discharged from hospital would benefit considerably from a period of 'rehabilitation' to speed recovery of function and confidence, and to allow for realistic planning of return to work. The benefits to the individual patient from such a rehabilitative period are complemented by the economic advantage to the community.

Rehabilitation after injury

If the patient has a residual disability, discussion between the doctor (either hospital or general practitioner) and the employer, directly or through a medical social worker or Disablement Resettlement Officer, is often sufficient to enable the patient to return to work. But too often, the appropriate decisions are not taken, or decisions depend too much upon personal idiosyncrasies or variations in organization of the local medical services.

Uncomplicated appendicitis is characterized by rapid and smooth recovery, but traditions, the patient's domestic convenience, the whim of the individual surgeon and the hospital bed state are the determining factors influencing the length of the patient's stay in hospital. For example, the period before returning to normal activities after uncomplicated appendicitis varies considerably: 10 days for housewives, 14 days for schoolchildren, and up to 70 days for insured men.

Fractures of the wrist or hand are relatively minor injuries, rarely associated with complications, requiring only a short period of immobilization of the hand and wrist and resulting in little interference with function. After such fractures, patients in manual work usually have considerably more time off work than those in sedentary occupations, and although litigation may be involved in about one third of the cases, there may be little evidence of impairment of motivation to return to work.

Although some patients could manage while in plaster, they often do not return to work as they may feel, not unreasonably, that the wearing of a plaster might interfere with work and render them unacceptable to an employer. Indeed, it seems clear that it is part of the hospital doctor's duty to dispel these doubts and make an authoritative recommendation as regards the patient's fitness for work. When such action is taken, there is a need for close and rapid communication between hospital and general practitioner so that the GP can back up the hospital's recommendation for return to work.

If rehabilitation is taken to mean the promotion of maximal possible recovery, then whenever there is a patient with a physical disability, appropriate physical rehabilitation service must be provided. In this context, one must not forget that recovery depends on the patient's mental concentration, endurance and motivation almost as much as his physical capability, and it is usually necessary to stream patients so that the elderly, frail and those with chronic disability are separated from the young and vigorous with temporary disability.

Rehabilitation and medical conditions

Stroke patients and patients with rheumatic disorders make up a high proportion of those with chronic physical disability. The physical management of these patients differs from the rehabilitation of patients with injury both in tempo and in pattern of activity, and because their numbers are so large, they have shifted the emphasis of physio and rehabilitation departments from corrective treatment to preventive and restorative management.

In the case of rheumatoid arthritis, it has been shown that with early diagnosis and treatment and regular follow-up and intensive care during remissions and exacerbations, a high proportion of patients can be kept independent at home and at work.

In a retrospective survey of results of treatment in one Rheumatology Centre, over 60 per cent of the patients remained fit for full or restricted work over a follow-up period of 6 years. The majority of the patients with rheumatoid arthritis could be improved functionally by planned rehabilitation, although the men were often unable to continue in either heavy manual work or very skilled work. With increasing advances in surgical techniques for the management of rheumatoid arthritis, the proportion of patients remaining at work should increase (*see* Chapter 4).

Stroke is one of the commonest causes of locomotor dysfunction. With adequate rehabilitation, about 20 per cent of stroke patients will return to full work and a further 30 per cent will make a useful contribution about the home. Thus, approximately 50 per cent of those affected can achieve a working status. It is the impairment of intellectual function and speech defects which are usually the stumbling blocks to resettlement, and these are related (as with head injuries) to the extent of the original lesion and the subsequent brain damage (*see* Chapter 10).

Rehabilitation of amputees

The rehabilitation of the young patient with amputation of the lower limb presents problems which are usually readily solved or ameliorated (*see* Chapter 12). Nowadays, however, over 60 per cent of all amputees are over 60 years old and suffering from peripheral vascular disease; unfortunately, amputation is often carried out as an ablative procedure after many other procedures directed towards saving a gradually dying limb. The patient, being elderly, often responds poorly and is resigned to a severe physical handicap. A better approach would be to accept amputation as the first stage in regaining active function and as a necessary preliminary to satisfactory limb-fitting in all but the very senile.

The use of 'early walking aids' enables many lower limb amputees to be mobilized as early as possible while still in the surgical ward. With such aids, many patients can be returned home walking a few weeks after amputation.

A well-organized, integrated limb-fitting service, backed by the rehabilitation services, can ensure the provision of the appropriate appliance or prosthesis at the right place at the right time (*see* Chapter 13).

A similar dynamic approach can be applied to upper limb amputation. Intensive rehabilitation instituted soon after amputation, together with the use of temporary training devices, leads to early return to work and a greater acceptance of functional artificial arms.

Rehabilitation after surgery

Rehabilitation after surgery or amputation, or reconstructive orthopaedic surgery, is an accepted part of patient care. But there are many other surgical patients for whom the need for rehabilitation is less obvious. The rehabilitation services they require include counselling, provision of appropriate appliances and training in the use of these appliances. Two particular groups of patients for whom these services are essential are women who have had a mastectomy, and patients who have been given an ostomy.

Mastectomy is often as distressing as an amputation of a limb, and much of the distress and embarrassment can be avoided by understanding preoperative discussion with the surgeon or ward sister; immediate post-operative provision of a lightweight prosthesis which can be worn over dressings, and early referral to the Appliance Service for a more permanent breast prosthesis.

Ostomies too often are also the source of distress and embarrassment. Once again, early counselling, both general and detailed factual, is the basis of rehabilitation. Early fitting of the appropriate appliance and training in its use are the foundations of post-operative management. Some hospitals and some manufacturers employ a 'stoma therapist' who is usually a nurse specially trained in stoma care. Some areas have a panel of ex-patients with ostomies who will act as a source of information and help to potential and actual ostomates.

Training in management of the appliance, care of the skin and control and understanding of the behaviour of the gastro intestinal or urinary system are essential.

After an ostomy the patient needs understanding, efficient equipment, and considerable encouragement to achieve return to optimal independence in daily living.

Rehabilitation of spinal injuries

Spinal injury units were established because of the need to assess, treat, rehabilitate and initiate resettlement of patients suffering from paraplegia and other disabilities resulting from spinal injury. The clinical and rehabilitation needs of these patients were such that an integrated spinal injury organization was a natural solution.

Since the institution of Spinal Injury Centres, the results of treatment and rehabilitation have steadily improved, and now some Centres claim that 40–60 per cent of paraplegics return to work or domestic independence. Achieving these results depends on a high standard of initial definitive treatment and a co-ordinated and intensive period of rehabilitation; this involves training in bladder care, skin care and a wheelchair existence, and usually extends over a period of 6–9 months.

Ideally these Centres should be sited at District General Hospitals with adequate supportive facilities, and should form a focus for much of the rehabilitation services of that particular District General Hospital.

Head injuries

The majority of patients with head injury suffer a minor injury requiring only simple treatment. Good initial assessment followed quickly by a period of attendance at the rehabilitation department of the District General Hospital is all that post-concussion syndrome requires.

The more severe head injury patient requires a sophisticated system of progressive care involving physical rehabilitation together with educational, speech and behaviour therapy. Intellectual impairment with loss of memory, loss of concentration, loss of sense of responsibility, and emotional lability and depression are the main adverse features.

There is considerable pressure for the provision of special Head Injury Rehabilitation Centres in association with Neurological and Neurosurgery Centres. Such Centres require residential accommodation and a high ratio of staff to patients.

Some patients with head injury tend to be aggressive and require close collaboration between neurological, psychiatric and rehabilitation staff. In severe cases, the process of rehabilitation may extend over many years; but with good facilities for physical, psychiatric and industrial rehabilitation and follow-up, many patients with head injury can be returned to work in the community.

RESETTLEMENT IN WORK

Resettlement may be defined as the process of returning the patient to the most appropriate social situation. Planning resettlement must start as soon as the immediate definitive treatment is under way, with the aim of returning the patient to his original work and way of life, while overcoming any residual disability as far as possible and reducing the handicap to a minimum.

Resettling a disabled patient in work depends on many factors besides the severity of the disability. Among such factors are: the age of the patient, the nature of the work, the patient's education and domestic background, together with social and economic factors. One of the most relevant points affecting the success of resettlement is the time elapsing from the onset of disability until the definitive plans for return to work or training are brought into effect.

For some patients, return to their original work is not possible, and a detailed reappraisal of their working capability is necessary as a preliminary to retraining and re-employment.

In 1974 the responsibility for the country's employment and training services was transferred from the Department of Employment to a public authority—the Manpower Services Commission (MSC); it had, until April 1978, two executive arms: the Employment Services Agency (ESA) and the Training Services Agency (TSA). Thereafter they became operating divisions of the MSC. The Employment Service Division is responsible for about 1000 employment offices and job centres; within this organization are about 500 full time DROs, all of whom have been trained as executive officer employment advisers (up to 25 weeks) followed by 10 weeks special training. During the past few years a limited number of DROs have been attached full time to hospitals. The DRO's main task is to place disabled people in suitable work, if necessary after employment rehabilitation or vocational training. He is envisaged as playing the key role, acting as an intermediary between industry and the client and as an employment adviser to the disabled person in co-operation with the health services. There has been some pressure for integrating the work of DROs within the health and social services, but the current policy is that they should be part of the MSC staff who take up the resettlement of disabled people as a temporary role. Their success will depend upon early intervention to help prevent the disabled person relapsing into attitudes which delay return to work and employers from developing resistance to re-employment of the employee as a disabled person. But it is equally important that the DROs advise the clinical and social team about the possibilities and suitability of employment for the patient, and this will depend upon factors far beyond the clinical one – e.g. the patient's work record, job availability, and work requirements of specific jobs. The great advantage of the DRO system is that it could provide the vital link between patient, health services and industry, but currently it only provides this in a very limited capacity.

Unemployment in 1976 increased continuously at 10 000 per month and in June 1977 the seasonally adjusted figure reached the highest figure since the war at nearly 1.3 million in a total working population of about 22 million.

In 1977, the ESA, through its resettlement service for disabled people, with its staff of about 1800 placed about 50 000 disabled people in employment. Through the employment rehabilitation service, about 14 000 undertook courses of training at 26 centres (Brown, 1977). At the same time, 13 000 employees were in sheltered employment (MSC, 1977). It is difficult adequately to evaluate the effectiveness of this system for the ESD are now begining to take a more detailed look at the workings and aims of ERCs and are improving the follow-up of trainees. Most patients have temporary disabilities and those hospitals with access to well developed rehabilitation services usually succeed in getting patients back to their own jobs or other jobs closely related to the previous work. When necessary they re-assess, organize training, and arrange placement, seldom finding it necessary to call upon the full panoply of the ESA services. However, the patient who fails to respond, the patient who drops out from hospital rehabilitation services, patients who are not under close hospital supervision, the patient with major psycho-social problems, and the patient with a disease of chronic unpredictable course, are the most likely ones to be referred to the ESA service. Many of the patients representing a high proportion of those remaining unemployed at follow-up, are those with chronic low back pain.

The great value of the ERC is that it can provide a more realistic work simulation than a hospital rehabilitation department, and can offer an assessment of work readiness which cannot otherwise be obtained except by sending the person into open employment. These advantages are particularly relevant to the rehabilitation of the psychiatric patient (Spry, 1977). But for both psychiatric patients and those with chronic physical disorders, a close integration between medical and industrial rehabilitation programmes is essential. Much depends on the individual patient's attitude towards work. It is often suggested that even for the most severely disabled person work is valuable in bringing him into a 'normal' environment and allowing him to consider himself as part of the community. Even tedious repetitive work such as sorting small components – the type of sub-contract work carried out at work centres – has a 'therapeutic' or self-satisying effect. But for others, even highly paid repetitive work is 'soul destroying'.

REHABILITATION DEPARTMENTS

Good rehabilitation requires careful organizing, and each District General Hospital should provide a rehabilitation service.

Patients will initially be the responsibility of consultants of many different disciplines, but when the immediate (definitive) care is over, facilities for long-term management are often best handled by the co-ordinated efforts of the general practitioner and his team of paramedical workers in co-operation with the social services.

A Department of Rehabilitation should:

(1) Be an organization for the provision and co-ordination of the physical therapy services of the hospital and its dependent clinics.
(2) Be an advisory service on all problems of rehabilitation and resettlement:
   (a) By direct clinical referral of patients to the consultant in charge of the Department.
   (b) By referral to clinics devoted to special aspects of rehabilitation: e.g. Functional assessment unit; Wheelchair (and other appliances) clinics; and Resettlement clinics for advising and co-ordinating medical, social, industrial and training aspects of a patient's return to work.
(3) Co-ordinate and correlate all services concerned with rehabilitation and resettlement in the community.
(4) Provide a continuous programme of teaching and research into problems of rehabilitation and physical handicap.

Such a Department requires some beds, at least of a hostel nature, if it is to serve its purpose adequately.

SPECIAL REHABILITATION UNITS

There will always be a need for some specialized units for managing the more severely disabled (for example, patients with head injuries, spinal cord lesions, or the very severely disabled), and these are likely to be organized on a regional basis, drawing patients from a group of District General Hospitals. At these units, there will usually be a consultant who devotes all or most of his time to medical rehabilitation.

Apart from providing special facilities for management of the more severely disabled patients, a regional residential rehabilitation unit might be expected to provide all or some of the following facilities:

(1) Short-term in-patient rehabilitation for patients unable to return home immediately because of social problems or travel difficulties.
(2) Detailed functional assessment and long-term supervisory care of the severely disabled.
(3) Development and manufacture of special appliances and equipment for the severely disabled.
(4) Accommodation of patients needing prosthetic services, including amputees for limb-fitting and rehabilitation.
(5) Facilities for assessment and training of disabled persons and their relatives.
(6) Wheelchair appliance service.
(7) Information service dealing with all aspects of equipment and facilities for the disabled.
(8) Advice, help and training for professional workers on rehabilitation or resettlement.
(9) Facilities for early industrial assessment and retraining.

THE CONSULTANT IN CHARGE OF REHABILITATION SERVICES

The clinician directing rehabilitation services must be first and foremost a physician. He must be able to unravel the complexities of physical disorders of the locomotor system whether neurological, rheumatological, orthopaedic or psychological. Whilst not required to be a diagnostic virtuoso, he must have a working understanding of these specialties which can only come from a thorough grounding in internal medicine and orthopaedic medicine. Without such a grounding, his collaboration and consultation with colleagues, and his ability to derive the optimal return from the rehabilitation services will be restricted. In these circumstances, he will tend to become an administrative technologist rather than a consultant adviser with wide-ranging interests; for the management of patients must always be comprehensive and include the use of drugs, physical treatment and appliances. Full rehabilitation implies clinical, functional, social and welfare assessment and a co-ordinated approach to the patient's total management.

A consultant with responsibilities for directing the rehabilitation services of a District General Hospital should have his own particular clinical interests. Often he will be concerned with the diagnosis and treatment of rheumatic disorders, but he may well have other clinical interests such as neurology or orthopaedics. He may also collaborate very closely with colleagues in geriatric medicine and mental subnormality, where there is a pressing need for rehabilitation services.

The prescribing of physical therapy can be as precise as the prescribing of drugs, but detailed prescribing pre-supposes detailed knowledge of the agencies employed, and a willingness to monitor the patient's progress very closely and to re-prescribe at very frequent intervals, for response to physical treatment can vary considerably and rapidly. This entails frequent attendances by the patient at out-patient clinics or frequent visits by the doctor to the physiotherapy department in the hospital and is time-consuming to both.

A possible and probably more logical alternative is to encourage the physical therapists to develop a deeper understanding of their subject and so to become more able to assume a greater responsibility for the day-to-day variations in therapy, and for the management of the departments in which they work. The training and experience of physical therapists varies considerably, and indeed the training given in different countries also varies considerably, particularly in the proportion of practical to theoretical knowledge imparted. In the United Kingdom, the training is orientated towards the practical aspects of physical therapy, and the qualifications to practise this are granted in a Diploma. In many other countries, although the therapists complete a Degree Course, their practical experience may be very much less.

As a general principle, physical therapists should be primarily practical in their approach and their training, and their work should be directed towards practical assessment and practical treatment. The patient's individual response to the therapist determines the therapist's choice of treatment and the response she expects from the patient. The clinician's function is to establish the overall guidance and direction of the patient's management.

The consultant in charge of rehabilitation can give the therapist the best chance of achieving the results he wants by:

(1) giving an accurate diagnosis;
(2) giving clear indications of the aims of treatment;
(3) giving a clear indication of the likely outcome;
(4) specifying where drug therapy or disease characteristics may necessitate particular care in the administration of various treatments.

He should remember that short, intensive periods of therapy are more likely to have a therapeutic value than the prolonged intermittent attendances for palliative treatment which rapidly become more of a social outing than a therapeutic activity.

He should encourage the therapist to record details of the nature and effect of treatment so that feed-back information from her trained observations may substantially influence future management and enable her to contribute fully to its outcome.

SUMMARY

The foundations of good rehabilitation lie in good medicine—accurate diagnosis, careful prognosis, and early, appropriate and adequate definitive care. The superstructure of rehabilitation depends considerably upon the bricks of physical therapy: physiotherapy (including remedial exercises); occupational therapy; industrial rehabilitation; and the various aspects of the social services.

Unfortunately, responsibilities tend to become separated, and it is often necessary to have one consultant who can bring about the integration of the provisions of the Department of Health, the Department of Education, the Department of Employment and Productivity, the Local Authorities and any other organizations involved. This integration calls for good organization and management and clearly defined lines of communication and areas of responsibility.

There is a need in every hospital for one consultant to be responsible for co-ordinating these services. In some instances, he will undertake this only in a supervisory role, but in other instances, particularly where the rehabilitation service plays a large part in the hospital activities, he may make this his special interest. As a corollary to this approach, the paramedical professions should be more closely concerned with the management of rehabilitation services and take a greater part in the co-ordination of various aspects of rehabilitation.

BIBLIOGRAPHY AND REFERENCES

Brown, A. W. (1977). 'The employment service agency'. *Proc. Roy. Soc. Med.* 70, 9, 647

Buckinghamshire County Council (1970). Report of the Working Group on Services for the Physically Handicapped and Rehabilitation in Milton Keynes

Department of Health and Social Security (1972). Statement by the Committee on the Remedial Professions. London: HMSO

Department of Health and Social Security (1973). 'The remedial professions.' A report of a Working Party set up in March 1973 by the Secretary of State for social services. London; HMSO

Ministry of Labour and National Service (1956). Report of an enquiry of the rehabilitation, training and resettlement of disabled persons. London: HMSO

McKenzie, M., Weir, R. D., Richardson, I.M., Mair, A., Harnett, R. W. F., Curran, A. P. and Ferguson, T. (1962). *Further Studies in Hospital and Community.* Oxford; Nuffield Provincial Hospitals Trust

MSC Review and Plan (1977) Manpower Services Commission

Nichols, P. J. R. (1969). 'Physical medicine.' *Br. J. Hosp. Med.* 2, 1152

Nichols, P. J. R. (1974). 'Rehabilitation in the reorganised National Health Service.' *Occupational Therapy* 37, No. 7

Oxford Regional Hospitals Board (1973). *Community Hospitals Research Programme: Day Care in the Community Hospital*

Scottish Home and Health Department: Scottish Health Services Council (1972). *Medical Rehabilitation: The Pattern of the Future.* London; HMSO

Spry, W. B. (1977). 'Problems in the rehabilitation of psychiatric patients.' *Proc. Roy. Soc. Med.* 70, 658

2 Physiotherapy

INTRODUCTION

The origins of physical therapy are shrouded in antiquity, and many forms of treatment referred to in the earliest medical records include the use of heat and hydrotherapy for the alleviation of discomfort from diseases of the locomotor system. Over the years, the pattern of medical practice has changed considerably, as more and more specific treatments have been discovered. Before the discovery of specific treatments such as antibiotics, the only available therapy for many patients was palliative and supportive. As the effectiveness of therapy has advanced, so early mobilization and early discharge of patients have become the rule, and the pattern of hospital in-patient physiotherapy has changed, with less treatment of patients in bed and a wider use of mobilizing techniques and general rehabilitation.

Treatment evaluation

Most physical treatments involve dramatic situations – electric currents, heat, light and direct personal contact of patients with the therapists. Such conditions favour the placebo factor, and the role of the physical therapist is partly to exploit the empirical placebo response and partly to apply rational remedial therapy.

Many of the conditions traditionally treated by physical methods are degenerative, chronic and episodic. They are also subject to unpredictable remissions and exacerbations. No treatment is likely to produce dramatic results in the chronic degenerative locomotor disorders, but most of the patients respond to care and attention. This is what so many physiotherapy departments provide. Unfortunately, there has been remarkably little scientific evaluation of either the disorders or the treatments. It has been well shown in other fields that it is only when clinical problems are correlated with their underlying pathological mechanisms that therapeutic advice can be given on a rational basis. At the present time, there is still too much that is taught and practised in physiotherapy departments which is based upon an amalgam of tradition, personal experience and subjective patient response. Consequently, physiotherapy in the chronic locomotor disorders has remained until recently a part of medical practice has built up its own folklore and pseudo-science.

11

Trends in physiotherapy

Gradually, the mysticism surrounding physiotherapy is being cleared away, and the rehabilitation concept of progressive patient care is being more widely introduced. Many physiotherapists are challenging traditional methods and are seeking to widen their theoretical understanding of the techniques they use and to become partners in planning and organizing therapy with clinicians of all specialties.

Physiotherapists are concerned with the maintenance of total body function during acute illness, as well as the maintenance of joint range and muscle power of the limbs. They are also concerned with early mobilization and short-term rehabilitation after illness or injury. For long-term patients, physiotherapy is concerned with the assessment for many aids and appliances associated with locomotor function, such as splints, calipers, artificial limbs, wheelchairs, hoists and so on, and with training in their use.

More and more clinicians and therapists believe that if a patient needs physiotherapy he needs it frequently (i.e. daily), at least in the early stages of treatment. Intermittent, palliative, passive treatments are expensive in terms of the time of the department and of the cost and time spent in travelling to and from hospital. Such treatments contribute little to the patient's management.

Physiotherapy and occupational therapy

Occupational therapists are, in general, more concerned with functional activities than with locomotor capability, but their interests will, of necessity, frequently overlap those of the physiotherapists, and a combined approach will achieve the optimal result.

From time to time there may appear to be a conflict of interest between the physiotherapist and the occupational therapist. For example, the physiotherapist may train the patient with rheumatoid arthritis to work with sticks or crutches, but the patient may be unable simultaneously to undertake any domestic activity such as carrying a saucepan or teapot. The occupational therapist can teach the patient to be independent in the kitchen by using a wheelchair which she can propel with her hands while carrying domestic equipment on a tray; or 'paddle' with her feet, leaving the hands free. The conflict between the use of crutches or wheelchair is apparent rather than real and is easily resolved when *optimal* rather than *maximal* total functional efficiency is sought.

Collaboration, based on a full clinical, functional and social assessment, will enable the clinician to direct the most appropriate balance of activities to give the best functional recovery consistent with the patient's clinical condition.

Within the rehabilitation team there must also be close collaboration with the speech therapists, social workers, clinical psychologists, and all the other professions supplementary to medicine which are involved in the total management of a patient in the community. Without close collaboration under clinical direction, individual effort can often be dissipated, with consequent frustration to all concerned, including the patient.

Types of physiotherapy

It is conventional to describe the physical techniques under the separate headings of *active* and *passive* procedures. Passive physical treatments are mainly based upon the administration of soothing, pain-relieving applications of heat and the use of massage in various modes and mixtures. Active physical treatment is largely based upon exercises, ranging from minimal movements of single muscles to encourage recovery after paralysis or injury, to intensive exercise routines akin to the circuit training practised by athletes.

This classification is useful for the construction of an academic syllabus and for descriptive purposes but is virtually meaningless in the treatment of patients, as we hope to show in subsequent chapters.

The physiotherapist

The physical rehabilitation of a patient is a continuous process, from the onset of disability to the achievement of optimal rehabilitative potential, and the physiotherapist may employ many different techniques to achieve the end result. Frequently, it will be necessary to use different methods to achieve similar results. The art of physiotherapy lies in selecting the appropriate technique for a particular patient at a particular time. Furthermore, the quality of the physiotherapy depends almost entirely upon the quality of the physiotherapist. The quality of the physiotherapist depends upon her personality, her understanding of the patient and his disability, and her ability to contribute to the overall rehabilitation of the patient. In addition to having a detailed knowledge of all available techniques of physiotherapy, the physiotherapist must have a sound understanding of general medical and surgical care, of the availability and use of aids and appliances, and of the available resettlement facilities provided by the statutory and voluntary bodies. The physiotherapist must be trained to play an important role in the assessment of physical disability and in the instruction of techniques by which a patient can overcome or adjust to that disability. It is only by using this overall approach to rehabilitation that she can make an optimal contribution.

PASSIVE PROCEDURES

Heat

Heat has been used as a treatment for musculo-skeletal pain since time immemorial. There is no doubt that for many conditions giving rise to pain within the locomotor system, heat does have a palliative effect.

Heat may be applied to the body by changes in the environmental temperature, by contact with warmed substances, e.g. warm water, hot water bottles or wax baths, or by the radiation of energy into the body.

Hot water is probably the most widely used agent for conductive heating either as warm baths, hot soaks or compresses, but this is too commonplace a form of therapy to be acceptable to many patients (and their physicians) as a treatment in a hospital physiotherapy department, however often and effectively it is used in the home.

'Wax baths' are a convenient form of applying direct heat to the extremities. Paraffin wax used for treatment is solid at room temperature and melts at $130°F$ $(54°C)$. Once melted, it remains liquid at a temperature of about $120°F$. Melting is achieved in an electrically heated bath. The wax is then applied to the skin — either by immersion of the part or by application with a brush at $118°–120°F$ $(48°–49°C)$. The wax is easily peeled off after a treatment period (usually 20–30 minutes with 6–7 coatings of wax) and is returned to the stock for re-use. The heating effect is mainly due to the latent heat of solidification and to the specific heat of the wax. There is no evidence that immersion in wax is of any more benefit than immersion in warm water.

Electromagnetic radiations have two main properties which may be significant:

(1) The wavelength.
(2) The intensity.

In general, the hotter the source, the greater the proportion of shorter wavelength emission, and the shorter the wavelength the more easily the radiation is absorbed by water or dispersed. Radiant heat lamps are a convenient and relatively cheap source of heat in a dispensable form. The heat provided is no different from that of an electric fire. Electric pads and infra-red lamps provide heat mainly of a longer wavelength. They have a disadvantage in that they take longer to heat up − in fact some infra-red lamps need about 10 minutes to heat up and to reach an even temperature − and thus can be time-wasters in a busy department.

From the therapeutic point of view, the value of these lamps is probably two-fold. First, there is local warming. The emissions penetrate through the skin and into the subcutaneous tissue with consequent peripheral vascular dilation. Second, the patient has time to rest and relax before the next part of the treatment.

Temperatures developed in the tissues are the product of the pattern of heating, the characteristics of the tissues being treated, and biological factors associated with the organism as a whole.

The patterns of relative heating are an expression of the energy available for heating, determined by dielectric constants and conductivities of the tissues traversed by microwaves. The value of the specific heat of each tissue layer determines the temperature increments over a period of time; therefore, 'instantaneous' temperature distribution might be very different from one resulting from exposure over a period, depending upon biological factors such as blood flow and muscle contraction.

Skin and fat are poor conductors of heat. The skin temperature rises rapidly when in contact with the heat source, but the underlying tissues show a temperature rise of a lesser degree depending partly on the heat dissipated on the skin surface (by sweat and convection) and partly on the conductivity of the subcutaneous tissue (thickness of fat) and the amount of heat dissipated by the circulating blood. Muscle and joint temperature is not altered by heat conduction; but both tissues may show a delayed rise in temperature if a large area of the body is heated for 20−30 minutes, and this is associated with an overall rise of body temperature of 1−2°C.

The subcutaneous blood flow follows the skin blood flow, and when the skin temperature is raised, the skin blood flow increases by several hundred per cent. Thus both are increased by local or general heating of the body. However, surface heating is limited by the direct effect of heat on the skin tissue. A skin temperature of over 109°F (43°C) is associated with pain and a temperature of over 113°F (45°C) will rapidly produce arteriolar flare and a wheal.

Because of the problems of 'conducting' heat to deeper tissues, many techniques have been devised in an attempt to produce 'deep heat'. This work assumes that deep heat will have a therapeutic effect − as yet an unproven theory. In particular, it is assumed that heat will increase the flow of blood in the deeper structures.

The only published investigations on this subject indicate that although local and general heat will increase the blood flow through the skin and subcutaneous tissue, there is a much less impressive and often unreliable response in the deeper tissues. An increase in the muscle temperature may be associated with an increase in blood flow, but this is only of a limited amount compared with the increased flow through the skin. Any increase which does occur is quite insignificant compared with that which occurs in association with voluntary muscular contractions.

Short-wave diathermy

Much has been written about short-wave diathermy and there is a widespread belief that this form of electrical treatment will produce deep heat (the word 'diathermy' means 'heating through').

The heating effect is produced by placing the patient within an electric field created by a high frequency, alternating current. In effect, the patient forms part of the secondary circuit of a high frequency generator. It is impossible to measure the input into the patient, and the only control of the field's intensity depends on the patient's skin sensation of heat and its level of heat tolerance. If the tissues were homogeneous, short-wave diathermy would heat through them. If there were no conduction to untreated parts, then heat loss would eventually be determined by the temperature at the surface and the boundaries between treated and untreated tissue. In practice this does not often occur, for tissues are not homogeneous. Therefore it is impossible to achieve an even heating effect in the body. The highest current density will be at the surfaces, and heat will be dissipated by circulating blood and by conduction to surrounding tissues.

These effects are minimized by crossfire techniques or combining plate electrodes with conduction cables. However, it is impossible to record the true effects of the various techniques of administering this form of treatment, since the introduction of any form of thermocouple or recording device deforms the existing electrical field. Studies on blood flow and radioactive isotope clearance have failed to demonstrate that short-wave diathermy has an appreciable advantage over conventional heat radiators.

Ultrasound

Sound waves with a frequency of over 20 000 cycles per second are undetectable by human ear and are referred to as 'ultrasound'. High frequency ultrasound (800 000–1 000 000 cycles per second) produced by applying a high frequency current to a crystal is now used in many physiotherapy departments. The therapeutic machines produce vibrations of approximately 800 kHz with an output limited to 3 W cm^{-2}. The effects of the variations are mechanical, heating and chemical. Animal experiments have shown, however, that ultrasound given in therapeutic doses can accelerate healing and regenerative processes. Under certain circumstances, ultrasound can produce 'standing waves' in blood vessels, with 'banding' and stasis of red cells, which have obvious theoretical dangers.

The physiological effect of therapeutic heat is by no means clear. It certainly brings about a temporary easement of pain in some patients. However, muscle spasm is not necessarily painful and muscle spasm is not necessarily relaxed by heat. Indeed, in some patients, spasm and pain may be exacerbated by heat.

As with all forms of physiotherapy, the therapist should be allowed to use heat at her discretion, as required, and to employ whichever techniques of heat administration she considers most appropriate.

Ice

Pain and stiffness of musculoskeletal origin may well respond to heat, as indicated above, but they are also often considerably reduced by the application of cold packs.

The relative value of applying heat or cold has been argued for centuries, and currently, cold applications (e.g. ice packs, iced baths and cold compresses) are gaining considerable vogue. There is mounting physiological and clinical evidence to show that the therapeutic use of ice by local application, or by immersion in ice and water, can decrease the spasm of spastic muscles and also produce a vasodilation in deep tissues.

Ice therapy is now widely used in the mobilization of two main groups of patients.

(1) Those patients with pain and oedema associated with recent trauma or surgery or an exacerbation of arthritis.
(2) Patients with spasticity (e.g. hemiplegia or paraplegia).

This form of treatment has been reported as being particularly helpful in the management of the acute painful shoulder, whether idiopathic or associated with stroke or injury; for post-operative management of patients after patellectomy carried out for generalized osteo-arthritis of the knee; and for the painful spasm associated with spinal cord lesions.

Electrotherapy

Direct current – iontophoresis

Electrical currents applied directly to the tissues of low intensity have been used therapeutically to induce chemical changes resulting in an increase in skin blood flow, and also to introduce substances such as histamine into the skin so as to accentuate these vascular changes. This process is known as iontophoresis and is certainly effective as an irritant. Both histamine ionization and the application of direct current on its own are thought by many to cause increased circulation and therefore an improvement in the nutrition of the tissues in the path of the current.

The main effect of both direct current and histamine iontophoresis is superficial, neither technique producing consistent circulatory effects deep to the skin. Both techniques are, however, capable of giving counter-irritation, a method of treatment practised since time immemorial, and more cheaply produced by flagellation with nettles or the application of histamine ointment.

Interrupted direct current will stimulate muscle fibres or nerve fibres depending upon the intensity of the current and its duration. Muscles can only be stimulated directly by long-acting current (100 ms).

Short duration and long duration currents can be applied in many ways with various patterns of rhythm and superimposed surging and diminution. The currents therefore impose a variety of sensory effects and patterns of muscle contraction.

Such techniques have been employed as a means of maintaining active muscular contraction of denervated muscles. Some orthopaedic surgeons insist that recovery after denervation is improved by regular stimulation with 'galvanic' currents, whereas others believe that regular, frequent mobilization of the flail joints and the rigorous prevention of postural oedema is as effective a method of preventing contractures and a poor end result.

Short duration direct current (less than 1 ms duration) or 'Faradic stimulation' has two effects:

(1) Stimulation of sensory nerves.
(2) Stimulation of muscle via the motor nerves.

The discomfort produced by the stimulus is such that the contraction produced is rarely more than 30 per cent of that which can be produced voluntarily. There is no satisfactory evidence that muscle power can be improved by electrical stimulation and certainly any reported effect is insignificant compared with the increase in power which appropriate exercises can produce.

However, electrical stimulation can be of considerable value in those conditions in which voluntary contraction is apparently 'inhibited'. For example, when a joint is acutely inflamed, either as in a traumatic synovitis or an acute arthritis, the muscles acting on that joint will waste. This is certainly true as far as the knee is concerned, in which increased tension in the joint may be produced by an effusion and will induce a positive inhibition and rapid wasting of the quadriceps muscle. Similar inhibitor mechanisms may well exist for other muscles and joints.

A similar, effective use of electrical stimulation of muscle is in the treatment of flat feet, when the patient is unable to demonstrate active contraction of the intrinsic muscles of the feet. Once again, a short course of frequent electrical treatments (two to three times daily for several days, using small individual electrodes and stimulating the intrinsic muscles alone) will often enable the patient to gain adequate voluntary control to continue with the essential 'foot shortening' intrinsic muscle exercises.

A third area of use for electrical stimulation lies in the retraining of muscles after surgical transplantation. Sometimes patients have difficulty in achieving adequate contraction in the newly sited muscles, and electrical stimulation helps to improve an activity pattern leading eventually to the establishment of satisfactory voluntary control.

EXERCISE THERAPY

Exercise therapy occupies about 60 per cent of the physiotherapist's training time and nearly 70 per cent of her working time.

Of all the physical methods of treatment available, exercises have probably been subjected to more statistical evaluation than any other, but the true value of the application of various techniques of exercise is still by no means clear. There are almost as many exercise routines as there are physiotherapists and remedial gymnasts.

There are innumerable reports in the medical and physiotherapeutic literature extolling the virtues of specific techniques, routines and types of apparatus. As yet no report has failed to prove that a particular technique of routine gives good results, but as yet there is no *controlled* clinical trial in which various techniques and routines are compared under adequate controls. Until an authoritative comparison is produced, each practitioner will tend to develop a routine from her own experience, and providing she believes in her routine and can inspire the patient to follow it, her results will usually be to her own satisfaction. One of the reasons for this unclear state of affairs is that 'muscle strength' is the usual criterion for assessment and measurement, but this is only part of the story, for a muscle's function depends on its strength, endurance, speed of action and co-ordination with other muscles.

Muscle strength can be defined in two ways:

(1) The power which a muscle can develop instantaneously in an attempt to overcome an imposed load, either in lifting a weight (isotonic) or during static (isometric) contraction against a fixed resistance.
(2) The power which a muscle can develop in resisting an applied load. (This will usually be assessed by a 'break' or 'yield' test which will give consistently higher than the isometric contraction.)

Muscle endurance is the capacity to maintain or repeatedly develop a certain degree of tension. Strong muscles are at an advantage if expected to perform prolonged exercises at a low level of activity as inevitably their endurance will be greater than that of weak muscles.

Speed of contraction is a function of the rate of increase in tension of muscle fibres, the resistance to be overcome, the number of times the fibres contract, and the range of motion which each contraction imposes.

Co-ordination is the ability of the muscles to act together in correct sequence at the appropriate speed and tension, and is more a function of neurophysiology than muscle physiology.

It is generally agreed that the only way to increase muscle strength and endurance is by active voluntary exercise. Furthermore, when the strength and bulk of a healthy muscle is increased by active exercise, other muscle groups — particularly the antagonists and the contra-lateral muscles — also become stronger.

Exercise has local effects on the joints and muscles exercised, and it also has secondary effects upon the body as a whole. Thus, exercise therapy may be directed towards the local effect — increasing the function of a specific muscle group — or it may be directed towards the effects upon the body as a whole in terms of general fitness, including the improvement of cardiac function.

The local effects of muscular exercise and thus the functions of exercise therapy may be prophylactic or therapeutic. They are to:

(1) Preserve muscular function during a period of immobilization of any joint, preventing atrophy, fibrosis, venous and lymphatic stasis, and maintaining joint mobility above and below those joints immobilized.
(2) Strengthen weak muscles and mobilize stiff joints.
(3) Re-establish neuromuscular co-ordination.
(4) Prepare for functional activity (practice of skills).
(5) Encourage the patient by the regular demonstration of his increasing ability to perform the exercises demanded of him.

Assisted movements
These involve the active collaboration of the patient, who contracts certain muscles, while the therapist assists his movement. This type of exercise is particularly useful during early recovery after paralysis, and also in early mobilization of joints after injury or operation when movements are inhibited by pain as well

as weakness. As the patient progresses, movement may be achieved without assistance from the therapist.

Free movements
Such exercises may be undertaken with the assistance of slings or in water, to eliminate the effects of gravity. As joint range and muscle power increase, so the resistance may be increased in an effort to further increase muscle power. There are many techniques for introducing and increasing resistance to muscle action. The resistance may be supplied by the physiotherapist's direct manual resistance, by gravity, by weights, by springs, by simple or complex combinations of resistances imposed by many different types of apparatus, or by using the physical properties of water as in the practice of hydrotherapy.

Isometric and isotonic exercises
Physiologically, muscle contractions can be classified as:

(1) isometric – increasing muscle tension without altering the muscle length; or
(2) isotonic – exercises performed against a steady load with joint movement occurring.

Isometric exercises
Simple isometric exercises are usefully performed when a joint is immobilized. This type of exercise is particularly applicable to limbs immobilized in plaster casts, whether because of fractures, orthopaedic procedures, or joint inflammation, e.g. quadriceps setting exercises with a fully extended knee when a leg is in long leg plaster. There is good evidence that even in acute arthritis from whatever cause, e.g. trauma, rheumatoid arthritis or haemo-arthrosis, muscle bulk can usually be maintained and wasted muscle encouraged to increase in bulk by isometric exercises, provided the joint is adequately splinted and acute muscle inhibition is overcome initially by a few treatments of electrical stimulation. It is important to stresss however, that in certain circumstances acute arthritis may well be aggravated by isometric exercises even if the joint is adequately splinted, and the management of such cases requires considerable skill and experience.

Isometric exercises can also be given to any muscle groups acting across a joint which is not splinted by applying supramaximal load, but care must be taken to ensure that the load is not able to act and suddenly produce joint movement when the muscle is relaxed.

Isotonic exercises
Isotonic exercise is often used for building up muscle power after injury by applying predetermined weights and requiring the patient to perform a predetermined number of resisted movements. There are many differing techniques, some with the same load, some with increasing loads, some with decreasing loads. There are many rules for determining the load and the number of contractions, but no real guide as to the method of determining the most effective technique of exercising.

Considerable evidence exists to show that the isometric exercises can induce as much, and probably more, improvement in muscle power as isotonic exercises, and that active isotonic movement should be directed towards gaining joint movement rather than increasing muscle power.

In practice, resisted exercise routines involve combinations and modifications of these two main types of muscle contractions.

Exercises with apparatus

The use of apparatus has two advantages: it enables a physiotherapist to supervise several patients at a time and thus get through more work, and when weights or spring balances are used, it enables accurate records to be maintained.

Weights are often cumbersome, noisy, and uncontrolled. Because free exercises involve movement, exercises with weights are neither isometric nor isotonic.

Spring balances, provided they are well designed and allow little movement, are of much more use than weights in providing either a true isotonic or a measured isometric contraction. Recording has a further value in that it gives the patient an incentive with *every* contraction.

However, there are many disadvantages. Patients left to their own devices often cheat or develop trick movements. Some pieces of apparatus are positively dangerous if inadequately supervised, for the apparatus is not immediately adaptable when troubles arise and uncontrolled weight-resisted activities may well give rise to exacerbations of synovitis or injure already damaged ligaments.

Spring balances form the basis of most 'dynamometers'. With a few spring balances and a set of wall bars for their fixation, any physiotherapy department can have a 'dynamometer' for exercising and recording the contraction strength of any muscle group.

However, there are disadvantages in using springs, for the resistance increases as the movement proceeds, and the muscle becomes less able to overcome the resistance. Similar criticism can be levelled against exercises carried out on slings with gravity only as the resistance.

Techniques can be devised where the spring balance is used to assist rather than resist. For example, in re-education of the calf muscles after fracture of the tibia and fibula, an overhead spring balance can be used to assist the patient to 'lift' on the weak plantar flexors. As the muscle power increases, the poundage recorded on the spring balance decreases.

As a basis for planning exercise therapy, the following points can be assumed:

(1) Strength is built up in a muscle most effectively by resisting the movement the muscle produces – maximum resistance allows no movement, and the contraction becomes isometric.
(2) Repeated resistance exercises are believed to improve muscle endurance.

However, there are many other variations in the exercise routines commonly prescribed. Some authorities start with a high resistance, reducing throughout the exercise sessions. Others reverse this procedure, gradually increasing resistance. Others still believe in 'power exercising' with no variation in resistance, but there is no adequate comparative evaluation to guide the clinician or therapist.

Proprioceptive neuromuscular facilitation

Recently techniques have been introduced under the general classification of *proprioceptive neuromuscular facilitation.* First, it is believed that there are certain patterns of mass muscle movement, and that by performing multiple joint movements in these patterns, there is greater physiological facilitation of all muscles in the appropriate group; thus one or more small muscles may be 'called in' as part of the movement pattern when it would be impossible to obtain an isolated contraction, resistance being given to stronger muscles in the correct sequence of movement before 'pivoting' to the weak muscles. Second, by employing resistance, stretch reflexes and peripheral stimuli (i.e. by stimulating the proprioceptors in the muscles and joints), the demand made on the neuromuscular mechanism can be increased and its response facilitated.

The principles of proprioceptive neuromuscular facilitation are:

(1) Maximal resistance applied by the physiotherapist's hand.
(2) Proprioceptive stimuli induced before and during contractions by:
    (*a*) Skin pressure.
    (*b*) Stretch before contraction.   }   all supplied by the
    (*c*) Traction and compression of the joint. }   physiotherapist's hands.
(3) Set movements performed in diagonal or spiral patterns.
(4) The patient always just 'wins', that is to say movement in the pattern is always allowed.

There are two main advantages over other methods. First, the *movements* and *resistance* are at all times in the physiotherapist's control. Second, no apparatus is required. Unfortunately, these techniques are time consuming for physiotherapists because it is a case of one patient — one physiotherapist. Also, for the first time in the history of physiotherapy there is now a tendency for the physiotherapist to show greater signs of fatigue than the patient. However, those experienced in these techniques are convinced that they far exceed the effectiveness of all other techniques for the building up of strength in weak muscles.

Mobilizing exercises

Mobilizing exercises aim at increasing joint movement and are usually introduced when there is no evidence of active joint disease. They may have to be regulated by the recurrence of joint symptoms or by the evidence of adverse joint reaction. Pain or effusion or loss of range are immediate indications of the need to reduce the range of movement employed in the exercises.

These exercises are often preceded by the application of heat or ice packs, or they may be performed in water (hydrotherapy), in suspension apparatus, or using gymnasium apparatus (wall bars, parallel bars), the technique depending on the particular clinical situation, the facilities available, and the prejudices and predilections of the therapist or clinician. The physiotherapist responsible needs guidance regarding the restrictions necessary and the degree of response to activity which she may expect from the demands made of the patient.

As recovery proceeds, the specific exercises should give way to more purposive and functional activities. Walking, getting in and out of bed or on and off the lavatory, dressing and the gradual increase of activities up to the level of normal living and working are all purposive exercise activities and entail close collaboration between physiotherapist and occupational therapist.

Fitness training

For some patients, a high level of physical fitness is necessary, and rehabilitation should be taken to a level little short of the training programme necessary for sport. For others, there is no need for such intensive rehabilitation, and a rapid return to normal or near-normal living and working conditions will provide the necessary exercise.

For the first group, remedial games and athletic training are the relevant exercise activities; for the second group, functional activities are more appropriate.

The various systems of exercise introduced for specific muscle groups can be adapted to general physical training and incorporated into the technique known as 'circuit training'. Circuit training is a grouping together of a set of exercises designed to:

(1) Exercise the main muscle groups with consequent increase in strength and endurance.
(2) Obtain maximal general effect and improve general stamina.
(3) Improve certain skills by practice.

Circuit training is the logical final stage of any exercise programme. It not only aims at a functional end result, but also requires that the individual patient compete against his own capability initially and eventually adapts the exercise programme for non-specific exercising and the maintenance of general health.

The intensity and duration of exercise and activity routines employed vary considerably with the clinical problem. Many physiotherapists and remedial gymnasts will be more concerned with short-term effects of injury, and they will bear the particular responsibility of ensuring that patients return to maximal function in the shortest possible time. Regular, frequent, intensive exercise in the immediate post-injury period may well prevent prolonged morbidity. For example, most patients with simple fractures of the lower limbs can well return to work while still immobilized, provided they have first been taught to walk properly in plaster of paris and have been indoctrinated with the need to exercise immobilized muscles adequately, using isometric techniques.

Functional activities may encourage a patient to greater effort than repetitive exercises in the gymnasium and enable all concerned to obtain realistic assessment of the patient's capabilities.

PASSIVE MOVEMENTS

Passive movements are the movements of joints and muscles produced by a therapist unaided by the voluntary contraction of the relevant muscles by the patient. They help to maintain proprioceptive sense in the excessively weak or paralysed muscles. Such movements also help to maintain joint mobility or to re-establish mobility in joints which have stiffened up. They are particularly useful in the early phases of management after paralysis from any cause, but the need for a prolonged programme of passive movements in conditions such as brachial plexus lesions has probably been exaggerated.

In the acute early stages of hemiplegia, passive movements of the arm as a whole, and the shoulder in particular, are important in preventing the common and disabling complication of 'frozen shoulder'. Passive movements of the leg help to prevent flexion deformities of the hip and knee and an equinus deformity of the foot. Similarly, during the period of early flaccid paralysis following spinal cord lesions, passive movements of the legs are important to prevent the development of deformities. However, when spasticity develops, great care and gentleness is needed to carry out adequate passive movements without causing any soft tissue damage. Patients may be unconscious or suffering from diminished or absent sensation, and the usual protective mechanisms are absent.

In a number of patients with strokes or spinal injury, periarticular calcific deposits appear, particularly around the hip joints. These deposits are sometimes judged to be akin to traumatic myositis ossificans and are associated with over-vigorous passive movements or injudicious attempts to achieve the full range of joint movement while muscles are in spasm. The fact that similar deposits are rarely encountered after flaccid paralysis indicates that the muscle spasm has a part to play in the aetiology. For these reasons, adequate relaxation achieved by hydrotherapy, hot packs, adequate anti-spasmodic drugs, or the appropriate injection of local antispasmodics (45 per cent alcohol or phenol) provides an important prelude to passive movements and the ensuing re-educative physiotherapy when recovery begins.

TRACTION

Limb traction
As a brief surgical manœuvre, traction is used to reduce a fracture or dislocation. Continuous traction applied to the limbs is used to relieve pain, secure rest and overcome painful muscle spasm, to gain and to maintain anatomical alignment, and to prevent or correct deformity.

Such forms of traction may be 'fixed' traction, e.g. Thomas' splint, 'balanced' or 'sliding traction', or a combination of fixed and balanced traction.

The physiotherapist's concern is to understand the principles of traction and of counter-traction so that she can maintain joint mobility and muscle power within the restrictions of the traction and its consequent immobilization. In addition, the orthopaedic physiotherapist will be concerned with the pressure areas and the state of the skin, which is often at risk during prolonged traction. These techniques are, however, special ones, usually restricted to orthopaedic hospitals and accident departments, and are not a particular concern in this book.

Spinal traction
Traction has been used in the treatment of neck pain and backache for many years, and, as with many other forms of physiotherapy, there is a mass of reported personal experience, dogma and folklore. Unfortunately, there has been little scientific investigation and few authenticated therapeutic trials.

The only effects which traction can be expected to achieve are some distraction between vertebrae at the intervertebral disc and apophyseal joints, tensing the longitudinal ligaments of the spinal column (particularly the posterior common ligament), and some slight widening of the intervertebral foraminae. These effects can only be expected to occur while the traction is being applied. Continuous traction might be employed also to achieve effective immobilization of a patient in bed. There is some evidence to suggest that acute lesions of the neck and back respond to more vigorous manipulative procedures whereas the less acute lesions tend to be self-limiting. Those that persist with considerable general limitation of movement appear likely to respond to traction or immobilization. Persistent pain, associated with restriction of specific movements, may also respond better to mobilizing techniques.

Some authors argue that traction is a form of manipulation or a *part* of manipulation, or a preliminary to manipulative procedures. Many authorities advise a combination of treatments, particularly the use of a support (cervical collar or lumbosacral belt) in association with traction. A well-fitting support often seems to prove beneficial after a short period (20–30 minutes) in traction, and to prolong the symptomatic improvement achieved by traction.

Manual traction is traction applied by the physiotherapist's hands, usually only for brief periods, often combined with lateral and rotational manœuvres (the entire procedure being under the therapist's direct control), and is really more properly classified as a manipulation. The best results are usually obtained in the presence of acute symptoms.

Continuous traction is applied through some form of harness and continued for 24 hours or longer. The forces used are relatively small and the treatment is used mainly as an in-patient procedure, and usually reserved for severe, intractable root pain.

Sustained traction is a technique of traction usually applied for 20–30 minutes.

Intermittent traction is similar to sustained traction but applied intermittently, the traction being alternately applied and withdrawn, the pulsation being applied by various mechanical devices.

Sustained and intermittent traction are applied through harnesses. In the case of cervical traction, the patient's body weight provides adequate counterweight. For lumbar traction two sets of harnesses are usually used, providing a symmetrical pull on the torso.

The force used may be large, from about 15–25 lb (6.8–11.3 kg) for cervical traction, to 40–50 lb (18.2–22.7 kg) for lumbar traction, but under careful control, cervical traction may be increased to 40–50 lb and lumbar traction to between 70 and 150 lb (31.7–68.1 kg).

The angle of traction, the position of the head and neck, and the weight applied are usually achieved by trial and error. Indeed, the position and weight which produce relief of pain vary from patient to patient, and for each patient they may vary considerably from day to day. Most patients with neck and arm pain respond to traction, but most also respond to simple positioning or to the application of a firm collar. However, most physiotherapists believe they can achieve best results by a combination of these techniques, varying their treatment according to the patient's response. Because of the variability of the response, it is unwise to be too specific when prescribing such treatments. Indeed, it is more appropriate to give the physiotherapist latitude of approach, and if the patient does not respond to traction, it should be discontinued and other measures tried until relief from pain is achieved. Often patients with an acute lesion respond badly to sustained traction as they are particularly prone to rebound pain when traction is relaxed.

There seems to be little theoretical reason for expecting traction to be effective in degenerative spondylosis of the cervical spine, any more than it is likely to be effective in osteo-arthritis of a limb joint. Traction will reduce the natural cervical lordosis (with a pull of 20–25 lb (9.1–11.4 kg) and a separation from C2–C7 of 3–14 mm can be demonstrated to occur at a pull of about 45 lb (20.4 kg). However, there is evidence that the first radiological indication of cervical spondylosis is a loss of cervical lordosis, and thus traction might well be expected to reproduce and exacerbate the early changes and the accompanying symptoms in some instances.

In the lumbar spine, traction has been demonstrated to produce a separation of about 2 mm at each disc space; but such separations are unstable and reversible.

Therapeutic trials of traction have been inconclusive, and mostly without adequate controls, but there is adequate physiotherapeutic folklore to encourage physiotherapists to master the techniques; to use them for patients with persistent pain; to learn to assess the patients; and to retain an inquisitive, objective and sceptical attitude to both treatment and patient.

Perhaps the only absolute rule about the use of traction in the treatment of skeletal pain is that it should never be used unless an absence of bony metastases has first been demonstrated by radiological investigation.

MANIPULATIVE PROCEDURES

There is much controversy about manipulative procedures, most of which is engendered by lack of understanding, imprecision of diagnostic terms and valueless speculation about the pathology of undefined clinical syndromes. In the commonly held view, a manipulation is a passive movement restoring range of movement to a joint which is 'stuck' with intra- or periarticular adhesion, 'subluxated' or in some manner restricted in its movement. The procedure is usually regarded as being instantaneous in imparting relief, forceful in character and often accompanied by a 'snapping' sensation or sound. It is also widely believed that the technique is understood only by a small group of physicians, osteopaths and chiropracters.

During recent years, however, many of the techniques previously restricted to such practitioners have been rationalized and are being taught to large numbers of physiotherapists. In the professional sense, the term 'manipulation' can be used to describe any procedure applied passively to a relaxed part of the body for the purpose of restoring joint range and functional activity. Force and flamboyance are usually unnecessary, and sudden dramatic manœuvres are not always associated with dramatic recovery.

Certainly, the popular medical literature and the folklore of patients is full of personal histories of dramatic cures, but the scientific literature is surprisingly void of authenticated studies detailing diagnostic criteria, relapse rates and adequately controlled trials.

Physiotherapists are experienced in handling stiff and painful joints, and now that they are being more widely encouraged to learn and to practice manipulative techniques, these can be included in the normal physiotherapeutic repertoire and should also be introduced into the controlled clinical trials which are beginning to play an important part of physiotherapy training and practice.

Radiological examination of a joint is an essential preliminary to manipulation. Spinal manipulation should never be undertaken if there is evidence of vertebral fragility or instability, nor in the presence of neurological signs of cord compression or irritation.

Careful, passive examination of the joint is the beginning of the manipulative treatment. The full examination of a joint's passive range cannot be separated from the initial exploratory passive treatment by stretching and manipulation. Modern physiotherapeutic manipulation consists of a repeated sequence: examination, followed by exploratory passive increase in mobility range, then by re-examination and recording of the range attained. Forceful procedures only follow on after a similar procedure with less force has achieved an increase in mobility range, which is retained. Such gentle techniques require considerable practice and sensitivity. They are gaining considerable support from physiotherapists. They are more properly referred to as 'mobilizing techniques', whereas 'manipulation' is probably more correctly restricted to those manoeuvres involving a sudden, high velocity movement. These latter techniques also require much skill and practice, yet their complexity is not necessarily reflected in their usefulness.

To summarize, both 'manipulations' and 'mobilizations' are techniques of increasing joint range by passive movements. The former are based on single quick movements and are often less controlled than the latter repetitive, gentler movements. It is claimed that because mobilization is more 'controlled' it can therefore be more localized, particularly in relation to spinal joints.

Although there is a considerable volume of anecdotal case law, there are as yet no acceptable clinical trials, nor long-term follow-up studies. Both these forms of physiotherapy deserve a more detailed scientific and unemotional appraisal than they have so far been subjected to.

BREATHING EXERCISES

Medical conditions

Depending upon the needs of the individual patient, the physiotherapist treating a medical condition may seek, by breathing exercises, to:

(1) Maintain chest wall mobility, e.g. ankylosing spondylitis.
(2) Compensate for weakness of muscles of respiration, e.g. tetraplegia, anterior poliomyelitis, myasthenia gravis.
(3) To assist patients to expectorate sputum.
(4) To alleviate the effects of bronchial obstruction or spasmodic constriction, e.g. chronic bronchitis, bronchial asthma.
(5) The counteract the increase in Pco_2 which occurs with inadequate alveolar ventilation.

There is some evidence that breathing exercises can be helpful in the agitated patient. They seem to allay anxiety and they can be a useful adjunct to the treatment of cardiogenic dyspnoea or insomnia.

Surgical conditions

In treating patients undergoing surgical procedures, the physiotherapist teaches breathing exercises pre-operatively when possible, so that in the early post-operative days, which are not conducive to learning new procedures, the exercises may be remembered and used as needed.

The value of breathing exercises has never been clearly established, but they have become traditional in many hospitals. Indeed, such techniques may occupy the attention of 10–20 per cent of the available physiotherapy staff of a District General Hospital. Recent studies indicate that much of this activity is of little value, and the physiotherapist would be better employed in undertaking the energetic treatment of 'at risk' patients before surgery, and in contributing to the care and management of the chronic bronchitic (see Chapter 15), rather than attempting to give breathing exercises to all pre-operative and post-operative patients.

Respiratory complications of surgery

The common post-operative chest complications are likely to derive from blockage of the smaller branches of the bronchial tree by secretions. This leads to infection and local areas of collapse. Expulsion of the secretion by coughing and drainage is the most effective method of prophylaxis and treatment. The overall incidence of these complications has remained virtually unchanged in spite of advances in surgery, anaesthesia and chemotherapy. Patients undergoing abdominal operations are more at risk than patients having operations on the limbs, and upper abdominal operations are more prone to such complications than lower abdominal operations. Such complications appear to be associated with the almost invariable sharp reduction in ventilatory function which follows upper abdominal surgery and which is probably due to temporary diaphragmatic inhibition.

The inhibition of ventilatory function in itself may not be particularly dangerous, but patients who are elderly, who have a history of chronic bronchitis, and who are cigarette smokers are particularly at risk. Pre-operative physiotherapy, associated with an intensive 'no smoking' campaign, can reduce the likelihood of clinically significant post-operative complications.

Patients with chronic bronchitis are considered at special risk, and whatever the operation they are undergoing, if a general anaesthetic is given then post-operative breathing exercises are mandatory. Apart from daily or twice daily sessions with the physiotherapist, such patients should be instructed pre-operatively in relaxation and controlled diaphragmatic breathing and required to take a number of deep breaths every houe. It is customary to recommend a minimum of 10 deep breaths during the hour, but there is no scientific basis for this specific recommendation.

Patients undergoing thoracic surgery, upper abdominal and major spinal surgery are also at special risk of developing post-operative pulmonary collapse. For them, too, regular deep breathing at hourly intervals with the operation wound supported, when possible, by pressure from the hand of the physiotherapist, the nurse or the patient himself, is essential. Assisted coughing, regular postural drainage and regular suction may also be necessary post-operative measures to ensure efficient pulmonary ventilation, encourage expectoration and promote venous return, and in this way discourage the development of pulmonary collapse and infarction.

If such complications arise, then physiotherapy directed towards assisted expulsion of bronchial secretions (while supporting the surgical wound) is often dramatic in its effect. Thus, the problem of the post-operative chest is mainly one of selecting 'at risk' patients before surgery, and treating them vigorously.

Circulatory complications

Post-operative physiotherapy is also directed towards improving venous return from the legs in order to prevent the development of deep venous thrombosis. Considerable scepticism now exists concerning the development of post-operative deep vein thrombosis. Indeed, it is now evident that, in many instances, the thrombosis occurs during a long period on the operating table. In some centres, active measures are in use to prevent the development of thrombosis during this time. These may involve electrical or mechanical stimulation of the calf muscles while the patient is unconscious during the operation. The mechanical measures consist of devices which move the foot through a range of movements at the ankle joint, alternately stretching and relaxing the calf muscles. Electrical techniques consist of the application of an interrupted electrical stimulus to produce intermittent calf-muscle contraction. The calves are usually encased in a bandage or gaiter, for passive movement of the calf without such a constrictive gaiter would be less effective in promoting venous return. Such devices may be left on the patients until they are able to co-operate by performing frequent active movements of the legs. This approach to the prevention of deep vein thrombosis is apparently much more successful than conventional post-operative physiotherapy, which may well be unnecessary for those without a deep vein thrombosis and too late for those who have developed it.

Physiotherapy in intensive care units
In an intensive care unit, it is necessary to distinguish between the need for elective, prophylactic and therapeutic procedures, which are properly the role of the physiotherapist, and the emergency care of an 'acute chest', which all personnel in the unit should be trained to treat. Some patients in intensive care units will be paralysed and will require passive movements for the limbs; others will be recovering from cardiac conditions and will require gentle encouragement to move their limbs under the guidance of the cardiologist; others will be recovering from multiple injuries or major surgery, and their recovery will be a matter of graduated activity determined by their general clinical status. A proportion of patients in intensive care units require intensive respiratory care, and it is these to whom physiotherapeutic techniques—in particular the 'bag-squeezing' technique combining assisted coughing, drainage, and suction—can be life-saving.

Patients in respirators because of severe paralysis, and patients with chest injuries, present special problems of acute physical care, which are not properly the concern of this book.

Breathing exercises as a relaxation technique
During the recent re-awakening of Western interest in Eastern customs, exponents of Yoga and Karate have demonstrated anew the importance of effective voluntary breathing control in exercise performance and in mental and physical relaxation. Surveys currently being carried out appear further to indicate that voluntary control may also be learned and temporarily applied to certain processes normally controlled by the autonomic system, such as heart rate and blood pressure.

Despite these indications of the far-reaching effects which learned voluntary control can have on essential body functions, the term 'breathing exercises' is still used in a mildly derogatory fashion by those doctors who have not needed them for themselves or their patients. Even so, if breathing exercises are correctly taught, and correctly used, they appear to be of value.

When teaching relaxation technique, each physiotherapist uses the method of tuition which she has developed to suit her own personality and modifies it to suit the personality of each individual patient whom she teaches.

Most physiotherapists check that the patient is lying comfortably, and ask him first to contract the muscles of the upper limb and then relax them, and finally to relax the muscles completely without preliminary contraction. This sequence is repeated for the muscles of the lower limbs and abdomen and the thorax, in this order. To help them relax, many patients need the assistance of evocative images–such as lying in a warm bath or bed on the first day of the holi-day, or lying on hot sands listening to the sound of the surf–derived first from the physiotherapist's voice and then from their own minds. It is important that once the technique of relaxation at will has been mastered, it should be practised regularly in the several position in which any particular patient is likely to experience respiratory distress, and that such practice should become an important part of the programme of daily living for patients with chronic respiratory dysfunction.

When the patient can relax at will, he then learns first the 'awareness' of the various muscles, particularly those of respiration, and then the 'control' of the duration and power of their contraction. Against the resistance of the therapist's hand, and progressively against the resistance of his own fist, pillows or belts, he develops increasing strength in these muscles. He then learns how to control the timing and depth of breathing until the duration and volume of expiration and inspiration can be varied at will.

The need for the acquisition of breathing control is common to all conditions involving respiratory dysfunction. It is the optimal timing and mode of application of this control which is highly individual to each patient and his particular situation.

HYDROTHERAPY

Hydrotherapy has been a standard form of treatment for many diseases for many years. However, it is usually regarded as mainly being of value for rheumatic disorders and for patients with paralysis following poliomyelitis. For this reason, treatment pools were installed in the physiotherapy departments of hospitals specializing in these problems. Because most of the patients were severely disabled, the classical approach was to install a *small* pool, and hydro-therapy apparatus, such as a Hubbard tank, became the standard fitting. The emphasis in all this type of work was on individual passive treatment.

In the rehabilitation of lower limb injuries, following limb operations and in the general care of the arthritic patient, this 'classical' approach is exactly the opposite of that which gives the best results. A large heated pool, although an expensive item of equipment, provides a wide range of active therapy for a wide range of patients, and is a very adaptable piece of apparatus which should repay its cost in its general usefulness.

It is usual to regard hydrotherapy as providing buoyancy and thus assisting movement for weak muscles and damaged joints. It was this particular attribute which aided in the management of poliomyelitis and gained a high repuation for hydrotherapy. In fact, however, it can provide many other forms of activity, ranging from total suspension of the severely disabled to strong resistance exercises for those approaching the final stages of rehabilitation. This variation is provided by simple techniques involving either working with the water or against the water.

The assistance provided by the buoyancy of the water and the resistance which it offers can be enhanced by the use of flotation devices. These may be in the form of inflated cushions or rubber rings attached to the arms and legs. They can also be made from buoyant materials such as polystyrene.

Flat walking areas in the pool can provide the simplest form of graduated partial weight-bearing for re-education in walking after injuries or surgery of the lower limbs. The patient starts off in relatively deep water, where most of his weight will be taken by buoyancy, and graduates to shallow water as his condition improves, finally progressing to full weight-bearing outside the pool.

In some centres, the areas of different depth are separated by internal walls or rails, whereas at others, small pools of different depths are provided as 'annexes' of the main pool.

The warmth and the effect of the water are an exce.ent basis for mobilization of stiff joints. The only contra-indications to intermi·tent hydrotherapy, apart from patients encased in plaster of paris, must be incontinence and open or infected wounds. It is evident that this form of treatment could be used to advantage for a large number of patients of any rehabilitation unit.

In general, the best size for a treatment pool suitable for a major rehabilitation unit or department would be 40 ft by 20 ft (12.2m x 6.1m) (18 ft x 14 ft is the recommended minimum size). It should be maintained at a temperature of 90°– 95°F. There must be easy access into the water via shallow steps, and for the more severely disabled, appropriate hoists should be installed. Preferably, there should be graduated levels of depth from 3 ft to 4 ft 6 in (91.5–137.2 cm) or if it is not possible to provide graduation, a pool of constant depth of about 2 ft 6 in to 3 ft (76–91.5 cm). If the edge of the pool is raised above the floor of the department by 2 ft to 2 ft 6 in (61–76 cm), it facilitates transfers to and from wheelchairs and it is more easily supervised by instructors outside the pool.

Finally, there must be adequate changing room accommodation to allow for continuous use of the pool while patients are preparing to enter the pool and, later, drying and dressing after treatment. Indeed, the surroundings and necessary associated services are almost as important as the pool itself, and although they certainly add considerably to the space and cost involved, they contribute significantly to the efficiency of the department as a whole.

There are many practitioners experienced in rehabilitation who would be prepared to forgo almost all the other facilities normally present in a physiotherapy department if they could retain a good, well-appointed hydrotherapy department.

The Spas in particular have flourished upon the reputation of hydrotherapy, although this is by no means the full extent of the medical service which these centres customarily supply.

Natural hot springs are reputed to have a number of properties associated with medical effects which are not present in heated mains water. There is, however, no scientific evidence that there is any effect other than warmth and buoyancy. The effectiveness of spa hydrotherapy treatment cannot be separated from the people who dispense and prescribe it, nor can it be considered apart from its surroundings. There is undoubtedly a very large placebo effect from physical treatment, which is enhanced by the traditional setting of the spa, but what probably contributes most to the efficiency of spa therapy is the overall regimen (the rehabilitation approach) which is imposed upon the patient. Those spas with a positive approach and good overall medical supervision can provide an excellent rehabilitation service for patients with locomotor disorders.

BIBLIOGRAPHY AND REFERENCES

General
The Physical Medicine Library (1969). S. Licht (Ed.). Connecticut; E. Licht
    Volume 1: Electrodiagnosis and Electromyography.
    Volume 2: Therapeutic Heat and Cold.

Volume   3: Therapeutic Exercise.
Volume   4: Therapeutic Electricity and Ultraviolet Radiation.
Volume   5: Massage, Manipulation and Traction.
Volume   7: Medical Hydrology.
Volume   8: Medical Climatology.
Volume   9: Orthotics, etcetera.
Volume 10: Rehabilitation and Medicine.
Volume 11: Arthritis and Physical Medicine.

Ultrasonics
Bierman, W. (1954). 'Ultrasound in the treatment of scars.' *Archs. phys. Med. Rehabil.* 35, 210
Dyson, M. and Pond, J.M. (1970). 'Effect of pulsed ultrasound on tissue regeneration.' *Physiotherapy* 56, 136
Dyson, M. and Pond, J.M. (1973). 'The effects of ultrasound in the circulation.' *Physiotherapy* 59, 284
Summer, W. and Patrick, M.K. (1964). *Ultrasonic Therapy.* Amsterdam; Elsevier

Exercise therapy
De Andrade, J.R., Grant, C. and Dixon, A.St.J. (1965). 'Joint distension and reflex muscle inhibition.' *J. Bone Jt Surg.* 47A, 313
Gough, J.V. and Hadley, G. (1971). 'An investigation into effectiveness of various forms of quadriceps exercise.' *Physiotherapy* 57, 356
Leach, R.E., Skyker, W.S. and Zohn, D.A. (1965). 'A comparative study of isometric and isotonic quadriceps exercise programmes.' *J. Bone Jt Surg.* 47A, 1421
Lenman, J.A.R. (1959). 'A clinical and experimental study of the effects of exercise on motor weakness in neurological disease.' *J. Neurol. Neurosurg. Psychiat.* 22, 182
Salter, N. (1967). 'Exercise therapy.' *Ann. phys. Med.* 4, 81

Hydrotherapy
Bolton, E. and Goodwin, D. (1967). *Introduction to Pool Exercises* (3rd edn). Edinburgh and London; Livingstone
Davis, B.C. (1967). 'A technique of rehabilitation in the treatment pool.' *Physiotherapy* 53, 2, 57
Duffield, M.H.T. (1969). *Exercise and Water.* London; Bailliere, Tindall and Cassell
'Planning of hydrotherapy departments' (1965). Report of a Conference at the Hospital Centre, London. *Br. Hosp. J. Soc. Serv. Rev.* 75, 2289

Manipulative procedures
British Association of Physical Medicine (1966). 'Pain in the neck and arm: a multicentre trial of the effect of physiotherapy.' *Br. med. J.* 1, 253
Cyriax, J.H. (1971). *Textbook of Orthopaedic Medicine.* Vols 1 and 2 (5th edn). London; Bailliere, Tindall and Cassell
Maitland, G.D. (1964). *Vertebral Manipulation.* London; Butterworths
Maitland, G.D. (1970). *Peripheral Manipulation.* London; Butterworths
Stoddard, A. (1959). *Manual of Osteopathic Techniques.* London; Hutchinson

Traction
Matthews, J.A. (1968). 'Dynamic discography. A study of lumbar traction.' *Ann. phys. Med.* 9, 275
Powell, M. (1970). *Orthopaedic Nursing* (6th edn). London; Livingstone
Yates, D.A.H. (1972). 'Indications and contraindications for spinal traction.' *Physiotherapy* 58, 2, 55

Breathing exercises
Nichols, P.J.R. and Howell, B. (1968). 'Routine pre- and post-operative physiotherapy: results of a questionnaire.' *Ann. phys. Med.* 9, 264
Nichols, P.J.R. and Howell, B. (1970). 'Routine pre- and post-operative physiotherapy: results of a trial.' *Rheum. phys. Med.* 10, 321

3 Occupational Therapy

INTRODUCTION

Occupational therapy offers a service designed to help the patient to return to his former occupation, or, when necessary, to help the patient to adjust to an adapted or new occupation.

The term 'occupation' implies more than a person's actual work, whether that of a bricklayer, bank manager, housewife, student or schoolchild. It implies the role normally associated with the person's work in the person's own environment. It must also imply a sufficient degree of mobility, personal independence and psychological maturity to maintain that role.

Thus, occupational therapy may be defined as a paramedical service with the function of assisting the patient's return to the fullest possible physical, psychological and social competence both in his former occupation and in his customary role in life.

To this end, the occupational therapist is increasingly concerned with the assessment of the patient's physical capabilities, the exploitation of his residual skills, and the planning of the retraining of patients with a permanent disability. Practical assessment should precede the final stages of rehabilitation and settlement, and repeated assessment can provide objective records of a patient's progress. There is no other profession supplementary to medicine so aptly suited to help the patient bridge the gap between physical disability and functional capability.

Occupational therapy training includes considerable study of psychology and at least 6 months' work in psychiatric hospitals prior to registration. The therapist therefore has an awareness of the closely interwoven psychological and physical factors in illness and disablement and of the impact of these factors upon the patient, his family and his social environment. The therapist's training enables her to offer some assessment of the patient's attitudes and social background, as well as his residual physical capability, and thus equips her to contribute to the planning of his rehabilitation programme and return to work.

Occupational therapists are taught the basic skills of home economics, wood and metal work, and heavy workshop techniques, together with creative work of all kinds, from painting and pottery to cooking and gardening, from typing and fretwork to bricklaying and house decorating.

When a patient is of normal retirement age, or is so severely disabled that it is impossible for him to resume work, the emphasis will be on finding positive and creative leisure interests that will bring him into contact with other people, so reducing the isolation which severe handicap inevitably brings.

Consequently, occupational therapy still carries with it the relics of the 'arts and crafts' image, and some of the practitioners and teachers unfortunately still place undue emphasis on training in traditional but superficial aspects of the work. These activities were never intended to be an end in themselves, but a means whereby the therapist could assess and train a patient's manual skill, range of joint movement, learning ability and work tolerance. Diversional and recreational activities have their place in the overall management of long-stay patients and patients with chronic disability, but in present-day rehabilitation, the emphasis on the importance of these aspects of occupational therapy has changed.

The most important contribution that the modern occupational therapist makes is in the assessment of a patient's actual and potential functional capability with or without aids and appliances. The design, manufacture and prescription of these aids and appliances is influenced by the informed opinion of the therapists who train patients in their use.

Although the complete functional assessment of a patient must include the social, clinical, educational and domestic implications, the functional capabilities must be expressed in a practical fashion in terms of normal activities, and this translation should be the occupational therapists' particular contribution. For these reasons, an increasing number of occupational therapists are employed in domiciliary work or are based in community services rather than hospital services. The occupational therapists working in a domiciliary setting are often attached to general practitioners and work in close co-operation with the Social Services at Health Centres and Community Hospitals and among patients in their own homes. The future trend would appear to be the further development of this aspect of the service as a link and extension of progressive patient care through hospital and out into the community.

PSYCHIATRIC PATIENTS

Although not the concern of this book, it is important to note that nearly half of all qualified occupational therapists work in psychiatric departments. As well as aiding diagnosis and helping to control symptoms through purposeful activity, a variety of situations are used whereby work, domestic, social and personal competence can be assessed. If necessary, modifications can be advised to prepare for return to normal life or at least to maintain as high a standard of functional integrity as is possible in those who suffer chronic and irreversible conditions.

Activities are carried out individually or in groups, according to each patient's needs. The therapy prescribed has several possible advantages – it may be of individual, group or social value and can also be designed to improve the patient's ability to form social relationships.

Creative activities give the patient means of expressing an emotion which would otherwise remain unrealized, or relieving an inhibition. Pottery and painting or musical and dancing activities are of particular value in this context. Apart from providing a means of self-expression, working with one's hands is a welcome diversion during a period of psychiatric treatment.

Similarly, the patient's capabilities for performing jobs and tasks can be evaluated. Initially this may be in clinical surroundings but may progress to assessment for employment in sheltered or open workshops. Coping at home may be difficult. Problems may arise in day-to-day activities such as cooking, cleaning and serving. These and other skills must be retaught, where appropriate; if possible, relatives and friends should be involved so as to encourage a cohesive family unit.

Contact with others may lead to control of expression or to an ability to express reasoned thought. It may also lead to an improvement in self-confidence and behaviour. It is important at this stage to maintain, encourage and improve the standards of personal care, fitness and hygiene. This will be by means of advice on diet, clothes, and care of the skin and hair, coupled with appropriate amounts of physical exercise.

OCCUPATIONAL THERAPY AND PHYSICAL DISABILITY

The occupational therapist has a role to play at many stages during the patient's development of and recovery from physical disability. By her assessment of his psychological and physical disability and handicap, she makes a major contribution to the initial understanding of his problems.

During treatment, she can contribute to the development of maximal functional capability through appropriate activities in relevant situations. At a later stage she can prepare the patient for return home to his particular social and economic situation.

The tools of the occupational therapist are the everyday activities of life:

Self-care activities   Dressing, washing, feeding, toiletting and grooming.
Domestic and child-care activities   Mainly for women but many can be usefully taught to men and should include house maintenance.
Work activities   Clerical work, wood and metal work, and light industrial work.
Leisure activities   Games, hobbies and gardening.

If the activity chosen has significance to the patient by relating to his intellectual level and social environment, it will gain and hold his co-operation, e.g. a repetitive packing job will have no significance to the middle-aged teacher, but will be a 'real' situation to a factory girl of 18.

The activity is chosen not to 'keep the patient busy' but because:

(1) It provides a medium for the occupational therapist's observation of functional performance and emotional reaction.
(2) It provides suitable physical exercise to build up precision skills, co-ordination and work tolerance.
(3) It provides suitable activities for training in the use of appliances, such as artificial limbs.
(4) It provides a means of assessing the patient's learning ability.
(5) It provides creative and expressive activities, e.g. art, music and drama, used in the diagnosis and treatment of mental illness.

Functional assessment
An essential preliminary activity and a necessary part of training is the assessment

of the patient's functional capability; such a functional assessment forms the framework within which rehabilitation plans can be realistically shaped. It is therefore as important to the patient's future activity as the assessment of *disability* has been to an understanding of his present state.

Functional assessment:

(1) Gives a base line, at any given time, from which future progress or deterioration in function may be measured.
(2) Gives a guide to any changes which need to be made in the patient's routine and functional techniques or to the need for provision of appliances, aids and equipment.
(3) Adds to the diagnostic data, e.g. in a patient with brain damage the area of visuo-spatial defect or the nature of a dysphasia may be defined by observing the patient's performance throughout a series of activity patterns.
(4) Gives some prognostic guide as to physical function, e.g. comparative functional assessment of a hand with and without a simple corrective splint will give an indication to a surgeon whether surgical reconstruction will give his patient fuller hand function.
(5) Gives some prognostic guide as to the patient's motivation and ability to benefit from a programme of rehabilitation.

Assessment is an ongoing process and repeated reappraisal is necessary to define the patient's current problems and to indicate necessary adjustments in the rehabilitation programme. The activities which it entails may be carried out in hospitals, special rehabilitation units, work centres, sheltered workshops or the patient's own home.

In the rehabilitation of the physically handicapped, the main function of the occupational therapist is to help the patient to reach and maintain his optimal physical, psychological and social competence.

The patient's activities with which she is mainly concerned are:

(1) Mobility.
(2) Personal care.
(3) Domestic activities.
(4) Work potential.
  (a) Manual skills.
  (b) Ability to use educational skills.
  (c) Work tolerance.
(5) Educational and recreational activities.

The activities involved in personal care (including feeding, washing, dressing), domestic activities, such as cooking and housework, and mobility in relation to domestic and work situations are referred to collectively as activities of daily living (ADL).

It is thus the occupational therapist who, by planned salvage operation, helps the patient to adjust to his new role occasioned by disability and who helps him to accept both the new role and a new environment, should this be necessary. Where disability exists, the occupational therapist first seeks methods and techniques to overcome the difficulty. Reorganizing of daily routine and minor adjustment of habitual methods either at home or at work are often all that is necessary. Some aids or equipment may be of help, but the fewer and simpler the better. Additional services, such as home helps and meals-on-wheels, are available and are recommended, when needed, by the assessing occupational therapist. Finally, particularly for the more severely disabled, complex devices or adaptations to house and home may be the only way of retaining some level of independence.

General principles

The basis of all modern occupational therapy is the functional assessment of the patient. Whereas the physiotherapist will be concerned with recording the range or strength of the movement, the occupational therapist is more concerned with the applied range, strength and co-ordination in the performance of essential activities. Following their individual assessments, e.g. on a patient who has had a hip operation, the physiotherapist will be primarily concerned with devising an exercise programme to re-establish hip mobility and the patient's ability to sit, stand and walk. The occupational therapist will be more concerned with improving his ability to dress and use the toilet independently (activities which involve sitting, standing and walking). This assessment of the patient's functional capacity cannot be considered in isolation. It must be part of a total assessment, including the clinical evaluation of status and prognosis and a study of the patient's domestic and environmental background. Other factors, such as the patient's age, attitude of mind and social circumstances, must be taken into account.

The occupational therapist's functional assessment can be of many different varieties, depending upon the clinical situation and the assessment situation. Usually she will start with a structured enquiry directed towards delineating particular areas of difficulty. The initial enquiry entails questioning the patient about activities of daily living, work and hobbies. This is followed by more detailed checks and cross-checks but always it is necessary to observe the patient undertaking certain selected tasks. Answers to questions are notoriously misleading, and many patients give answers calculated to avoid complications. For example, few patients readily acknowledge difficulties in coping with personal toilet, for such an admission may lead inevitably to authoritative decisions being made about their ability to continue living independently at home. Thus, close observation of dressing and toilet activities in hospital or in the occupational therapy department will give more realistic information than simple questionnaires.

The next stage of functional assessment is the use of clearly structured tests. These tests can be repeated at intervals and used as a measure of the patient's progress. When the structured tests are activities of daily living, then the tests themselves become a training exercise and lead, therefore, to the solution of some problems which present difficulty, finally enabling the patient to 'pass the test'. This sequence of exposing the problems, trying to overcome them and then retesting, forms the basis of the occupational therapist's functional assessment.

However, if the problem-solving is to be realistic, it is necessary to extend the assessment procedure to gain maximal information about the patient's real problems in his own environment. For example, assessing a patient's ability to bath herself is unrealistic if the house in which she lives has no bath. Although most occupational therapy departments have their own assessment forms, which vary in detail, the information required to highlight the main problem areas follows a common pattern:

(1) Home conditions:
   Type of residence,
   Accessibility (steps, etc.),
   Family and relatives or friends available for help;
(2) Mobility:
   Walking, use of aids and appliances,
   Steps, etc., to be negotiated,
   Use of wheelchair,
   Need for and availability of outdoor transport;
(3) Personal care:
   Washing, dressing, toilet and bath,
   Eating and drinking;
(4) Communication:
   Speech, telephone, writing and typing,
   Reading,
   Transport available,
   Shopping;
(5) Domestic activities:
   Meal preparation,
   Housework;
(6) Work:
   Problems of job,
   Problems at work (including housework),
   Schooling and education of children or training school for older children;
(7) Leisure and recreational activities and hobbies:
   Past and present interests and problems.

As part of her work, the therapist will learn much about the patient's attitude, reactions, dependence, co-operation and adaptability to disability. This contributes considerably to the overall assessment. Many departments use different check lists for different clinical conditions. Thus, a patient with a temporary disability only needs a short check list, related to the specific problem which his temporary disablement incurs, whereas patients with more severe and more chronic disability require more extensive assessment procedures.

The elderly patient who falls and breaks a wrist may need some help and advice while her wrist is in plaster. The assessment will consist of a few key questions, a simple test and a short explanation. Patients recovering after total hip replacement need a different approach—encouragement in regaining confidence and confirmation that they can manage normal activities, such as sitting on a toilet. Amputees present a much greater problem, particularly if they are elderly. They need a considerable amount of help which should include training in dressing, bathing and the use of a wheelchair (for those occasions when they are unable to use their artificial limbs).

For the more severely disabled, it is important for the occupational therapist to carry out her practical assessment in related sequence. While a patient may achieve washing, dressing, cooking and feeding when assessed separately, the full sequence, from starting in bed to eating a cooked meal, may require a level of activity beyond the patient's endurance or may consist of a sequence of manoeuvres which cannot be achieved in his particular domestic context. The determination of capability to achieve a continuous sequence of activities is particularly important in assessing the likelihood of the patient's return to work.

Thus, the occupational therapist working in hospital or rehabilitation unit requires considerable ingenuity in achieving realistic assessment and in inventing 'real life' situations corresponding to the patient's home or work. Without these practical tests, she is likely to make mistakes which can have considerable repercussions. For this reason, many forms of structured tests have been devised which duplicate domestic and work conditions. Many departments have an assessment kitchen or even a complete living area with bedroom, bathroom, kitchen and living room. Other departments have light and heavy workshops to provide realistic testing and training for industrial activity. All occupational therapy assessment and training, including leisure activities, should be related to activities useful to the patient.

These days there is more emphasis on getting disabled people out into the community and there are increasing opportunities for them to take part in activities such as swimming, riding and fishing.

Records and reports
It is upon the recorded information about the patient's disability that many complex, expensive and important decisions may be based. It is therefore incumbent upon the therapist to maintain careful and accurate records and to be able to present them in a clear and precise fashion. Verbal reporting is often called for within the team, but written records are essential for communication with others (e.g. from hospital to domiciliary staff) and for following progress over long periods of time. Here it cannot be over-emphasized that documentation of unsuccessful attempts and unsuccessful therapy can be more important in the long-term record than details of successful activities. Furthermore, it is essential to record *reasons* for decisions that are taken. If advice is given without explanations, or notes do not record lack of success, other therapists may waste many hours covering the same ground. Had such written information been available, changes in the situation might have been revealed on review or recourse to the records, which would otherwise have remained unnoticed. With carefully planned check lists and details of performance, the occupational therapist's records can be as precise and as valuable to the clinician as the muscle chart and joint range records maintained by the physiotherapist. Whenever possible, the tests should be presented in a form which is immediately intelligible and, when repeated, should indicate clearly whether improvement or deterioration is occurring. Furthermore, the tests should, whenever possible, be selected so that the results can be recorded accurately, even if carried out by different therapists.

OCCUPATIONAL THERAPY IN SPECIAL UNITS

District General Hospital
The occupational therapy department of a District General Hospital usually comprises heavy and light workshops, a clerical section, a quiet area for study, and a domestic unit including kitchen, bedroom and bathroom, for assessing and training in activities of daily living.

A comprehensive, modern occupational therapy department is able to provide an atmosphere closely approaching that in a normal home or work situation. The assessment and testing is almost surreptitious. The occupational therapist will note whether the patient is anxious, depressed, co-operative, alert, moody, aggressive, euphoric or unrealistic. Over a period of time she will be able to note changes in behaviour (improvement or deterioration). Through simple activities she will be able to note the patient's power of concentration and his 'distractability'. Indeed, the surrounding distraction can be graded by altering the place in which simple activities such as playing games are carried out and by altering the complexity of the recreational activity.

Many simple leisure activities can be used to test memory and the ability to carry out both verbal and written instructions. Gardening, cooking and model building are all examples of apparently diversional activities which provide material for very reliable assessments. The patient's initiative (verbal and physical), his reliance upon others, his 'fatiguability' and his personality can all be gauged by the therapist while the assessment is undetected by the patient. Indeed, the occupational therapist can assess the response to adverse situations by spoiling the patient's chances in a game or apparently failing to provide correct or adequate materials.

The therapist's personality clearly plays a large part in this type of assessment, particularly with brain-damaged patients. About one half of all occupational therapists work in psychiatric hospitals, and a considerable proportion of their training is directed towards this field. This gives them a wider knowledge and understanding of behaviour, behaviour problems and abnormalities than many other workers in the field of physical handicap.

On the physical side, the occupational therapist can provide graded activity designed to increase muscle power, joint range, co-ordination and balance. Her work complements that of the physiotherapist, and extends the use of the patient's limbs in functional activities relevant to daily living. She is able to provide additional stimulus and interest through constructive and creative activities, employing different aspects of motivation to achieve similar objectives. In specific instances, functional or diversional activities can be adapted to supplement exercise regimes already introduced by the physio-therapist. Patients with hand injuries may, for example, spend time in the physiotherapy department exercising their hands in hot water or after wax treat-ment. This can be followed by a period in the occupational therapy department playing 'draughts' with specially designed heavy draughtsmen or playing a form of blow football using hand-squeezed pumps to blow the ball.

It is often argued that muscle strength, co-ordination and independence all improve simultaneously without specific therapy, but most patients do better and feel better if these activities are encouraged both by specific exercises (physiotherapy) and general or specific functional activities (occupational therapy).

Medical Rehabilitation Unit

When the emphasis in a Medical Rehabilitation Unit, whether out-patient or residential, is on active restoration of function and progression to a full day's work for the patient with a temporary disability, the occupational therapist's role will be mainly therapeutic. This will be achieved through her selection for each patient of appropriate activities calling for a repetitive movement of the injured part, and through the programme she devises in which a working activity involves progressively longer periods of standing, walking and co-ordination.

Much of this activity will be supplementary and complementary to the general and specific exercises and activity given by the physiotherapist.

Prior to initiating the treatment programme, the occupational therapist investigates the patient's work potential and any relevant problems of mobility. The aim must be, if possible, to return the patient to his or her employment. If this is unrealistic, consideration must be given to transfer to an industrial training centre or to sheltered employment.

The occupational therapist will provide an assessment of the need for help and training with personal care and activities of daily living, and such training may well prevent further deterioration in the patient's condition.

Adult Training Centres, Sheltered Workshops and Work Centres

An Adult Training Centre usually consists of a Sheltered Workshop and a therapeutic Work Centre. Where possible, these are situated in an industrial trading estate, where a variety of small contract work is available from local firms, and the handicapped workers have daily contact with workers in adjoining industries.

A Sheltered Workshop is subsidized by the Department of Employment and Productivity and referral is usually through the Disablement Resettlement Officer. In these Workshops, the permanently handicapped who can cope with an 8-hour day, 5 days a week, but who are too disabled to compete in open employment, are able to earn a small wage. They are usually expected to travel to work independently.

Many disabled people cannot work at this level, and they may be referred to a Work Centre catering for the severely disabled who can benefit from regular work and who may progress to sheltered open employment. Such patients receive National Health Insurance or Unemployment Benefit, but are usually restricted in how much they are allowed to earn. When necessary, transport is provided. Attendance may be for part or all of the working week, according to the patient's capacity.

The occupational therapist can contribute much to the Work Centre in co-operation with the Industrial Manager. She can assess the handicapped person's ability by a series of aptitude and work potential tests, advise the most suitable Centre for him, and adjust the work to his needs.

An atmosphere of realistic work and progress should be built up within such Centres and by frequent reassessment the opportunity should be open for a patient to progress to a Sheltered Workshop, though it is appreciated that there are administrative and financial difficulties involved in such a transfer.

A therapy area within the Work Centre can provide a quieter situation in which more help is available for the physically severely disabled and for mentally handicapped patients who need more supervision. Facilities for activities of daily living and social training should also be available within the therapy area, providing for individual help or work in small groups. Any workers needing this training would come out of the Workshops for short periods during the day.

All work facilities for the disabled should be closely associated with the clinical rehabilitation facilities and should be geared to allow the easy transfer of patients as and when their clinical and functional capabilities indicate that this is possible. This implies a level of collaboration, integration and interest between all departments concerned with the disabled which is not yet available, but which could develop with the reorganization of the National Health Service. Should regional 'rehabilitation' teams develop, they should include doctors concerned with occupational health and rehabilitation, the Workshop Manager, therapists, social workers, the Careers Advisory Officer and the Disablement Resettlement Officer.

Day Centres
In contrast to Day Hospitals which are therapeutic organizations, Day Centres are recreational and social and serve four main purposes:

(1) To 'maintain' the severely disabled and provide them with positive interests.
(2) To relieve the family of their care for short, regular periods.
(3) To provide social contacts and activities for the residents of Old People's Homes and Homes for the Young Severely Disabled.
(4) To provide a hot, nutritious meal (particularly important for those who live alone).

Ideally, patients would be referred to these Centres by the general practitioner and would be regularly reviewed by a visiting rehabilitation team. At present, Day Centres are run by the Social Services Departments of the Local Authorities, but after the integration of the Health Services in 1974, it is hoped that there will be closer collaboration between all the rehabilitation services concerned.

It is estimated that there should be one Day Centre for every 30 000 people. Each Centre should have a professionally trained supervisor, preferably from a paramedical profession, but would be largely staffed by assistants with lesser training and by volunteers.

An occupational therapist spending two or more sessions a week at the Day Centre can provide an extra service by advising on daily living problems and helping to organize a wide range of leisure activities catering for all intellectual levels.

Domiciliary occupational therapy
Visits by the occupational therapist to the handicapped person in his own home are necessary to assess his functional capability and to identify his problems in his own environment of house, family and community.

She should pass on relevant findings to the:

(1) General practitioner.
(2) Hospital — before the patient's admission or in preparation for his return home.
(3) Local Authority Departments concerned, including the housing department.

The occupational therapist will be able to:

(1) Continue activities of daily living training started in hospital and supply aids needed.
(2) Deal with difficulties of access and mobility.
(3) Assist the family and other helpers with difficulties in the care of the patient, and the social adjustment.
(4) Provide educational and recreational activities for those unable to attend the Day Centre.

In practice, the occupational therapist will often carry out the initial assessment and provide advice; the detailed activities are likely to be carried out by occupational therapy aids or Red Cross workers.

In practice, most patients are referred to the domiciliary occupational therapist by the general practitioner and do not reach a hospital department. The domiciliary occupational therapist of the future may be attached to General Practices, which can facilitate communication with all members of the primary care team.

A Disabled Students' Hostel, a Residential Home for the Young Disabled or an Old People's Home should all be considered in this context as the individual's home and should receive the services of a domiciliary occupational therapist.

The position of the occupational therapist in the team concerned with the rehabilitation of the severely disabled patient is well established. Less well recognized is the vital part which she can play in the rehabilitation of the temporary or moderately disabled patient, whether this disability is physical or mental in origin.

Temporary disability often means a loss of cash and convenience to the average patient. He often understand too little about the interrelationship of time and motion to be able to reorganize either himself or his surroundings to minimize the disabling effects of his condition.

The occupational therapist assists such a patient by making an accurate assessment of his personal and environmental needs and his executive potential, both at home and at work, and by formulating a realistic programme by which the two may be satisfactorily integrated. For both mentally and physically disabled patients, she attempts to delineate areas of actual or probable functional difficulty and to compensate for any effects of disability by promoting a more efficient use of residual ability. For example, wearing an appliance may give rise to a serious loss of immediate functional efficiency, whether it is a replacement prosthesis such as an artificial limb or a corrective, compensatory or stabilizing device such as a caliper or a splint. Using her professional skills to identify the occupations which will give him the necessary practice in prosthetic use, an occupational therapist can teach the patient the necessary expertise by which he can regain manipulative skill.

To anyone with a locomotor lesion, daily life in the home, at work or in transit between the two, may be fraught with many hazards and discomforts. By simple alterations in body posture and movements, by minor but strategic changes in the arrangement and use of necessary home and work equipment, fittings and furniture, the occupational therapist seeks to alter the patient/milieu relationship until the patient's occupation and surroundings can play a useful role in the therapeutic programme.

Children's Assessment Unit

Children's Assessment Units are being planned in many areas in association with school facilities for the physically handicapped. These Units may be centred on an educational site rather than on a hospital site, but wherever the situation, an integrated course of occupational therapy and training can be planned as part of the child's total programme. A multidisciplinary team will assess and review the physically disabled children and those with behavioural, emotional, learning and speech difficulties who are referred by the school medical officer, the general practitioner or the paediatrician.

The Assessment Unit will also provide a continuing counselling service for parents and will have the responsibility for bridging the gap between eduation and employment.

In this type of organization, the occupational therapist with specialized knowledge and experience of children's disorders is able to:

(1) Organize play therapy for purposes of observation and assessment.
(2) Assist in the testing of developmental level and ability.
(3) Assist in assessment of perceptive loss.
(4) Give training to children and parents in activities of daily living and general independence.
(5) Advise on any aids needed for school or at home.
(6) Inform the domiciliary occupational therapist concerned of the progress and relevant recommendations.

ASSESSMENT OF SPECIAL PROBLEMS

For the majority of patients, a simple functional assessment covering the activities of daily living is all that is required prior to returning home from hospital. However, the occupational therapist may be required to be more specific in the assessment. She may have to deal with problems created by the particular clinical condition, e.g. stroke or rheumatoid arthritis, or with particular activities of employment, e.g. clerical work or light engineering.

Activities of daily living
On admission to hospital, many patients with temporary or permanent disability and most elderly people will be found to have some impairment of function. Although not essential for their care, a careful assessment of their functional capabilities will reveal some activity or activities which could be achieved more easily. Many activities of daily living — getting in and out of bed, getting on and off the toilet, dressing, housework and leisure activities such as gardening — involve complex manoeuvres which become a burden for the elderly, arthritic or mildly infirm. A few simple changes of activity pattern or a few simple aids can often make life easier. The timely support of the social services through the provision of a home help or meals-on-wheels may enable the patient to retain independence at home for a longer period of time. Such an assessment service, coupled with provision of appropriate help, can contribute much to the quality of life. Assessment must begin as soon as possible. If the patient is in hospital, it should be initiated there but only in close co-operation with the community services. Provision and continuity of care must be fostered by means of good communications between hospital and community-based workers. The occupational therapist has a vital part to play in bridging the gap between the patient's clinical care and community care.

A major area of activity for many occupational therapists will therefore lie in assessing patients' aids to daily living, in providing these aids, and in training in their use.

The most frequently required aids are:

(1) Walking aids — frames, sticks and crutches.
(2) Bath and toilet aids.
(3) Simple dressing aids.

The equipment most frequently required includes:

(1) Hoists.
(2) Wheelchairs.

All of these items need individual assessment and practical trials. Thus, occupational therapists need to assess patients in all activities of daily living, determining the need for alterations to be made in the home, demonstrating the safest routines in the kitchen, helping with dressing, effecting necessary adaptations to clothes, re-enforcing speech training, and helping with difficulties in shopping, social activities and so on.

Patients in hospital will start this training in the hospital occupational therapy department and then continue in the home situation, if possible with the same occupational therapist. The integration of the hospital and domicilary service is a goal which might become possible when the Health Services are integrated, but is rarely possible at present.

Pre-vocational assessment

Ideally, the man with a disability should return to normal working conditions either full- or part-time. Apart from the financial benefits, he gains status, dignity and social contacts, together with the satisfaction which most men achieve from work. When this level of activity is not possible, a man may be able to earn a reasonable income by working in his own home or in a sheltered environment. This restricts his social contacts and limits his horizons but may nevertheless enable him to retain interest, dignity and status. For those who are unable to achieve a working status, a specific leisure activity may offer enough creative outlet − physical or intellectual − to enable a disabled person to lead a happy and surprisingly satisfactory life.

For a woman, a main aim is usually to be able to run her home and care for her children and husband, thus fulfilling her normal role in the life of the family. If this is not possible, the next level of achievement to be aimed at is the running of the home with help and assistance. Again, for the severely disabled, a specific creative activity should be the aim for everyone unable to achieve a level of domestic independence.

For children, the end result aimed at should be normal school life, even for the severely physically disabled. Only through as near-normal school life as possible is a satisfactory transition from school to work environment likely to occur. When normal schooling is impossible then special schooling may enable the severely physically disabled child to achieve a good education. However, integration into employment is likely to be more difficult, and the transition from school to community is often not achieved. For the very severely disabled, tuition at home may have to be instituted and can be very successful. Problems almost inevitably arise when schooling comes to an end or when family support is threatened by the parents' increasing age or ill-health.

Thus the early assessment of rehabilitative potential of a patient of any age may be a very important activity and may set in motion a chain of activities which can lead to success or failure in terms of a disabled person's ultimate integration or re-integration into the community.

An occupational therapist may frequently be the first person to broach the problem of a patient's possible return to work. This may be a simple matter calling only for a clinical decision to be made concerning the timing of return to work, or it may be a long and complex procedure involving a series of assessments and periods of training.

The initial pre-vocational assessment comprises a review of the clinical situation, the patient's general functional capabilities, previous employment, domestic situation, financial status and family responsibilities.

On a more specific basis, his attitude towards work, his learning ability and 'fatiguability' are important features which must be assessed. It is important to clarify the likely problems relating to domestic circumstances and the area in which he lives – the availability of employment and availability of suitable transport. With regard to physical disability, it is important to establish not only the patient's ability to work but his ability to cope independently with transport to and from work, and with feeding and toilet activities while at work.

Finally, a preliminary assessment of his level of physical activity in relation to past employment or other specific jobs can be established by a series of relatively simple tests.

Pre-vocational assessments of adults with a physical disability must always start from past experience in terms of education, training and work. Knowledge of local industries is of considerable help, and here the Disablement Resettlement Officer (DRO) should be of assistance. With the increasing establishment of hospital DROs, the resettlement of hospitalized adults will tend to become more of a routine activity of the hospital social worker and hospital DRO. Although the hospital occupational therapist and the DRO will clearly need to collaborate very closely, it is the DRO who is likely to take the initiative for the men with temporary and minor disabilities, whereas the occupational therapist is likely to take the initiative for the housewives and the more severely disabled men. Furthermore, she is likely to be concerned with providing some simulated activities at various levels of physical and intellectual activity which will enable the hospital DRO to make a realistic appraisal of the man's working capabilities. The increasing collaboration between the occupational therapist, the DRO and the assessment team of the Adult Training Unit gives considerable scope for development in the future. Unfortunately, at present these activities tend to be administratively and geographically isolated, but the modern trend is to bring the skills and expertise together, preferably in close proximity to the clinical situation. This ensures a rapid transition from hospital to industrial assessment and a unified collaborative approach towards return to work.

Clerical assessment

Aptitude and capability for clerical work can be readily assessed in an occupational therapy department. Preliminary tests involve writing, copy typing and typing from shorthand, graded spelling tests, reading lists and simple arithmetic. Progression from these involves reading aloud, discussion about the passages read and writing a letter on the subject discussed. The ability to use common reference books such as telephone directories or trade catalogues is also important. Simple office procedures, such as filing, answering the telephone and taking and passing on messages, can be simulated.

Tests of more advanced capability using adding machines, dictaphones or shorthand can often be found within the hospital, making it possible to achieve a realistic assessment.

Geriatric assessment

Elderly patients usually present a complex clinical problem, as they frequently suffer from a number of specific illnesses simultaneously. Many also suffer from some degree of intellectual deterioration, and this will have a significant effect on their capabilities.

Although many elderly patients will be able to accomplish many individual activities of daily living, their ability to return to some level of independence will depend more upon their memory, their ability to initiate action, their understanding of simple problems, their level of concentration and their degree of unimpaired judgement. These features can be assessed by simple tests involving memory, vocabulary, calculation and orientation in time and place. In addition, routine activities of daily living are designed to assess co-ordination, power and general physical capability.

Specific disabilities

Tests of general functional capability, by means of activities of daily living or pre-vocational assessment activities, are non-specific and are relevant to almost all physical disability. However, occupational therapists have a further part to play in devising and carrying out assessments relevant to specific disability. These assessments are used not only to clarify the degree of specific disability, but also to contribute to an objective evaluation of the patient as a whole, the effectiveness of treatment and the need for specific reconstructive surgery. Examples of such disabilities are rheumatoid arthritis, stroke and low back pain.

Rheumatoid arthritis

Rheumatoid arthritis provides a notable situation in which general assessment and specific assessment based upon occupational therapy are of considerable importance in determining the management of a patient.

The general assessment leads to a programme of instruction and training designed to help the patient understand and overcome his disabilities whilst yet preserving function, and to prevent unnecessary deterioration and deformity. Some stress on joints is inevitable during the activities of daily living, but by careful planning and reprogramming, many unnecessary harmful stresses can be eliminated or reduced. Aids and splints are used when it is not possible to overcome difficulties without them. For example, the use of drip-dry clothes and household linen eliminates the need for ironing, and a chair with a seat at an appropriate height minimizes the demands made on upper limbs for pushing up from a sitting to a standing position. Similarly, appropriate grab rails in the toilet and in the bathroom will reduce the repeated weight-thrusting stress sustained in the upper limbs during toilet and bathing activities. Naturally, there is considerable interest in and concentration upon the hands of the rheumatoid arthritic, and many occupational therapists have developed sophisticated tests for assessing hand function.

Hand function tests are usually constructed around the various types of grip:

Pin grip Adequate opposition of thumb; good intrinsic control; good sensation.
Key grip Strong intrinsic control, stable, terminal and proximal interphalangeal joints.
Knife grip As for key grip; good flexion of index finger.

Handle grip or power grip   Adequate adduction of thumb; good finger flexion; good power in long flexors of fingers and wrist dorsiflexors.

Tests can be devised to measure the individual grips and to record them in terms of power and precision. However, hand function only becomes of use if the hand can be placed accurately in space and is therefore dependent upon total upper limb function. Activities such as eating and writing must each be assessed as co-ordinated activity sequences and can also be graded in terms of applied strength and precision. In rheumatoid arthritis, the severely involved hand rarely approaches the strength recorded in normal hands, but the precision and functional ability which can be attained are often remarkable.

Hand function tests are of considerable value to the experienced team, and they provide the clinician with valuable information and insight into the need for and likely response to reconstructive surgery.

Strokes

Almost every occupational therapy department will have its share of patients with strokes.

The pattern of recovery is determined by the severity of the cerebrovascular accident. Functional assessment is often helpful in delineating those patients who have persistent defects of balance and those whose activities are hindered by residual sensory defects. It is important to reveal these features since they signify a poor prognosis as far as functional recovery is concerned. Patients who are unaware of their paralysed limbs are unlikely to co-operate in activities such as dressing, which demand acceptance of the disability. Much more investigation of hemiplegia needs to be undertaken to perfect techniques for teaching these patients to adapt to their disabilities.

Formal speech therapy for patients with dysphasia following a stroke is often only available for short, infrequent sessions. Within the occupational therapy department speech training can be extended into several hours a day. In addition to individual training, group activities can often help the dysphasic patient to relax and spontaneous speech sometimes occurs in such an atmosphere. Singing, in particular, is a great morale booster, and likewise the repetition of well-known things, such as the alphabet or nursery rhymes. Relatives may need help and may need to be taught how to talk to the patient, phrasing their questions so that a 'yes' or 'no' answer is possible. They and the patient often need reassurance that he is not insane or mentally retarded now that speech is lost.

If there is an overwhelming residual disability, an occupational therapist is often the person upon whom both relatives and patients can vent their feelings of oppression and depression.

Visual and sensory defects may lead to dangerous circumstances, and the patient and relatives need to be taught techniques which are safe in potentially dangerous situations, such as the bathroom, workshop or kitchen.

Back pain

Back pain is a symptom which is more often referred to a physiotherapy department than an occupational therapy department at the present time, but many hospitals are recognizing that the occupational therapist's approach has a lot to offer. The occupational therapist can often analyse an individual patient's living activities more thoroughly than a physiotherapist because she is more experienced in this form of assessment. She can then go through these activities and retrain the patient, particularly the housewife, to avoid provocative situations. This may entail reorganizing the way in which she carries out any particular activity, or it may involve the use of simple aids. Dealing with awkward cupboards, lifting children or heavy objects, and carrying out many routine household activities involving lifting and bending can precipitate the return of backache unless they are approached correctly. This is a particular area where collaboration between occupational therapist and physiotherapist can be of great benefit.

OCCUPATIONAL THERAPIST AS A TEACHER

The occupational therapist spends a great deal of her time in teaching patients. The teaching is based on assessment, but the logical outcome of assessment is a period of training (teaching). She teaches the patients individually and in groups to regain activities which have been lost or impaired by disability; to wear and use appliances; to use aids and equipment; to prevent damage and injury to affected joints; and to readjust to a changed set of circumstances. For these reasons, the occupational therapist needs a wide understanding not only of the disabilities, but also of the mechanisms of learning and the techniques of teaching. There is an increasing awareness that patients forget a great deal of what doctors and therapists tell them. Instructions and advice are more likely to be forgotten than other information. The more the patient is told at one time, the more he will forget. The relationship between anxiety and the retention of information is complex, and moderately anxious patients remember more than the highly anxious and more than those who are not anxious.

Therefore, the contribution of the occupational therapist is often a vital one in training the patient to put into everyday practice the advice which the doctor gives to the relative about the underlying clinical condition.

OCCUPATIONAL THERAPIST AS A COUNSELLOR

Much of rehabilitation and resettlement is concerned with disorders which have a chronic, variable and often unpredictable course. With such disorders there is frequently an associated major psychosocial component. The patients are often entitled to a wide range of benefits including: supplementary benefits, sickness benefit, invalidity pension, invalidity allowance, disablement benefit, mobility allowance, invalid care allowance. Many patients want advice on their domestic (including sexual) problems or vocational problems.

Much of the help they require can be supplied through a variety of professionals, including doctors, nurses, psychologists, social workers, resettlements officers; however it is often a therapist, working with the patient in the context of assessing their activities of daily living, who perceives the need for further advice, counselling or training.

Frequently the therapist will need to act as a counsellor in one of many aspects of daily life, and help the patients pick their way through the maze of sources and legislation to achieve the appropriate help and guidance, or indeed to supply such direct counselling herself.

BIBLIOGRAPHY AND REFERENCES

Goble, R.E.A. (1967). 'The role of the occupational therapist in disabled living research'. *Am. J. occup. Ther.* **23**, 145

Macdonald, E.M., Maccough, G. and Murrey, L. (1970). *Occupational Therapy in Rehabilitation* (3rd (edn). London; Balliere and Tindall

Milton Keynes Report of the Working Group on Services for the Physically Handicapped and Rehabilitation (1970). Buckinghamshire County Council

Mountford, S.W. (1965). *Towards Rehabilitation: A Study of Widening Horizons.* Edinburgh and London; Livingstone

Mountford, S.W. (1971). *Introduction to Occupational Therapy.* Edinburgh and London; Livingstone

Occupational Therapist Board (1972). 'Future education and training of occupational therapists.' London; Council for Professions Supplementary to Medicine.

White, A.S. (1972). *Easy Path to Gardening.* London; Readers Digest (in association with the Disabled Living Foundation)

4 Rheumatoid Arthritis

INTRODUCTION

Among patients who suffer from diseases of the locomotor system those with rheumatoid arthritis rank numerically second only to patients with degenerative joint disease.

In the United Kingdom, rheumatoid arthritis affects about one million women and hearly half a million men. The importance of the disease derives from its natural history, its high incidence among younger people, its associated systemic effects and its involvement of multiple joints in a progressive inflammatory, and later, degenerative condition. About half the patients seen in hospitals or special rheumatology units will improve with care and treatment and about half will deteriorate almost inexorably. Many patients, however, have mild rheumatoid arthritis only and never become ill enough or disabled enough to be referred to hospital.

There is increasing evidence that with a period of intensive in-patient therapy followed by careful out-patient supervision and readmission when necessary, many patients can be maintained in a good state of health and may remain actively employed for many years. With close collaboration between rheumatologists, orthopaedic surgeons and rehabilitation services, both in the hospital and in the community, even the most severely disabled patients can be improved and the majority of them can be helped to retain a good functional level and to remain independent in their own homes.

The intensive management in special units with the high staff/patient ratio advocated by some workers is well justified by the long-term results. Some of the most important contributions of these units are the accurate assessment of the patient's disability and handicap and the establishment of clear indicators of disease activity and progress. From these baselines it is possible to form realistic therapeutic aims and detailed, agreed plans for management in terms of drugs, surgery and rehabilitation.

Rheumatoid arthritis presents a challenge in general and specific management and illustrates the need for close collaboration between physician, orthopaedic surgeon and all those concerned with rehabilitation. The general pattern of care has five main aims:

(1) Relief of pain.
(2) Prevention of deformity.
(3) Correction of existing deformity.
(4) Improvement of functional capability.
(5) Control of systemic manifestations.

In order to achieve these aims, a balance needs always to be maintained between rest and activity, and no less fine a balance between medical and surgical intervention. The supervision of medication must be continuous and close, and is the combined responsibility of general practitioners, rheumatologists and surgeons. Splints can be used to provide rest, to correct deformity and to aid function of permanently damaged joints. Conventional passive physiotherapy has little place in the rehabilitation of the rheumatoid patient, other than as a palliative treatment. Passive movements usually evoke pain and muscle spasm, but carefully controlled static and resisted exercises can build up the bulk and strength of wasted muscles. Patients vary in their opinion as to whether heat or cold give most relief to their symptoms.

Occupational therapy is of help in assessing the functional capacity of patients and in training them to cope with the difficulties of daily living. Reassessment prior to return home, and pre-vocational assessment prior to resettlement in employment are other valuable contributions of the occupational therapist.

Stress has a definite effect on this disease and social adjustments and welfare care play an essential part in the general rehabilitation.

It is most important the the interrelationship between medical treatment and the activities of daily living be clearly established at the first meeting of the clinician and patient. Rehabilitation is not a series of regimes, supplemented by a selection of appropriate mechanical aids, which an occupational therapist or a physiotherapist grafts on to the final stage of the medical treatment of a patient. It embraces the total therapy offered to a patient with rheumatoid arthritis and aims at restoring him to normal active daily life. In this process it must never lose sight of the importance of the relief of pain. A patient in pain is worn down mentally and physically. He may well become depressed, choosing inactivity, even though he is irked by it, in an effort to minimize his discomfort. Therefore, one of the earliest and most important steps in the rehabilitation of a patient with rheumatoid arthritis is the institution of an adequate regime of medication employing drugs which are both anti-inflammatory and analgesic, or, if necessary, the carefully monitored use of gold, chloroquine or penicillamine. The use of simple analgesics alone does not produce relief of the inflammatory condition in the joint which gives rise to much of the pain, nor does it relieve joint stiffness. When the pain load is reduced to its lowest level by appropriate drugs, the real personality of the patient emerges, and he is able to co-operate in the struggle to attain maximal independence.

An explanation of the difficulties which exist in the constant attempts to reconcile long-term and short-term aims is also essential in the case of each patient. While the attainment of the maximal degree of pain-free mobility and independence in the fastest possible time is the main object of every patient, it is important for him to realize that the level of mobility attempted at any one stage of the disease must be influenced by the effect which it must have upon mobility in the future. Thus, a patient may be advised to avoid walking with the assistance of elbow crutches to the limit of his endurance, since he may well exacerbate pain and precipitate deformity in his shoulders, hands and wrists. Similarly, a patient with active arthritis of shoulders and hands may be advised to avoid hand propulsion of a wheelchair and to accept a powered chair as a substitute in order to conserve function of the joints of his upper limbs. An explanation of the 'substitution value' of upper and lower limbs will enable a patient to realize that his upper limbs can give him movement even when his lower limbs cannot, and will make him less likely to over-use or badly use his arms and hands in an effort to regain or retain mobility.

CARE IN THE EARLY ACUTE STAGES

The primary objectives of treatment are the reduction of inflammation and pain, the preservation of function and the prevention of deformity.

The essentials of treatment of early acute rheumatoid arthritis are (1) supervised rest, (2) the administration of anti-inflammatory drugs, and (3) gentle physical therapy.

How these components of treatment are blended must depend upon the needs of the individual patient and the opinion of the doctor who supervises his care.

In-patient care
As has been said earlier, follow-up studies indicate that rheumatoid patients are best managed in an independent unit, where medical care is integrated with physiotherapeutic skills and where the slowness of the patient's rate of progress is not accentuated by the faster recovery of patients with less chronic medical conditions. Within a rheumatology unit, the concept of total patient care for these patients can be realized in a manner which is impossible either in a mixed acute ward or an out-patient department.

A period of in-patient care offers the opportunity not only for rapid control of the disease, but also for detailed instruction and advice about the nature of the disease and its management by various members of the treatment team, and the responsible part that must be played by the patient.

Bed rest is used less than previously, as more powerful and specific drug therapy has reduced the need for physical control of the inflammation. Nevertheless, many rheumatologists believe that bed rest, often rigidly supervised, has a part to play, and certainly is important in those with severe, acute disease.

Drug therapy
The last decade has seen an immense change in the drug treatment of Rheumatoid Arthritis, as the development of new products both for the control of symptoms and the control of the disease has been matched by growing enthusiasm and skill of physicians.

Drugs must be used to control symptoms of pain and stiffness at all stages of the disease, while in a proportion of patients the progressive nature of cartilage erosions is an indication for more specific, disease-modifying therapy. It must be emphasized that these drugs are potentially very toxic, that they require careful supervision (often by a hospital department) and are effective in only some two out of every three cases. Thus they are not the treatment for all and certainly are not curative.

A simple plan for drug treatment would be:

(1) Analgesics on demand;
(2) Minor anti-inflammatory agents e.g. proprionic acids that have few side effects;
(3) The addition of Indomethacin at night for the control of residual morning stiffness.
(4) Major anti-inflammatories: the more toxic salicylate and Indomethacin in full dosage day and night;
(5) The addition to 3 or 4 of drugs that act over a period of 2—3 months to control the disease e.g. Anti-malarials, gold salts, Pencillamine, Levamisole, immuno-suppressives. These are potentially very toxic, must be carefully monitored but once found to be effective may need to be given for several years;
(6) Cortiosteroids: currently rarely used.

Physiotherapy
The physiotherapist gives treatment in the acute stage by immobilizing the patient's affected joints with splints, supervising the performance of static exercises and encouraging gentle activity and postural changes within the restrictions imposed by the splintage.

The bed used should have a firm mattress or bed boards under the mattress. The patient should lie flat with only one pillow for his head and *no* pillows under the knees. He may sit up for short periods for meals or toilet, using a firm backrest. At other times he should lie flat with a bed-cage and padded footrest. He should be prone for 20—30 minutes, two or three times a day to prevent flexion contractures of the hips. Splintage of the involved joints for periods of up to 3 weeks is now strongly advocated by some centres. Skin-tight plaster of paris splints holding the joints in functional positions are surprisingly well tolerated. The common ones are:

(1) Posterior shells for the legs, extending from gluteal crease to the heels with a right-angled foot plate and the knees in 3—5 degrees of flexion.
(2) Posterior arm splints from elbow to finger-tips with the wrist in mid-pronation and a few degress of extension. A band is usually added to hold the fingers in a few degrees of flexion and the thumb is usually left free. For the more deformed wrists or hands, an anterior splint is probably more satisfactory.

During the acute stage physical therapy has little place, but as inflammation subsides, activity is gradually introduced. Static exercises can be taught to most patients even in their splints, and the only guides at this stage are the tolerance of the patient and the experience of the therapist. Passive movements are best avoided altogether. Once it is realized that immobilization for up to 3 to 4 weeks can be safely employed without risks of permant loss of movement, the traditional urge to 'maintain mobility' can be ignored.

The stage at which static (isometric) exercises and gentle active exercises are introduced depends entirely on the patient's general and local response to the total treatment. Increasing pain and subsequent stiffness are important warning signs which must not be ignored but must cause the exercise programme to be reduced accordingly. In general, short (5 minutes or less) periods of activity spread at hourly or 2-hourly intervals are likely to be better tolerated and more effective than sessions of physical therapy of more traditional duration.

The performance of exercises can usually be facilitated by a preceding period of warmth, either from wax baths, heat lamps or warm water. For some joints, ice packs produce greater pain relief and better relaxation of the surrounding musculature, but individual response is so varied that it may be necessary to try several palliative measures for a patient before the most appropriate is found.

As the patient responds, physical activity can be gradually increased and the splints can be removed for increasing periods. Weight-bearing is introduced only when the muscles are clearly strong enough, and adequate appropriate walking aids are essential to provide graded weight relief. Other activities such as personal toilet and dressing are also part of the patient's graded exercise routine. At this stage, particularly close collaboration between physiotherapist, occupational therapist and nursing staff is essential to adjust a patient's activity level to his physical capability, while the patient himself gradually learns to undertake the responsibility of determining the pattern of exercise and activity necessary for his recovery.

This staged mobilization is an intensely individual procedure and may need to be revised from day to day.

RETURNING HOME

By the time the patient returns home, he has been taught to manage his life in such a way as to minimize his disabilities and to avoid aggravating his illness. The actual time at which he leaves hospital will be related to the suitability of his home conditions and his own ability to satisfy the demands made upon him by the architecture of his home and the behaviour of his family and friends.

The patient's overall care will then be the responsibility of his family doctor. Good liaison must exist between all concerned and clear recommendations as to future management should be passed on from rheumatologist to general practitioner. However comprehensive the recommendations may be, it is impossible to foretell the relapses and remissions which do occur in this disease. Unpredicted events may well take place and it would seem that, however competent the family doctor, the patient with a chronic, progressive and painful disorder is not satisfied unless he has access to specialist opinion.

All except the mildly affected should probably be reviewed occasionally by a rheumatologist, but it is important to avoid long ambulance journeys and lengthy out-patient waiting periods.

From his rheumatologist and family doctor the patient will have learned the natural history of his illness and of the need to remove stress and fatigue from his life by careful planning of his daily programme; to fragment and vary his routine on any one day according to his condition; to take rests when he needs them; to use the exercise regimes and postural habits taught by the physiotherapist; to employ the methods and aids for his daily living activities advised by the occupationa therapist. Before his regular routine of hand and foot exercises and quadriceps drill, supplemented by specific exercises for other affected joints, performed in several short sessions 5—10 minutes each day, he may somtimes use heating or cooling techniques. The heat may be from a hot bath or shower, an electric fire or domestic infra-red lamp. Alternatively, the patient may apply ice-filled bags to cool a joint, or submerge hands or feet in water in which crushed ice is floating.

Fatigue is to be avoided. The housewife should be encouraged to take a mid-day rest, to rest when joints are painful, and not to push resolutely on through pain. Hand and foot exercises and quadriceps drill must become a part of life.

The patient must come to terms with the practical aspects of his life at home and at work. Organization of daily life should be as simple as possible, following a programme of rest, work and exercise.

ASSESSMENT

The major aim of rehabilitation in chronic disorders is to attain a satisfactory state of equilibrium between the demands made on the patient by his work, his home and his family, and his physical ability to meet those demands. No equilibrium can be obtained without an accurate knowledge of the factors concerned in both, and this demands an accurate assessment of the patient and his milieu. Rheumatoid arthritis is a progressive disease, and the clinical condition of the patient tends constantly to change; thus, many repeated assessments of disease activity and functional capacity are needed if the medical, surgical and rehabilitative aspects of his management are to be appropriately blended. The chronicity of the disease is great, and its effects are so far-reaching that such assessments must be total, combining the specialized opinions of clinician, physiotherapist, occupational therapist, medical social worker, clinical psychologist and nursing staff. Repeated assessment enables a knowledge of a patient's physical state, intellectual and psychological make-up and present and future situations to have an appropriate influence on his overall management.

As some aspects of care call for a reversal of approach, collaborative assessments and detailed consultations are necessary at all stages so that a change from conservative care to a more aggressive surgical approach, or a decision to reduce activity and rely more upon aids and appliances can be discussed frankly with the patient. At all times, the patient's complete understanding of his disease and realistic aims for his treatment are essential to his management.

Functional assessment
The total assessment of the rheumatoid arthritic patient provides information on a number of separate features:

(1) General disease activity.
(2) Local joint disease activity.
(3) Degree of deformity and consequent functional disability.
(4) Extra-articular features and complications.
(5) Concurrent illness, both physical and psychological.
(6) Family, work and social state, and ability to fulfil commitments at home, at work and in society, with delineation of specific difficulties.

These functional assessments provide pertinent summaries of a patient's disabilities. Clinical examination will provide details of muscle power and joint range, but what matters to the patient is the combination of joint and muscle action used in his everyday life. What he wants from those who give him care is the expertise which enables them to detect and rectify a breakdown or threatened breakdown in his personal equilibrium of real need and functional ability. Repeated assessments can do just this.

For the less disabled patient, whose management is largely in the hands of his family doctor, regular enquiry to ensure that daily living activities can be adequately performed will often suffice, although ideally, regular visits by a domiciliary occupational therapist to a patient in his own home would provide more accurate information about the patient's true functional balance. A patient in hospital, or at an out-patient clinic, often tends to put the best face on things — from a desire to please or to avoid 'fussing', from courtesy, or from embarrassment — and he may give a highly inaccurate account of himself. In his own home he ceases to 'put on an act' and discrepancies between his capabilities and his home circumstances become apparent. It is what he does do, rather than what he can do, which counts.

For the more severely disabled patient, repeated and detailed functional assessments are even more important. The employment of standardized methods of enquiry and recording enable estimations of improvement and deterioration to be made and accurate plans for future management to be outlined.

Method of functional assessment
Functional assessments rely partly on standardized questioning by the therapist and partly on her observation of the patient's performance of relevant daily living activities.

A preliminary scanning enquiry made by the occupational therapist into the activities of every patient attending a rheumatology out-patient clinic can focus the attention of the clinical team on the spheres of activity at risk. For in-patients a more detailed functional assessment is the usual practice.

In such an enquiry, the occupational therapist questions the patient about difficulties in:

(1) Personal care:
   Washing,
   Toilet,
   Feeding,
   Dressing;
(2) Mobility:
   Walking,
   Wheelchair,
   Transfers;
(3) Dexterity:
   Reaching,
   Lifting,
   Carrying,
   Handling;

(4) Home conditions:
    Structure of house,
    Housework,
    Shopping,
    Cooking,
    Cleaning,
    Clothes maintenance;
(5) Hobbies/recreation;
(6) Outdoor activities;
(7) Work;
(8) Communication;
(9) Personality and mental state:
    Positive or negative attitude,
    Quick or slow reaction,
    Anxious or relaxed,
    Co-operative or resentful,
    Dependent or independent.

The more detailed enquiry analyses the patient's ability to perform specific actions and tasks. Assessments of mobility bear a relationship to trunk and lower limb function, whereas dexterity provides an estimate of upper limb power, co-ordination, range and speed of movement. Information of this sort is increasingly important as a prelude and a sequel to joint surgery.

MANAGEMENT AT HOME

The majority of patients with rheumatoid arthritis can live a relatively normal life in a normal environment, providing they observe certain general rules and remain under constant clinical review. In the domestic situation control is one of the key words in the patient's management of his disease, for it is only by controlling the precipitating factors that the exacerbations of rheumatoid arthritis may be minimized. Broadly speaking, anything producing physical, mental or emotional strain can precipitate an exacerbation, since rheumatoid arthritis, whatever its initial cause, behaves like a stress disease once it is established. Patients should therefore be counselled to live a balanced existence, aiming at:

(1) Sufficient sleep.
(2) Sufficient rest periods during the day, thus avoiding over-activity to the point of fatigue.
(3) Sufficient food of nourishing variety. Over-eating and obesity should be avoided and excess weight removed by dieting, when necessary.
(4) Sufficient fluid intake — bearing in mind the likelihood of renal damage from many of the drugs used in the therapeutic treatment of rheumatoid arthritis.
(5) Sufficient exercise of a moderate sort, which does not precipitate the pain in the joints but prevents them from stiffening.
(6) Suitable work where the physical and mental demands are within the patient's capabilities.

(7) Regulation of bowel action. It is possible that regular administration of analgesics may induce constipation, and if this is so, the introduction of increased roughage or a bulk-producing laxative may be necessary.

(8) Maintenance of good posture and good joint position at all times.

(9) Control of the tendency to anaemia deriving both from the rheumatoid process and from gastro-intestinal haemorrhages due to the drugs used in the disease. Women with rheumatoid arthritis who suffer from heavy menstrual flow should have the severity of the periods controlled by regular hormonal therapy or be considered for hysterectomy.

Family relationships

Many patients with rheumatoid arthritis are 'crotchety' because of their persistent pain and frustration at the limitation it imposes. Naturally personal relationships tend to suffer both at home and at work. Adequate supression of pain is important from every aspect of the patient's general management. All members of the family need to understand the nature of the disability.

When a man is affected, it may be necessary for him to change employment and to accept a somewhat reduced financial reward. This can lead to domestic stress, and the wife may have to take on a more dominant role in the partnership. When a woman is the patient, then her role in holding the family together may tend to suffer. Certainly rheumatoid arthritis, whoever the sufferer, will have a noticeable impact upon any family. Domestic routines will need to be adapted and the general standard of living may be reduced. Loyalties become divided, and both patient and partner may show real evidence of reactive depression. Such stresses should be guarded against, allowed for, and treated when present.

Need for aids and appliances

Patients with rheumatoid arthritis are faced with the limitation of function imposed by pain and physical disability. Most patients want to retain maximal independence and are reluctant to sacrifice this, even gradually. However, the struggle to retain independence often precipitates further pain and physical limitations. Rehabilitation aims at helping people to think and plan ahead with a realistic attitude to the situation involved. When possible, it forestalls the limitation of function. If restriction of bodily activity is unavoidable, or desirable, good rehabilitation should counsel its acceptance and its circumvention by means of aids and appliances.

A physiotherapist may be able to keep a man walking by exercising and splinting his legs and providing sticks, crutches and walking aids. But should she? An occupational therapist may be able to keep a man independent by teaching him how to dress himself. But should she? By accurate assessment, it becomes apparent at what point in time the therapist is jeopardizing the function of the upper limbs by permitting them to over-compensate for the dysfunction of the lower. It is then that the need for a wheelchair existence is established. By accurate assessment, it becomes obvious when the exertion and pain of dressing becomes so great that it reduces total function by the extent of the fatigue which it induces. It is then evidence that help must be accepted with this one activity to enable other activities of daily living to be accomplished.

In general, the majority of disabled patients manage to continue to live an active life without any aids, apparatus, appliances or special equipment and it is often more important to spend time advising them how to do without such aids, than prescribing them. Physical disability does not necessarily mean absolute handicap, for functional handicap is usually relative to architectural, mechanical, domestic, social and financial limitations.

In order to retain *optimal* rather than *maximal* independence, objective assessment and objective discussion with patient and family are essential.

It is necessary for the patient to learn that no lasting good can derive from endurance of a high level of unnecessary pain. For example, a rheumatoid arthritic with involvement of the hip joints can reduce his pain on walking by using crutches, but if he persists in walking the same distance on crutches as he did before he developed rheumatoid arthritis, he is courting disaster. By reducing the weight on his hips, he is increasing the weight on his hands and wrists, and by using them in an abnormal manner he is increasing their chance of becoming painful, inflamed and later deformed. Thus, when walking becomes painful, and it is inappropriate to prescribe further analgesics or to recommend surgical procedures, the patient must come to accept one of the following alternatives:

(1) He can plan his daily living activities to avoid undue walking.
(2) He can use some walking assistance, such as crutches, sticks, quadrupeds, tripods or walking aids. If he does use these, however, and his hands, wrists and elbows are affected, he should use gutter crutches to reduce the strain taken by these joints. He should avoid axillary crutches, which have a detrimental effect on the shoulder joints, and also elbow crutches if their use exacerbates the pain in any of the joints of the upper limb or if there is active arthritis in these joints. Nor should he utilize the assistance so much that the structure and function of his arms and hands are prejudiced, and use of assistance *must* be coupled with an overall reduction of the day's activities.
(3) He can use a wheelchair. If the patient's hands are unaffected or relatively unaffected, then propulsion of the wheelchair by his hands is acceptable. If they are potentially or actually severely affected, he may propel with his feet or else resort to a powered chair. In this way, his hands and arms may be saved pain and later dysfunction.

Too many arthritics believe that they are 'giving in' if they resort to a wheelchair, but a wheelchair can so often be a prophylactic measure and could be more widely used with advantage to decrease the demands on a patient's limbs.

There are many simple aids and devices available from hospitals, local authorities and voluntary bodies which enable patients to use unmodified everyday articles. These are mainly personal aids, and those most commonly supplied are:

Bath aids Bath seats, non-slip mats, safety handles.
Toilet aids Raised WC seats, commodes.
Eating aids Adapted cutlery, plates and cups.
Dressing aids Elastic shoe laces, stocking aids and adapted clothing.
Walking aids Sticks, frames.
Household gadgets Pick-up sticks to increase reach, adapted kitchen and cooking gadgets to compensate for weak muscles and diminished range of movements, key and tap turners to increase the leverage applicable by weak and painful upper limbs.

For the more severely disabled, larger articles may be supplied to assist function. These pieces of equipment include:

Wheelchairs Self-propelled, attendant propelled or electrically propelled.
Beds Mechanical, electrical and tilting.
Hoists Portable or ceiling tracked.
Chairs Adapted or special design.
Kitchens Adapted equipment and/or specially designed working surfaces.
Reading aids Talking book library, bookrests, page turners.
Writing aids Electrical typewriters.
Intercommunication devices Call systems, adapted telephones.

For the very severely disabled, there are complex sophisticated devices available (e.g. Patient Operated Selector Mechanism) to enable the patient to retain some control over his environment.

Walking aids

Many patients with rheumatoid arthritis will feel the need to resort to some form of weight-relieving assistance early on in the disease when lower limb joints are affected. Initially, a walking stick will help to relieve some of the weight transmitted by a painful swollen knee joint or hip joint. Many patients will ultimately need to use crutches, but as has been said earlier, axillary crutches should be avoided whenever possible because of their potentially harmful effect on the gleno-humeral joints and brachial plexus. Elbow crutches and gutter crutches are more acceptable alternatives but the arm-pieces and forearm gutters often need padding applied to overlap sharp edges. Ideally, handgrips of crutches should be purpose-built for each patient from a mould of the patient's grip with his hand in a position of comfort. When facilities for making individual grips do not exist, the handles of the crutches may be bound with foam rubber to widen them or, alternatively, a foam rubber pad attached to a velcro strap may be worn around the palm of the hand. These manoeuvres enable the crutches to be gripped firmly even when the hands are severely affected.

At a later stage it may become necessary to use a walking frame in preference to crutches. This should be of a height appropriate to the degree of involvement of the spine and upper limbs, with grips correspondingly sited in the vertical or horizontal plane. All walking aids, sticks, crutches or walking frames should be of the correct height. Sticks and frames usually should be held at the same height as the patient's greater trochanter when the patient is standing upright in shoes. All walking aids should have good broad-based ferrules which should be replaced as they become worn (*see* Chapter 16).

Wheelchairs

Wheelchairs can provide a means of independent progression for those with severe functional impairment of their lower limbs as well as a means of transport of considerable assistance to friends and relatives who manage the general care of the elderly and infirm.

The type of wheelchair required by any one patient needs careful assessment. The specifications may need to be different depending on whether the chair is for indoor or outdoor use, for self-propulsion, or for attendants to push. The final choice of chair depends as much on the home conditions as on the clinical needs. Often the needs cannot all be met in a single chair because of the difficulty in designing a wheelchair which is at once comfortable, light, robust and adaptable. Many of the more disabled wheelchair users will therefore require more than one wheelchair, e.g. one for work and one for home use, and these may be of different design. The design of most standard wheelchairs attempts to embody a compromise between the needs of the patient and his helpers and the demands of his home, his surroundings and his mode of outdoor transport in a composite structure of durable materials and reasonable cost. Since each patient has individual problems, modifications may occasionally be necessary, particularly for the more seriously disabled patients who may have involvement of all four limbs and trunk. Foot plates may need to be extended or built up; armrests, headrests or one or more padded, elevating legrests may be needed. However, as with all appliances, it is necessary for the patient to accept some restriction of his functional capabilities.

In recent years there has been an increasing use of electrically powered indoor wheelchairs for the more severely disabled; for some patients such a chair can prove to be the key to their resettlement.

Although the criteria for eligibility for a powered indoor wheelchair have been an inability to walk coupled with upper-limb disability so severe as to make hand-propulsion impossible, the conditions for supply are gradually changing. Long-term observation of disabled patients, particularly those with rheumatoid arthritis, strongly indicates that the stage of the disease at which they *should* not propel, comes long before the stage at which they *cannot* propel. The prescription of powered indoor chairs at this former stage is a prophylactic measure to prevent accelerated degeneration of the joints of the upper limbs through over-use. Not only does the issue of such a chair produce a considerable gain in functional efficiency in the immediate present by reducing pain and fatigue, but it also leads to prolongation of functional independence in personal care and daily living activities.

Often the conventional modes of controlling standard, powered indoor chairs will need modification to permit their use by the severe rheumatoid arthritic. However, head, chin and 'suck—blow' controls, as well as modified hand-controls, are now offered as alternatives for most standard powered chairs, and one of these is usually found to be suitable.

Outdoor transport

Public transport in Britain is of a high standard of frequency and availability compared to that of many other countries. Such comparison is of no comfort to the rheumatoid arthritic patient who, on a bad day, cannot walk a hundred yards to the bus stop, cannot tolerate the wait in the cold, cannot grasp the grab rail to pull himself on to the bus platform. Even with help he may be unable to flex his hip and knee sufficiently to climb on to the bus. Even if he can manage this, he will probably find that ankylosed or arthrodesed knees are difficult to pack in between the seats. Even more acute is the problem when a further walk awaits a working man at the end of his bus ride before he can reach his place of work, or if a woman has to attempt to carry home a heavy shopping bag while supporting herself on elbow crutches.

To the patient who is moderately disabled, but must still earn his own living or do her own housework, and to the more severely disabled patient who would otherwise be confined to the house, suitable outdoor transport may well be the essential factor in maintaining outdoor independence.

There are several alternatives open to a patient who wants to drive, and those alternatives depend partly on the distribution and severity of his arthritic involvement, and partly on his income.

A mildly disabled patient with rheumatoid arthritis who drives his own car can increase his comfort and efficiency by installing in his car the following pieces of equipment:

(1) A panoramic mirror, an extra inside mirror and an extra wing mirror, to help minimize the amount of neck movement needed.
(2) A headrest integral with the car seat to reduce the chance of whiplash injury.
(3) An adequate heater to keep the car at an even temperature.
(4) A cloth or leather cover for the steering wheel to reduce the discomfort of gripping a rigid, cold, plastic surface with stiff fingers.
(5) Windshields for the windows, to decrease draughts.
(6) A special car seat or a special cushion to avoid backache.
(7) Extra large control knobs.
(8) Automatic transmission.

A more severely disabled patient with stiff, painful lower limb joints can have various hand controls fitted, depending on the nature of his disability. Thus, accelerator, brake and clutch may all be hand-operated with the brakes servo-assisted, so that a light touch can call forth an intensified response. The fitting of automatic transmission is also helpful to an arthritic patient with considerable involvement of the hands. The elimination of the effort of gear changing and clutch operation reduces the multiplicity of minor traumata to the fingers and left foot and prevents the infliction of pain which constant rapid changes of position and grip may precipitate.

As a patient becomes progressively more disabled, provided he has the money to pay for them, a large number of possible conversions can be fitted to the controls to compensate for specific disabilities. A disabled driver must, however, register his disability when applying for his next licence and should take the opportunity of belonging to the Disabled Drivers Association. Membership entitles a person to a sticker for his car and to the club magazine which publishes articles of interest to disabled drivers. Regular social events for members widen the horizons of the disabled driver and enable him to visit places and attempt activities which he might well avoid without the moral support of other disabled people. A disc which he can display will often enable him to park in places prohibited to the general public, so that he is within easy reach of his destination. This can be obtained from the local Social Services Department once he has been registered as disabled.

A patient with rheumatoid arthritis wanting assistance with transport from the Department of Health and Social Security, under present regulations should obtain a Mobility Allowance Request Form from a Post Office, National Insurance Office or Integrated Social Office of the DHSS. This form he fills up himself, and then dispatches to the Mobility Allowance Unit at Norcross, Blackpool. A general practitioner living in the vicinity is requested by Blackpool to visit and assess the patient's disablement and the degree to which it affects his walking. The decision to award or withhold the allowance is made by Blackpool, on the facts submitted by the examining doctor.

The allowance is granted to those who are unable or virtually unable to walk, and to those who suffer an unacceptable degree of distress or endanger their health by attempting to walk. A patient may contest the decision to refuse him the allowance at an independent tribunal.

There is no condition attached to the usage of the Mobility Allowance, which may be put towards the purchase of a car or an outdoor powered chair, or used for taxis or the maintenance of an existing car. Currently it may also be used to rent a car on the Motability Scheme, in which the MA is paid over to any one of a group of firms involved, which provides a car for use by the patient for four years. After this the car is returned to the suppliers, and another new car is substituted. The patient never actually owns the car, which is always the property of the supplying firm.

The DHSS does not produce or provide three wheeler motorized vehicles any longer. These are being gradually phased out of existence. A patient already possessing such a vehicle is offered the alternatives of:

(1) Exchanging the vehicle for Mobility Allowance.
(2) Keeping the vehicle. In this case it is repaired and replaced by the DHSS until existing stocks of three wheelers are exhausted.

No further three wheeler cars are being manufactured for the DHSS.

Currently, all disabled drivers suffering from progressive disorders (such as rheumatoid arthritis) and possessing Department vehicles are required to report for a yearly medical check-up of their fitness to control their vehicle, followed, if necessary, by a practical demonstration of capability in front of the Department's Technical Officer. This is a wise modification of the old regulations which did not call for regular review and under which it was possible for a patient to deteriorate to a state at which he was unfit to drive without any knowledge of this reaching the supplying Centre.

Hoists
The more severely disabled arthritic patient may need hoisting to enable him to get in and out of bed. The choice lies between a hydraulic portable hoist and an electric hoist.

The hydraulic hoist has the advantage that it can be moved to operate in several places and it is less expensive to buy.

The electric hoist is easier to operate and can be operated by the patient himself. The installation of electric track hoists is expensive and many houses and flats are not sufficiently strongly constructed to bear the combined weight of the equipment and the patient. Freestanding electric hoists which are attached to an overhead gantry supported on four legs are easier and cheaper to provide. Such a hoist usually remains sited over the patient's bed so that he can be transferred from bed to adjacent wheelchair or commode.

The electric hoist is usually chosen for a small helper who is hoisting a tall, heavy, arthritic patient. For such a patient/helper combination the provision of a hydraulic portable hoist is an economy potentially dangerous to both parties. It demands too much physical effort on the part of the small helper who still has to push the heavily loaded hoist from place to place. It may also subject the patient to possible trauma from door frames, walls and furniture as the helper will be unable to push the hoist along and steady the patient at the same time.

DESIGNING AND ADAPTING THE HOME

Many of the day-to-day difficulties of the disabled stem from the structural design of their home, its fittings and furniture. Sensible reorganization and, when necessary, replacement or redesign, can make the life of an arthritic much less difficult and play a large part in maintaining his active involvement in the community.

Sitting and dining rooms
The sitting and dining rooms used by a rheumatoid arthritic patient must:

(1) Be easy to enter and leave.
(2) Be uncluttered to allow easy circulation within them.
(3) Leave room for the equipment of the patient, e.g. wheelchair or crutches.
(4) Possess at least one easy chair of such a height that the patient can get up and sit down unaided.
(5) Have a table of a suitable height so that a patient with stiff spine and upper limbs may use it in comfort.
(6) Have a carpet rather than a series of rugs on a polished floor, and carpet of such a pile it does not make it difficult to walk using crutches or other walking aids or to propel a wheelchair.
(7) Have windows and doors which are easily opened and shut.
(8) Have enough space to allow for elevating legrests on a wheelchair or the presence of a long stool of appropriate height so that the patient can sit with his feet up in comfort.

The elderly and disabled tend to spend much of their time sitting down. Selecting a suitable easy chair for them is often difficult. The chair must be of a suitable height so that they can sit down and get up from it without undue effort or discomfort. It must be robust, for such patients tend to 'drop' into the chair and 'lever' themselves out of it, imposing unusual stresses upon it. It must be stable, as the user often tends to slump when sitting and to rock forwards, backwards and sideways in the chair when changing position. The back must be set at a good angle and high enough to give support to the shoulder and head. The seat height is critical and may need to be adjusted by means of four wooden blocks attached to the chair legs, or else by a firm cushion placed in the seat of the chair. It is possible to buy chairs whose legs can be shortened as well as lengthened by means of telescopic 'over legs'. The height of the arms of the chair needs to be such that the patient can push himself up or ease himself down with maximal efficiency and the least possible pain. A patient with stiff, weak hips and perhaps a stiff knee may need a spring-loaded ejector seat for his chair to help him get out of it, or failing that, an ejector seat operated by an air pump or electric motor. Usually, however, precise adjustment of the height of the seat and arms will enable all but the most severely disabled patients to transfer independently.

The shape and contours of a chair contribute more to its overall comfort than the softness of the cushion. There are several chairs marketed for 'geriatric' or hospital use which are likely to be suitable for arthritics, and these are usually available for trial in hospital and residential institutions.

For an arthritic patient with a stiff or fixed hip, sitting can be made more comfortable by using a cushion with a groove cut in the appropriate side. This can be made from plastic foam 3 in (7.5 cm) thick and cut to the shape of the chair seat. A groove is cut 6 in (15.25 cm) wide and 2 in (5 cm) deep on the side corresponding to the patient's affected side and tapered to fit the individual patient. A sheepskin-covered cushion or a sheepskin laid over the standard chair cushion can increase comfort considerably for the patient with very restricted mobility.

Kitchen layout and equipment

A kitchen specially designed or adapted for an ambulant woman with rheumatoid arthritis will differ from that designed for a woman who is chair-bound. For the former, the kitchen will be designed to reduce floor space so as to lessen the distance which the patient must walk; for the latter, the floor area will be large enough to permit a wheelchair to be manoeuvred easily between cooker, sink, refrigerator and working surfaces. In both kitchens, the heights of the fixtures, the ease with which they can be utilized, and the dimensions and weights of the utensils they contain are equally critical.

In order for the patient to avoid lifting or carrying heavy saucepans, all the working surfaces should be of the same level, so that pans can be slid to and from the stove, working surface and sink. Split-level cookers are helpful and a trolley with one shelf flush with the oven allows oven-cooked food to be slid in and out without lifting. Such a trolley is invaluable, for it can be pushed around the kitchen or even the house, and its many tiers can carry food, cutlery and cleaning equipment from place to place. It also acts as a walking aid when equipped with handles and two rubber-tipped legs in addition to its castors or wheels. By doing triple duty as an extra shelf, equipment carrier and walking aid, it saves space in the house which might tend to become cluttered with equipment.

A sink needs to be the exact height at which a woman can stand and work without getting backache, and should, whenever possible, be installed by the plumber with the patient standing beside him to indicate the exact height needed for her comfort. Similarly, the working surfaces should not only be flush with each other, but also of a suitable height for the rheumatoid patient to use them either from her wheelchair or working stool.

Kitchen floors need a surface which is non-slip and easily cleaned, such as plastic tiles or vinyl sheet flooring.

Cupboards and drawers need to be sited at a convenient height calculated to avoid undue stooping and stretching. Doors should open easily and runners should glide smoothly.

Where possible, taps should be fitted with lever handles and sited in whichever position is best for the patient, possibly at the side rather than at the back of the sink. If the kitchen is not purpose built, or structural alternations are not possible, the use of a long-handled tap turner makes the use of standard taps much easier.

Laundry

Washing presents great problems to the rheumatoid arthritic patient, especially when she has a young family. An automatic washing machine, with a tumble drier, is an expensive but justifiable piece of equipment. If a non-automatic machine and spin drier are used, the use of a rotating clothes-line enables the patient to peg out her clothes while sitting on a stool or in her wheelchair.

Ironing is another chore calculated to cause pain in many affected joints of the woman with rheumatoid disease. If it is done from the sitting position, at a table or board of the right height, using a lightweight iron, much of the effort and consequent pain and stiffness may be avoided. Whenever possible, clothing and household linen should be drip-dry and the total amount of ironing reduced to a minimum.

Heating and electrical supply

Solid fuel heating is contra-indicated for a patient with rheumatoid arthritis unless someone else is responsible for bringing in the coal, and making up and cleaning out the fires. Even then, the use of coal fires should be avoided and a more even temperature aimed at by adopting some form of central heating, boosted when necessary by gas or electric fires. It matters not whether the central heating is gas-fired, oil-fired or all electric, provided it is adequate and economical. If cost is an important factor, the use of night-storage heaters, which use electricity at off-peak times, may prove an economy.

Electric power plug sockets should be installed at waist level and the on/off switches chosen for ease of manipulation.

Bedroom

Bedroom furniture should be stable and strategically placed to provide support and yet permit easy passage around it. A bed which backs on to a wall allows transfers to be made from either side, although it is sometimes preferable to place on one side of the bed against a wall so that it is extra stable when it is necessary to push on the bed to stand upright from the seated position. Height is also important when difficulty is experienced in transferring from bed to chair, wheelchair or the standing position, and wooden blocks of the appropriate height, with recesses for the legs of the bed, can be used to raise or lower it to the desired level. A firm mattress, either laid on a hard-based bed or supported by a board beneath it, makes it easier to move within the bed as well as to and from it, and is of prophylactic value in that it discourages spinal and hip deformity. For people with stiff hips, the adjustment of bed height may be critical; but to retain independence for transfers in and out of bed, patients may need more than this adjustment. The use of a bed-ladder facilities sitting up in bed for those with stiff, weak spines and hips. Such a ladder is made from two lengths of rope or heavy sash cord which are threaded through holes in steps made from short lengths of wooden broom handle and knotted between the steps. One end is attached to the bed rail above the bed-clothes. The patient hauls on the far end, and by climbing the steps with his hands gradually pulls himself to an upright position.

Continental quilts (duvets) or cellular blankets of man-made fibre are lighter than the conventional woollen blankets, and patients may prefer to use them in order to reduce pressure on weak and painful limbs and make turning in bed easier. If traditional heavy bed-clothes are used, a bed cradle may be helpful.

Toilets and bathrooms

Ideally, bathrooms and toilets should have their fixtures specially sited for patients disabled with rheumatoid arthritis. In actual practice, this seldom occurs, and most arthritic patients must manage in rooms of conventional design. There are several relatively minor modifications which can be made to facilitate their use. Often it is only necessary to ensure that the toilet seat is raised to the correct height for the arthritic patient concerned so that he is immediately able to use the toilet without difficulty. In addition, it may be necessary to fit grab rails at appropriate positions on the toilet wall or to fit a standing rail beside the pedestal to make it easier to sit down or rise up from the toilet seat. The toilet door-handle may need alteration, as may the key or bolt, to enable them to be manipulated by the arthritic patient with deformed fingers.

Toilet flush levers are notoriously stiff, and the standard toilet chain may be difficult to reach and painful to pull. The addition of a large knob-like handle whether to the lever or the chain and the extension of the latter to bring the handle to a position which can easily be reached by the patient prevents toilet flushing being an exercise in ingenuity and pain endurance.

The type of toilet seat-raise advocated depends on the needs and wishes of the family, as well as those of the patient. Plastic overseats of several types are available commercially, with special modifications for the person with an arthrodesed hip. These have the advantage that they can accompany the patient when he goes to other houses (suitably transported in a light suitcase). More comfortable and stable for the average patient is a fixed wooden, box-like seat reminiscent of Victorian toilets and easily constructed by a local carpenter to fit over the existing pedestal and seat. The top of the overseat is hinged to allow cleaning of the flush pedestal.

Getting in and out of the bath is difficult for the arthritic, and because of the hard, wet surfaces, the activity is potentially dangerous. For the more severely disabled, the elderly and the frail, some assistance from another person for undressing and entering the bath, and for getting out and dressing is more sensible than trying to arrange wall rails or hoists.

The most useful and simple bath aid is a bath seat, and the most useful bath seat is one which fits firmly into the bath at one end and which extends to form a bath-side stool. A second seat, attached and placed in the bath, can be used either as a 'half-way seat' before actually sitting in the bath, or can be used to sit on for the bathing process. Wall rails should be used in conjunction with the bath seat or on their own, but they must have a non-slip surface and must be fitted at the position and angle most useful for the individual patient.

Whenever possible, a practical assessment by an experienced occupational therapist should be carried out in the patient's own home.

It is likely that a combination of bath board, bath seat and wall rail with non-slip surface, together with a non-slip mat in the bath will make bathing an easier and safer activity for the arthritic patient. Whenever there is doubt about the patient's capability, it is wisest to advise that bathing should only be attempted with the assistance of a competent helper.

For the very severely disabled, it is possible to use a hoist, either portable or attached to a ceiling track. If this is not possible, then arrangements can be made for the patient to be given a regular bed bath or to attend the local hospital or day centre when bathing can be carried out by skilled personnel.

MENSTRUATION, CONTRACEPTION AND MARRIAGE

The management of the menstrual cycle and pregnancies of a woman with rheumatoid arthritis occupies an important part of the total management of the disease.

Menstruation

No patient with rheumatoid arthritis who still has persistently heavy periods following treatment of her rheumatoid condition can be considered as fully rehabilitated if rehabilitation is considered as 'return to as full and normal an everyday life as possible'. Anaemia secondary to heavy menstrual loss can be debilitating in any woman but may be particularly so in a woman with rheumatoid arthritis, exacerbating her fatigue and depression and aggravating any anaemia due to the disease itself.

In the investigation of the cause of such heavy periods, a blood count and a gynaecological examination, possibly followed by a dilatation and curettage are essential.

Depending on the result of these procedures, appropriate surgical treatment such as polypectomy or myomectomy may be advised, or even hysterectomy.

More commonly menstruation is regulated by administration of progestogen or combined oestrogen/progestogen therapy, unless this is contraindicated by the patient's condition.

Marriage

When possible, it is desirable that a doctor should discuss the difficulties of a marriage in which one of the partners has rheumatoid arthritis, with both of the partners concerned. The fact that malaise and pain can seriously inhibit both the wish and the ability to make love must not be construed as coldness on the part of the affected partner.

If long continued pain or deformity of the lower limbs makes intercourse in the customary position impractical or impossible, the timely instruction of the husband and wife in alternative postures for intercourse may save the marriage from tension and collapse. Many orthopaedic surgeons now accept that inability to have normal intercourse is a strong indication for corrective surgery, and total hip replacement to permit hip abduction may be undertaken for this reason.

Contraception

In the presence of abnormal periods, hysterectomy may be indicated to prevent both unwanted periods and unwanted pregnancies. When the periods are normal, however, other methods of contraception may be indicated. At the present time there is no evidence that the use of the contraceptive pill is any more risky than for a non-arthritic woman. Indeed it may be the contraceptive method of choice, for a cervical cap or diaphragm may be difficult if she also has involvement of the joints of her lower limbs. Alternatively, tubal ligation is a relatively simple operation, which can be done under local anaesthetic, and provides an effective and permanent method of contraception. The insertion of an intra-uterine device is an alternative method but may cause a painful and heavier menstrual loss and may not be feasible in a woman with painful stiff lower limbs and spine.

When the male partner of the marriage has rheumatoid arthritis, it is appropriate that it should be he who adopts contraceptive measures, when no further children are wanted, by procuring a vasectomy. During intervals in which temporary contraception is employed during acute phases of the disease in either partner, the use of a penile sheath by the husband is probably the simplest procedure.

It is a matter for discussion with the family whether contraception is best practised by the wife or the husband. Should it be necessary to use a contraceptive method which could lead to sterility, it has been suggested that there might be good psychological reasons for the affected person, rather than the healthy person, to adopt this. The reasons underlying this view are that disability in one partner often induces resentment in the spouse. Should the spouse be expected to accept sterility as well as a disabled partner, the resentment may well be considerable. However, as with physically able-bodied couples, discussion with a doctor experienced in family planning can help to resolve many of the difficulties. Certainly. a woman with rheumatoid arthritis can be saved the risks of the pill and the difficulties attendant upon other forms of contraception if her husband agrees to vasectomy.

Pregnancy

It is impossible to lay down hard and fast rules about the most desirable number of children in a family in which one of the partners has rheumatoid arthritis. The final choice must lie with the affected partner, and the doctor can only help by advising accurately about the factors involved in the choice. It must be made clear to both parents how essential it is to avoid physical and mental strain, and the family should be limited to a size which is unlikely to produce such strain either in the mother who cares for it or in the father who earns for it.

Women with rheumatoid arthritis are often very well during their pregnancy. Symptoms are reduced and disease activity apparently slows down. This often makes them reluctant to accept advice about limiting the size of the family. However, it is necessary to discuss frankly with her and her husband the advisability of having a family, emphasizing that young children can be a considerable physical burden.

In a woman with severe rheumatic arthritis, when birth must be by Caesarean section because of pelvic abnormalities or severe hip involvement, it may be considered advisable to follow the second Caesarean by bilateral tubal ligation or by hysterectomy.

WORK AND LEISURE

Planning for return to work

In rheumatoid arthritis, as with other disabilities, resettlement in work depends on many factors other than the severity of the disability. The nature of the work, the patient's education and domestic background must all be considered together with social and economic factors. Early planning must be the responsibility of the consultant in charge of the patient, and early decisions can be helped by an efficient rehabilitation and resettlement organization bringing about the necessary integration of the provisions of the Department of Health, Education and Productivity, and Local Authorities.

The majority of patients with rheumatoid arthritis are able to pursue their usual activities in the early stages of the disease process, and many are able to continue in their chosen employment until normal retiring age. However, most patients are faced with some limitation in their physical activities. This limitation may interfere with employment if it cannot be overcome by some mechanical aid or device and a planned approach to the total management of the disease.

The manual worker and the housewife with a large family will almost certainly have to accept some restrictions. For the housewife, these restrictions in physical activity may usually be offset by the use of appropriate aids and appliances, but the unskilled manual worker may well need to change his employment for something less physically demanding. Office and sedentary workers will usually be able to continue in their previous employment, providing the mode of travel to and from work is well within their physical capabilities.

Some skilled workers may have to change their employment if their hands are severely affected or if their work demands awkward positions, prolonged standing at a work-bench, or over much walking when there is severe involvement of weight-bearing joints.

It is often difficult for the employer to understand the complexity of establishing a realistic prognosis either in terms of persistent handicap or rate of deterioration. It is only by accurate assessment of a man's work potential that a basis for retraining or reallocation of duties can be found. The importance of this assessment cannot be overemphasized and will depend upon a careful appraisal and recording of:

(1) The patient's symptoms, particularly morning stiffness and joint pain.
(2) His functional capabilities as determined by objective trials wherever possible.
(3) The number of joints involved and the severity of their involvement in terms of pain, reduced range and instability.
(4) Functional expressions of joint rage and muscle power in terms of mobility and dexterity.
(5) Clinical tests, e.g. of the sedimentation rate and haemoglobin level, and quantitative tests for rheumatoid factor.

Repeated, careful, quantitative assessments will indicate the rate of progress of the disease and so help the clinician to evaluate the patient's work potential.

Frank discussion between the clinician, patient and employer based upon these assessments will usually bring about a satisfactory readjustment of the patient's working conditions. When it is not possible for the situation to be resolved in this simple fashion, then there may be a need to resort to the official organization designed to resettle and, when necessary, retrain a patient for an occupation more appropriate to his disability.

It is important that the question of return to work should be considered as early as possible during the hospital admission of any patient, since concern about his future may be a potent cause of worry or even depression. In the first instance, return to a patient's last place of work should always be attempted and negotiations for his return to his previous job should be opened by the medical social worker or the patient himself. Failing this, the next best thing is to return to work for his old employers in another capacity. Only when these two possibilities have been adequately explored should re-employment or retraining be considered.

Resettlement in work
In the United Kingdom, there is a Disablement Resettlement Officer at each of the Employment Exchanges, and it is his special responsibility to find suitable work for disabled men and women. A Disabled Persons Register to which any person with a physical impairment can apply for registration, is maintained at every Employment Exchange and certain jobs can be reserved for those who are registered. So far, only passenger-accommodating electric lift attendants and car park attendants are so designated, but some firms employ more than their 'quota' of disabled.

There are approximately 30 Employment Rehabilitation Centres in the United Kingdom providing work assessment facilities. After a period of assessment lasting 6–7 weeks, full training in one of the 40–50 trades at a technical or commercial college or Skill Centre may be available.

Collaboration between hospital workers, social workers, Disablement Resettlement Officers, Adult Training Centres and Skill Centres must be very close if the disabled person is to be satisfactorily resettled. It is particularly difficult to match the physical capabilities and disabilities of the rheumatoid patient with the available openings in industry, while yet permitting the well-regulated home-based living which is so essential to the successful management of the disease.

For the more severely disabled patients, sheltered workshops provide work under conditions somewhat less stressful than those found in open industry, but the employees in such workshops still have to be capable of a level of productivity considerably less than that of open industry.

Occupational Centres provide diversional therapy and are the responsibility of the Local Authority. Patients attending these Centres receive a limited amount of financial recompense ('pocket money', not a wage). Some patients may achieve work at home (e.g. dressmaking, copy-typing or providing a telephone answering service), but this type of work is often poory paid and un-satisfying.

Hobbies

For those unable to work, hobbies can play a large and important part in their lives, as they may bring about social contacts and creative activities which compensate for the frustrations of disability. Previous training and interests influence the choice of hobby and leisure pursuits, but it is part of rehabilitation to explore the possibilities and to help the patient to develop at least one creative activity over and above his activities of daily living. Even when the disability is severe, with help and appropriate aids, many patients can develop surprising and worthwhile hobbies.

SURGERY IN RHEUMATOID ARTHRITIS

It is becoming increasingly difficult to consider the total care of patients with rheumatoid arthritis without close collaboration between physician, surgeon and general practitioner on both out-patient and in-patient basis. Therefore the aims of surgical treatment are threefold:

(1) Improvement in function.
(2) Relief of pain.
(3) Improvement in appearance.

As surgical procedures become a more frequent episode in the management of the disease, it is necessary to consider the part which rehabilitation services play both pre-operatively and post-operatively.

Firstly, a patient's response to simple rehabilitation can be an important measure of his 'motivation' and can indicate whether he is likely to respond well to major surgical procedures. Assessment of the patient as a whole — his personality, social background and attitude to his disease — is one of the important preliminaries to the planning of surgical treatment.

General considerations
Factors which must be considered before embarking on surgery include:

(1) The patient's general health.
(2) The patient's local disease.
(3) Wound healing.
(4) Drug therapy.

Clearly a patient whose disease is reasonably well controlled and who is neither anaemic nor underweight is likely to recover more rapidly from major surgery.

Although the local disease usually determines the joint selected for surgery, it is important to consider the patient as a whole. For example, it may be important to undertake wrist surgery before hip surgery so that post-operative rehabilitation can proceed smoothly.

Assessment of clinical condition
A general assessment of the patient's clinical condition is the second prerequisite to surgical intervention. If surgery is proposed for several joints, the surgical programme may be protracted and a long period of hospitalization must be contemplated. The physical stamina of the patient must be carefully evaluated and probable functional gains must be balanced against possible functional losses. Furthermore, any alteration in the functional capacity of one limb may have considerable repercussions on his overall activity. Thus, for example, it is unwise to plan reconstructive surgery of a lower limb if the severity of the involvement of the upper limbs completely precludes the use of walking aids. However, such lower limb surgery may be justified even when walking is not contemplated post-operatively if that surgery can offer either pain relief, a better sitting posture, or an increased mobility of some joint which will facilitate personal care or transfers. For example, the mobilization of extended adducted hips will permit comfortable sitting and easier perineal cleaning and toiletting.

As involvement of the cervical spine in the rheumatoid process is relatively common, pre-operative radiography of this region is essential to exclude atlanto-axial instability. The presence of such instability demands special precautions during anaesthesia. These include the use of an adequate collar throughout the period during which the patient is unconscious and the employment of particular care when the unconscious patient is transferred between bed, stretcher and operating table. Failure to take adequate precautions could be fatal.

Local disease
It is the severity and extent of tissue destruction which the disease causes in each locality that finally determines the choice of joint and type of operation to be selected for its repair. Assessment of the extent of the disease will depend upon:

(1) Pain and stiffness, swelling, loss of active movement, loss of range of passive movement and the joint stability.
(2) Radiographic appearance of joints.
(3) Assessment of the amount of joint destruction.

General indications for surgical intervention

Synovectomy is indicated when there is persistent 'boggy' swelling of one or two joints only. In addition to the reliable relief of pain and swelling, the operation may have a dual effect: it may be prophylactic against a more severe involvement of the joint operated upon, while also inducing remission in the general rheumatoid disease.

Some authorities advocate a radiation synovestomy – a procedure with a degree of success similar to that of a surgical synovectomy but using few hospital resources and carrying no post-operative morbidity.

Reconstructive operations – arthroplasties in various forms or surgical procedures involving tendons – are called for when the possibility of functional improvement exists. Finally, in the late stages of the disease when permanent deformity has supervened and the normal anatomical framework of the joints has been destroyed, salvage operations, often involving ablation of certain joints, with arthrodeses and excision arthroplasties of others, may give surprisingly good functional results.

In planning surgery, it is necessary to ask not 'what *is* the functional level' but 'what is the functional level *likely* to be'. The smaller the disability, the better the end result of its surgical treatment. Unfortunately, as patients with rheumatoid arthritis are continually adapting themselves to the slow progress of their disabling disease, they are reluctant to accept reconstructive surgery unless some major disability forces them to do so. In this way the most rewarding procedures are often left unperformed. It is important that patients with rheumatoid arthritis should be educated in the value of simple surgery with known good results and minimal need for rehabilitative treatment (currently the most effective operations in this category are excision of the lower end of the ulna and excision arthroplasty of the metatarsophalangeal joints).

The precise nature of the operation offered for any particular joint must be decided after careful analysis of the patient's functional capabilities and deficits. It aims most commonly at an end result which is a compromise between optimal mobility and optimal stability. Each surgical procedure needs to be followed by early ambulation, early mobilization of the affected joints, and rapid resumption of daily living activities.

The interrelationship between upper limb joints in particular needs careful study before operation is undertaken. A fixed elbow demands good forward flexion of the shoulder and palmar flexion of the wrist if the hand is to be able to reach the mouth during feeding. Loss of pronation and supination can be compensated for by abduction and rotation of the shoulder and, conversely, loss of shoulder range can be partly offset by re-establishing pronation and supination.

In general terms, surgery for a joint should be seriously considered when an adequate trial of conservative measures has been unsuccessful.

Surgery of the upper limb.

Shoulder

Primary involvement of the shoulder in the inflammatory polyarthritis of rheumatoid disease, or later secondary involvement following the development of a degenerative arthritis may both give rise to pain and restriction of movement which are distressing and disabling in their effect.

Nevertheless, provided a regular exercise regime is consistently followed and adequate medication given, in the majority of cases, joint function is comparatively well preserved, even in the presence of considerable structural damage. Local injection of corticosteroids is also helpful but should be used with discretion, since evidence in accumulating that bone erosion can follow its repeated use.

Acromionectomy has much to offer in joints in which upward humeral displacement has caused a severe and painful acromial reaction, but surgery on the glenohumeral joint has not provided consistent functional gain or pain relief. Although some centres are assessing total replacement with prosthetic devices, this technique has not yet had the success of total hip replacement.

Protection of the shoulder joint from over-use and misuse may be assisted by:

(1) Prescribing elbow rather than axillary crutches.
(2) Advocating wheelchair use rather than excessive crutch-assisted walking.
(3) Prescribing an electrically propelled chair when self-propulsion becomes painful.
(4) Prescribing a hoist when independent transfers demand excessive shoulder action and induce pain.

The elbow

Synovectomy and debridement with or without removal of the radial head may bring considerable relief from pain. Bilateral elbow involvement is very disabling and is an indication for arthroplasty on one side. Still's Disease is often associated with bilateral ankylosis, and excision arthroplasty of one elbow can restore considerable function. Bilateral excision arthroplasty is seldom performed, as the patient usually requires one stable elbow to push himself up from the chair seat, or to ease his position in a wheelchair. Internal prostheses are being developed which offer stability as well as mobility and are likely to be increasingly used in treatment.

For ambulant patients with elbow involvement, forearm gutter crutches help to distribute the load in a more acceptable pattern than simple elbow crutches.

The wrist

Arthrodesis of one or both wrists has been advocated for many years for patients with painful, unstable joints. However, the wrist cannot be considered in isolation. With restricted shoulder and elbow movement, wrist mobility may be the only movement which provides independence for feeding. Pronation and supination of the forearm can substitute for shoulder rotation and palmar flexion and dorsal extension of the wrist can compensate for loss of elbow movement.

Although popular in the past, arthrodesis of the wrist is seldom necessary. Should it be considered, a light-weight plastic splint will adequately mimic the end result, allowing the functional gains and losses to be assessed by patient and therapists. Excision of the lower end of the ulna often produces good results, but after this operation some patients require a wrist splint while working.

Synovectomy of the wrist joint and excision of the sheaths of tendons where proliferative tenosynovitis is endangering the integrity of the tendons are two prophylactic procedures which may be of great value in preserving hand function.

The hand

Much has been written on the details of surgery of the rheumatoid hand, but the purposes of surgical management can be summed up in two words — prevention and salvage.

Surgical management aims to prevent deformities by early synovectomy and decompression of affected joints and to restore function, particularly punch and punch grip, by a variety of stabilizing and reconstructive procedures. Synovectomy of the metacarpophalangeal joints is believed to have a valuable prophylactic effect when performed early enough.

Arthrodesis of the unstable, dislocating thumb, arthrodesis in flexion of a hyperextended proximal interphalangeal joint, and arthroplasty of subluxed deviated metacarpophalangeal joints are now routine procedures. Osteotomy may be necessary to convert ankylosed fingers from extension to flexion. Combined with soft-tissue surgery, such procedures can often convert the severely damaged hand into a useful prehensile organ once again, but careful evaluation of the probable functional gain to the patient must be an essential preliminary to the decision to operate.

Surgery of the lower limb

Although the main function of the lower limb is weight-bearing, enough mobility must be maintained to permit comfortable sitting and the performance of everyday activities (particularly toilet). Surgical procedures designed to regain mobility must also give relief from pain and yet retain a reasonable stability for the joints concerned.

Problems often arise later, as the disease progresses, or as degenerative changes supervene or some other disaster occurs. It is paradoxical but often true that in order to achieve walking independence, lower limb operations should aim at joint stability, whereas for a comfortable wheelchair existence, joint mobility is more important. Furthermore, for patients with progressive disease, walking sticks or crutches can be severely destructive for the shoulders.

If the patient is unable to achieve walking and has to remain in his wheelchair, the combination of restricted hip movements and stiff knees can often be disastrous. Inability to flex the knee and thus reduce the overall 'sitting length' make wheelchair existence in a normal house impossible.

Likely surgical procedures for the lower limbs are: excision of the femoral head, total joint replacement for the hip; synovectomy, joint debridement, patellectomy, arthroplasty, proximal tibial osteotomy, and arthrodesis of the knee.

The hip

When rheumatoid disease affects the hip, the resulting arthritis is usually painful and debilitating and leads to flexion and abduction deformity. Walking is voluntarily restricted to prevent the pain which weight-bearing induces, and the tendency to avoid activity by prolonged sitting further encourages the development of these deformities.

Excision arthroplasty of the painful rheumatoid hip should, nowadays, be reserved for the wheelchair-bound patient. For other patients, total hip replacement is the operation of choice.

For both these procedures and for soft tissue release operations, the best results are obtained when there is a good range of joint movement pre-operatively, and when a rigorous regime of post-operative exercises can be performed.

Arthrodesis of the hip is contra-indicated in the rheumatoid patient, both because of the progressive nature of the disease, which leads to increasingly severe involvement of other joints, and also because of the adverse effect which fixation of one hip inevitably has upon the spine and the other hip.

Total hip prosthetic replacement may present technical difficulties in the presence of osteoporosis and may be unjustifiable when many other joints are involved. Nevertheless, total hip replacement, is being increasingly used for the relief of pain and deformity of the rheumatoid hip. Painless movement is produced in 90 per cent of cases, although full range is seldom, if ever, attained, and there is often a residual limp.

Non-weight-bearing exercises are started on the first or second day post-operatively, using either balanced slings or else free movements and an abduction pillow. Although some surgeons permit immediate weight-bearing, many prefer to delay this for a few days. Strong abduction is essential, and abduction exercises must be practised assiduously. Flexion is promoted by use of a slippery board. Although most patients are allowed home 2 weeks post-operatively, there is a definite risk of prosthetic subluxation until adequate fibrous tissue has developed, and patients should be urged to avoid sitting on low chairs or stools which demand a squatting position and the provocative flexion/rotation movements of the hip.

The knee

The achievement and maintenance of full extension of the knee is the constant aim during all stages of rheumatoid arthritis. Without a straight knee, walking becomes increasingly difficult and painful. It is seldom that a rheumatoid patient can be bed-ridden for long without developing a flexion deformity of the knee, particularly if active preventive measures to avoid this are not taken during the period of bed rest, and if he has not subsequently returned to active life.

During the early stages of involvement of the joint, synovectomy is often undertaken to provide relief from pain and swelling. In about 90 per cent of cases, these features are considerably improved, although some loss of movement may result. Early mobilization is encouraged within the support of a firm supporting bandage.

During the later stages, when structural damage has occurred in the articular surfaces of the knee, reconstructive surgery may be indicated. For the moderately damaged joint, partial replacement arthroplasty by means of metal replacements for one or both tibial condyles (MacIntosh, McKeever) may achieve realignment, return of joint stability, and 90 per cent of flexion from full extension. For a more severely damaged knee, similar results may sometimes be attained by one of the total replacement techniques.

Early active movements are encouraged within the firm bandage which supports the knee post-operatively, and full mobilization follows suture removal.

Total knee replacement should always be considered as an alternative to arthrodesing the joint to relieve pain or restore joint mobility.

Arthrodesis of a knee certainly provides a stable and pain-free joint, but is only suitable for patients with limited involvement of other joint and as a last resort. In addition to causing 3–4 cm of leg shortening, it may exacerbate pain in the hips and spine if active joint disease is present in these regions. Without a good range of hip movement it may cause further disablement, and even when hip movement is adequate a stiff knee is a social handicap. Bilateral arthrodeses should only be undertaken in exceptional circumstances, since two stiff knees make sitting down and getting up independently almost impossible.

Post-operative care

Orthopaedic surgeons vary considerably in the post-operative rehabilitation programme which they advocate. After most surgical procedures, and particularly after synovectomy, early active movement is encouraged within 48 hours of surgery. Indeed, the general principles for physical therapy are not dissimilar from those described for the patient with acute early rheumatoid disease. Activity is gentle, non-resisted and encouraged in short, frequent sessions. The amount and vigour is largely determined by the patient's response to the activity. Passive movements and manipulative procedures are usually unnecessary and often contra-indicated. Total joint replacements are usually followed by early mobilization in the same manner, the surgeon giving clear guidance on the expected rate of recovery and a firm indication of any necessary restrictions on activity.

Many post-operative regimes will depend upon the availability of staff and facilities. Balanced slings and hydrotherapy will often be advised where they are easily accessible to the ward.

General surgical consideration

Arthroplasty by total replacement techniques and arthrodesis are the two forms of lower limb joint surgery which offer immediate post-operative freedom from joint pain.

Many rheumatoid patients have already had long and depressing histories of pain and systemic disease before they come to surgery, and therefore may not tolerate well the relatively long and demanding period of post-operative rehabilitation which some types of reconstructive surgery entail. Convalescence is often further complicated with osteoporosis, muscle wasting and soft-tissue contractures.

Despite the continued advances of surgical techniques, surgery can never be a substitute for suppressive and palliative drug therapy and the general medical care of the rheumatoid patient. It is against a background of well-planned medication that surgery stands its best chance of success. For this reason, the best form of hospital care is provided by special units where medical and surgical care can be shared by physician and surgeon, and surgical treatment and rehabilitation are completely integrated into the patient's total management.

CONCLUSION

Rehabilitation of a patient with rheumatoid arthritis is a complex exercise in general and specific management, requiring close collaboration between general practitioner, rheumatologist and surgeon, together with close understanding of the facilities available for helping the patient to obtain maximal functional independence at home and at work. The balance between rest and activity, the need for aids and appliances, and the timing of prophylactic or reconstructive surgery are all problems which require careful assessment for each patient.

The general clinical care and the physical management of disability cannot be separated, for each is independent on the other. The problems involved place a considerable onus upon the clinician, but he must not abrogate the responsibility if his patients are to achieve optimal function within the limits imposed by their disease. The rehabilitation of the rheumatoid arthritic must be part of the total patient care and for many patients is the major part of their management.

BIBLIOGRAPHY AND REFERENCES

Conaty, J.P. and Nickel, V.L. (1971). 'Functional incapacitation in rheumatoid arthritis: a rehabilitation challenge. A correlative study of function before and after hospital treatment.' *J. Bone Jt Surg.* **53A, 624**

Copeman's textbook of the rheumatic diseases. Ed. J.T. Scott. Churchill Livingstone, 1978 (2nd edn.) London/New York

Duthie, J.J.R. (1967). 'Medical management and prognosis in rheumatoid arthritis.' *Scott. med. J.* **12, 96**

Duthie, J.J.R., Brown, P.E., Truelove, L.H., Baragar, F.D. and Lawrie, A.J. (1964). 'Course and prognosis in rheumatoid arthritis.' *Ann. rheum. Dis.* **23, 193**

Mowat, A.G. (1970). 'Basic medical treatment in rheumatoid arthritis.' *Physiotherapy,* **56, 450**

Mowat, A.G. (1977). 'Rational approach to the use of non-skiordal anti-inflammatory·drugs.' *Advanced Medicine. Topics in Therapeutics 3.* Pitman Medical; London.

Mowat, A.G. (1978). 'Medical implications of orthopaedic surgery in rheumatoid diseases.' *Clinics in Rheumatic Disease,* **4, 249**

Mowat, A.G. (1978). 'Surgical treatment of rheumatoid arthritis' in *Copeman's textbook of the rheumatic Diseases.* Ed. J.T. Scott. Churchill Livingstone, 1978 (5th edn.) London/New York

Mowat, A.G., Nichols, P.J.R., Hollings, E.M., Haworth, R.J. and Aitken, L.C. (1979). 'A comparison of follow-up regimes in rheumatoid arthritis'. *Ann. Rheum. Dis.* (in the press)

5 Pain in the Neck and Shoulder

INTRODUCTION

A large number of the patients seeking medical advice complain of pain in the neck and arm, or of a painful stiff shoulder. An even larger number have these symptoms and do not consult a doctor. Of the latter group some consult various unqualified practitioners and other prescribe their own analgesics or palliative treatment. The total number of people involved is enormous.

Of those who consult their general practitioner, many are treated and cured, and it is only those with persistent, severe or frequently recurring symptoms who are referred for consultant advice. Such patients may be referred to medical, orthopaedic, neurological or rheumatological out-patient departments, and they certainly constitute a very large proportion of all patients referred for physiotherapy treatment.

The particular referral depends upon such factors as the frequency of the clinics, waiting list for radiological examination, waiting time for individual clinics, as well as clinical findings. The presence of neurological signs will tend to direct a patient to neurological or neurosurgical consultation, whereas a recurrent wry-neck is more likely to lead to an orthopaedic consultation. A painful stiff shoulder may be considered orthopaedic or rheumatological, often depending upon the waiting time for out-patient appointments.

In all instances there is considerable pressure for the provision of physiotherapy, for there is a general belief that physical treatment is helpful in these conditions.

There is however a wide range of clinical syndromes which present with localized or widespread pain in the neck and arm, with stiffness of the neck or shoulder, with paraesthesia in the arm, or with any combination of these symptoms.

In this chapter we discuss the two main groups of patients: those with a painful stiff shoulder and those in whom the symptoms appear to arise from degenerative changes in the cervical spine.

THE PAINFUL STIFF SHOULDER

General

Pain in the shoulder, with or without restriction of shoulder movements, is a very common symptom. Frequently it is considered to be an accompaniment of cervical spondylosis, although in retrospect the association may be shown to be fortuitous. The condition masquerades under names such as capsulitis, 'frozen shoulder', periarthritis and rotator cuff lesion. Too often authors use these names indiscriminately and as though they were interchangeable; others are precise in defining the different sumptoms and signs relating to different and sometimes hypothetical, soft-tissue lesions. Sometimes it is clear that pain in the shoulders is the result of cervical root irritation; limitation of neck movements, the association of paraesthesia with certain positions of the neck, tenderness in the supraclavicular fossa or along the major nerve trunks are all indications of the cervical origin of the symptoms. In all such cases, attention must be directed towards the neck. The majority of patients with shoulder pain appear to be suffering from one of a number of soft-tissue lesions which are self-limiting and rarely associated with prolonged serious disability, but it should be remembered that sometimes pain in the shoulder is a presenting symptom of a serious systemic disease. General limitation of glenohumeral movements, alteration in the scapulohumeral rhythm or limitation of abduction or adduction of the arm and localized pain associated with specific shoulder movements are all signs directing attention to the soft tissues of the shoulder joint. Localized tenderness and pain on 'springing' the acromioclavicular joint can draw attention to a localized and treatable arthritis of that joint.

Shoulder pain can arise from so many causes, the exact pathology of which has not yet been clearly defined, that unless there is definitive radiological or surgical evidence to establish a precise diagnosis, the indication for any particular form of physiotherapy must be correspondingly imprecise.

It is generally accepted that the painful stiff shoulder improves within a period of 9 months whatever the mode of treatment, and sometimes in spite of it. Worthwhile literature on the subject is scanty, the classification of the causes of painful shoulder are mostly unhelpful and the published trials of treatment frequently unacceptable. Diagnostic factors are debatable; the clinical features, the methods of examination and measurement, and modes of treatment are not amenable to standardization. The symptoms are often associated with an emotional response and influenced by psychological factors.

Rotator cuff lesions

Shoulder pain which is aching in character but which becomes acute when the patient performs certain specific manoeuvres is often loosely diagnosed as a rotator cuff lesion, or supraspinatus tendinitis. There are many different causes of this type of shoulder pain. Frequently the nature of the lesion is demonstrable by careful examination.

Supraspinatus lesions are characterized by a painful arc of movement in the mid-range of active abduction and adduction. Sometimes the lesion may be localized by tenderness on palpation along the length of the muscle.

There is some evidence that the critical zone of the rotator cuff, in which tears and calcified deposits tend to occur, coincides with that relatively avascular part of the cuff at which the anastomoses take place between the bloodvessels supplying bone and those supplying tendinous tissue.

Bicipital tendinitis can sometimes be diagnosed by elicitation of localized tenderness over the tendon of the long head of the biceps when the upper arm is externally rotated.

Both bicipital tendinitis and supraspinatus tendinitis often respond well to the local injection of hydrocortisone, although there is always a risk that this treatment may precipitate tendon rupture and that repeated injections may cause local necrosis.

Calcific deposits in the tendons of the supraspinatus, long head of biceps or subdeltoid bursa may produce an aching pain and stiffness of the shoulder so severe that surgical intervention becomes necessary. The calcified deposits are removed, adhesions divided, and any tendon ruptures repaired, resulting in considerable symptomatic relief.

Capsulitis

The condition in which pain in the shoulder is associated with gross reduction in all planes of movement of the shoulder joint is called capsulitis or periarthritis. Sometimes arising for no apparent reason, it may also be associated with a more sinister conditions such as:

(1) Angina or coronary insufficiency.
(2) Hemiplegia.
(3) Parkinsonism.
(4) Neoplasm of upper lobe of lung or bronchi.
(5) Neoplasm of breast.

The usual sequence of events in the natural history of capsulitis is one of pain, pain and loss of movement, relief from pain, then slow recovery of movement. The condition usually responds gradually to rest, simple analgesics and physiotherapy directed towards limiting the loss of movement. It may sometimes be accompanied by severe pain and systemic disturbances, and the patient may be found to have a raised erythrocyte sedimentation rate (ESR). Rest and salicylates are usually effective in controlling the condition, but a short course of steroids (7–10 days) has been advocated with a rapid reduction of the steroid dosage as improvement occurs.

Treatment of capsulitis, however severe the initial symptoms may be, must always aim at preventing the development of 'frozen shoulder'.

If conservative measures have not substantially relieved the patient's neck and arm symptoms, and if there is evidence of mechanical obstruction to the rotator cuff as it moves under the acromion, acromionectomy may offer a very successful solution.

Treatment for the painful stiff shoulder

Treatment has two main aims: the relief of pain and the restoration of normal shoulder movement. Treatments recommended include:

(1) Heat.
(2) Ice.
(3) Exercises of various types.
(4) Manipulation under anaesthetic.
(5) Manipulation without anaesthetic.
(6) Local or systemic steroids.
(7) Ultrasonic or x-ray therapy.
(8) Analgesics.

There is no general agreement as to the most effective treatment nor indeed whether any therapy alters the natural history of the condition.

Some patients are much relieved by heat in some form or another, whereas others tend to find that heat worsens their symptoms. Other patients find ice therapy, particular in the acute early phase of the condition, the most effective form of treatment.

Resting the arm in an elbow-supporting sling is usually followed by relief from pain, but it is important that the patient realizes the need for removing the arm from the sling several times a day to attempt a full range of hand and arm exercises.

The basis of physiotherapy lies in a judicious combination of rest and exercises within the painless range of movement.

Heat, ice, injection of hydrocortisone or of local anaesthetic may offer temporary relief from pain and allow the rest/exercise regime to be instituted. Usually, the symptoms slowly subside, and as the pain goes, so the painless range of motion slowly increases. Attempts to force the shoulder into the painful range, or over-activity of any kind, are usually followed by an exacerbation of pain and loss of joint range.

Not frequently, and particularly in the elderly, hydrocortisone injections are followed by some symptomatic relief followed by sudden loss of range of movement with or without pain. This is due to complete rupture of the suprasinatus tendon or biceps tendon, depending on the site of the injection.

Manipulation with or without anaesthetic may be needed if the symptoms are improving, but joint movement is not returning. This procedure is probably best avoided unless a full investigation has been undertaken, including electromyography of the appropriate shoulder muscles, to eliminate the possibility of an irritative nerve root lesion.

CERVICAL SPONDYLOSIS AS A CLINICAL SYNDROME

Introduction

There are two main groups of patients presenting with symptoms in the neck and arm:

(1) The young athletic person with an acute intense pain in the arm following sudden trauma, e.g. after a skiing accident, or a whiplash injury in a road accident.
(2) The middle-aged or elderly patient with a recurrent history of neck pain, limitation of neck movement, and brachialgia of root or partial root distribution.

The former is apparently due to a disc lesion and is characteristically made worse by coughing, sneezing and lateral neck movements.

The older patients with degenerative changes in the cervical spine (cervical spondylosis) characteristically complain of pain in the neck and shoulder-pain which is worse at night. Women are more often affected than men, and there is frequently a position of the neck which will aggravate the symptoms and another which will relieve them. General body posture also plays a contributory part in the aetiology of this type of neck pain and sitting long over the average-height desk or driving in an incorrect position are aggravating activities. Typical precipitating factors are playing golf, heavy lifting, and carrying.

It is often possible to differentiate between a neck pain which is due to a disease of the joints of the neck and neck pain associated with nerve root irritation, characterized by pain in the root distribution, paraesthesiae and referred pain. In either case the pain is usually most severe when the physical signs are least and often diffuse when the lesion is localized. This syndrome has been described repeatedly in the literature and been christened according to the changing theories of its aetiology. 'Acroparaesthesia', 'perineuritis', 'fibrositis', 'thoracic outlet syndrome', 'scalenus anterior syndrome' and 'brachialgia statica paraesthetica' are all terms given to a syndrome characterized by pain in the arm and occurring mainly in women aged 35–55 years. From time to time specific pathological conditions – such as compression of the brachial plexus at the thoracic outlet, cervical rib, scalene bend and compression of the medium nerve in the corpal tunnel – have been chosen to account for these symptoms in a small number of patients.

Sir Russell Brain described at length the condition of cervical spondylosis. He described radicular syndromes, acroparaesthesia, shoulder and arm pain of the referred type, 'frozen shoulder', and subacute multiradicular symptoms as all being associated with degenerative changes in the cervical intervertebral discs, and the osteophytic outgrowths on the adjacent vertebral bodies and posterior apophyseal joints.

Precisely what part cervical spondylosis plays in the aetiology of pain in the neck and arm (brachialgia) is unknown. It is generally assumed to be the commonest cause of pain in the neck and arm, and this assumption is based largely on the high frequency with which radiological changes in the cervical spine occur in patients with brachialgia. There is no clear correlation between radiological appearances of the cervical spine and the symptoms and signs which are present in any one patient. For this reason, some authorities have questioned the aetiological significance of cervical spondylosis, pointing out that almost all people over 50 years of age have radiological changes in the cervical spine characteristic of joint and disc degeneration. There is however some evidence to indicate that radiological changes in the posterior intervertebral joints are more likely to be accompanied by such signs and symptoms than are changes in the intervertebral discs.

A discrepancy between severity of symptoms and severity of radiological changes is a characteristic of osteo-arthrosis. It is often the soft-tissue reaction which both precedes and accompanies the joint degeneration which is instrumental in causing a variable degree of associated pain.

In the case of the cervical spine, it is not only bony overgrowth from the perimeter of the intervertebral foramen, but also perineuritic soft-tissue overgrowth within and beyond the foramina which causes the nerve irritation and pain. Of the two, it is probable that the inflammation and later the fibrosis of the meningeal perineuritic sleeve is responsible for the greater part of the pain induced by the radiculitis of cervical spondylosis, since actual mechanical pressure on the mixed nerve produces anaesthesia and weakness, with little pain, whereas irritation of the nerve due to inflammation of the perineuritic tissue is painful.

The persistent irritation of the nerve roots set up by the soft-tissue inflammation, bony outgrowth or joint malalignment of cervical spondylosis may well set up continued stimulationof afferent nerves, providing a background of subliminal sensory stimuli, and thereby increasing the central excitatory state. This would render the threshold for pain lower for other peripheral lesions in the same dermatome and would explain the apparent 'correlation' between 'tennis elbow', carpal tunnel or painful shoulder lesions and cervical spondylosis. It would also explain some of the discrepancies in the response of central and peripheral lesions to local treatment.

The presence of free intraneural circulation between nerve roots and the peripheral parts of the nerve may be responsible for the diffuse tenderness of peripheral nerves sometimes found in this condition, as well as for the variability in symptomatology, clinical picture, and response to treatment. It is conceivable that pathological changes in the soft tissues at the site of origin of the nerve roots could influence the vulnerability of the peripheral nerve to mechanical stress. Inflammation and later fibrosis associated with root irritation must diminish nerve sheath elasticity, thus increasing the tension which limb movements put upon it, and in particular predisposing to the sudden pain which patients often associate with certain movements of the neck or arm.

Because in very many people pain in the neck and arm are associated with radiological evidence of degenerative arthritis, cervical spondylosis has tended to become an accepted clinical diagnosis, whereas it is really a radiological diagnosis. Whether the symptoms are mainly pain, or paraesthesia, in the majority of patients, any one attack is likely to settle in 4—6 weeks. Only about one quarter of patients have symptoms persisting beyond 3 months.

With a natural history which is usually self-limiting, the syndrome of pain in the neck and arm is so common and its presentation so variable that it is often dismissed with minimal reference to a few key features. In order to rationalize the many treatments which are at present meted out without any apparent scientific basis for their selection, it is helpful to speculate about the clinical features of brachialgia, and much of this section is unashamedly speculative.

The joints most frequently involved in cervical spondylosis are those between the fifth, sixth and seventh cervical vertebrae, and the clinical features in any one patient vary with the level, type and degree of joint involvement.

Pain and paraesthesia

The common presentation is an attack of pain and paraesthesiae in the neck or arm. Some patients have difficulty in distinguishing between the symptoms, but usually there is a history of some neck pain preceding paraesthesia in the arm. Sometimes the pain is first felt in the muscles of the shoulder girdle, or it may radiate from the point of the shoulder down the lateral side of the arm to the elbow. Coughing, sneezing, active arm movements and active or passive neck movement may all accentuate the pain.

Paraesthesia often takes the form of numbness or tingling in the fingers, hand and forearm, coming on particularly at night. The symptoms are posture-related, and may be eased by deliberate changes in the position of the neck. One or both the limbs may be affected. Occasionally only the hand is involved, becoming cold and blue and feeling numb, although this may be confined to only one or two fingers or the thumb.

A patient, on being wakened in the morning, may complain of inability to use the affected hand, e.g. to turn off the alarm. By careful history-taking it is often possible to distinguish different patterns of presenting symptoms:

Recurrent attacks of shoulder pain: These may be induced by disproportionately slight effort and are frequently present on waking. They may be of maximal intensity then or may increase gradually throughout the day. Pain is maximal on rotation and abduction, but in severe attacks pain may increase in severity until all movement is inhibited. Examination may elicit tenderness over the long head of biceps, over the supraspinatus insertion, over either of the spinati bellies or the rhomboids, or at the insertion of the deltoid.

A gradual reduction of range of movement of the neck: This may occur over many years and is often accompanied by little pain.

Isolated or recurrent attacks of acute pain in the neck: These are sometimes induced by trauma and sometimes come on during unguarded movement, either during the night or during some apparently effortless occupation in the day. The neck is fixed in one position due to intense spasm of the cervical muscles, and voluntary movement is impossible or minimal.

Recurrent stiff neck: The patient may complain of recurrent attacks of neck pain and stiffness. Sometimes these attacks are associated with pain or paraesthesia in any of the dermatomes supplied by the nerves C1–7 and the first thoracic nerve T1. Symptoms are therefore located in the upper part of the chest and back, the shoulder, the arm and the hand, and the back of the head. Sometimes such attacks are associated with spastic paresis of the lower limbs caused by cord damage (cervical myelopathy, *see* p. 87).

Attacks of elbow pain: Pain in the lateral side of the elbow of the 'tennis elbow' variety and pain in the medial side of the elbow of the 'golfers elbow' variety, especially when recurrent and not attributable to severe unaccustomed activity involving excessive forearm use, may be indicative of cervical spondylosis.

Attacks of pain in the forearm, wrist and hand: Pain, paraesthesia, and stiffness of the hand, wrist and forearm may be due to cervical spondylosis. Symptoms referred in the distribution of the ulnar nerve or the median nerve must be distinguished from those arising from 'entrappement' of the ulnar nerve at the elbow or the median nerve in the carpal tunnel. When cervical spondylosis is present, minor trauma can precipitate a full-blown carpal tunnel syndrome.

Pain in the breast and axilla: Careful breast examination is necessary to distinguish this type of pain arising from cervical spondylosis from a similar type of pain arising from a neoplastic lesion of the breast with axillary gland involvement.

Pain in the front or back of the chest: Localized tender areas in the muscles of the upper limb and pectoral girdle occur frequently in cervical spondylosis and must be carefully distinguished from pain and tenderness in the same group of muscles of neoplastic, traumatic or inflammatory origin. A neoplastic chest lesion involving the upper lobe of the lung can present as shoulder or chest pain; so too can secondary deposits in bones of the thoracic cage. Pain in the upper part of the chest may also result from osteoporosis of the thoracic spine, from a peptic ulcer adherent to the posterior abdominal wall, from pathological conditions of the gall bladder, and from lesions involving the diaphragm.

Headache: When due to cervical spondylosis, this is always occipital on one or both side. It often spreads to, or involves independently, the forehead on the same side. It is associated with arthritic changes in the joints and soft tissues of the upper cervical spine but is not necessarily pure C1–C2 distribution. The headache may occur particularly in the mornings and is often associated with neck stiffness and pain incurred by faulty neck and head posture during the night.

Chin pain radiating to the arms: This is rare, but the lower part of the lower jaw and chin are partly supplied by C2—3 (anterior cutaneous nerve of the neck) and such a means of presentation is possible from upper cervical lesions.

Physical signs of cervical spondylosis

As with the symptoms, the signs of cervical spondylosis vary greatly with its phases of activity. Thus, although for the greater part of the time most patients with cervical spondylosis have only minor symptoms and few physical signs, when subjected to trauma, infection, prolonged exposure to cold, sustained posture or over-exertion, their symptoms and signs may rapidly become acute and severe.

During quiescent periods, there may be some limitation of neck movement and mild tenderness on pressure over the spinous processes of affected cervical vertebrae.

During active phases, or 'attacks', or in patients in whom the involvement of nerve roots, nerve cord, or cord vascular supply is permanently severe, the range of neck movement, and often shoulder movement, becomes drastically reduced and may be completely inhibited by pain and muscle spasm. The patient has a tense, apprehensive expression and the head is held in one position of relative ease by muscles whose spasm makes their outlines visible and palpable; the shoulder is held adducted to the body with forearm and hand in neutral position.

If neck movement is possible, the foraminal compression test will frequently be positive, i.e. downward pressure on the head when inclined to the painful side will cause pain in the ipsilateral arm.

Pain and fear of pain are the dominant features of both acute and chronic severe root involvement, but in addition, certain signs identify the source of the radiculitis. Thus, when the sixth cervical root is involved, the patient may complain of pins and needles in the thumb, numbness of the thumb, particularly the tip, and pain shooting down the arm and forearm into the thumb. Examination may demonstrate objective sensory loss in the radial aspect of thumb and forearm, and the tendon reflexes of biceps and brachialis may be weak or absent.

Some weakness of elbow flexion may be noticed, and of pronation, supination and occasionally some shoulder movements.

When the seventh cervical root is involved, pins and needles may be felt in the index, middle and ring fingers, and pain may radiate from the shoulder to these fingers. There may be diminished sensation over the back of the hand, the index and middle fingers, and the radial half of the ring finger; the triceps jerk may be weak or absent.

With involvement of the eighth cervical root and first thoracic, pins and needles and pain are located in the little finger, the ulnar side of the ring finger, and the hypothenar eminence, and there may be diminished sensation in the same areas. Weakness is usually confined to the small muscles of the hand, and patients complain of weakened grip and difficulty with manipulating small tools or implements.

Apart from shooting pains to the fingers, patients with severe or active cervical spondylosis complain of tender areas in the muscles innervated by the affected nerve roots. This applies especially to the trapezius, the spinati, the rhomboids, latissimus dorsi and pectoralis major and minor.

Sometimes the symptoms from the neck itself are less distressing than those from the shoulder, elbow, or wrist, and the diagnosis of 'frozen shoulder', 'tennis elbow', 'golfer's elbow' or 'carpal tunnel syndrome' may obscure the underlying lesion in the cervical spine. When a patent presents with symptoms and signs of these 'catch-phrase' diagnoses, cervical spondylosis should always be looked for as an underlying condition.

Differential diagnosis of cervical spondylosis

Because cervical spondylosis can cause referred pain in many distributions, it can be a considerable mimic of visceral disease. Also, because it is a commonly occurring degenerative condition, it may well be an incidental finding in association with other conditions. Thus, the diagnosis of cervical spondylosis is often one of elimination.

Visceral disease: Pain referred from pleura, pericardium or diaphragm, including carcinoma of the lung and myocardial infarction. It is particularly important to exclude polymyalgia rheumatica, which is a treatable condition.

Upper respiratory infections: Infections such as sinusitis or tonsillitis, with secondary adenitis of cervical and paratracheal glands, causing recurrent acute episodes of stiffness and pain in the neck.

Vertebral column lesions: Lesions such as rheumatoid arthritis, ankylosing spondylitis, spinal caries, neoplasms or fractures rarely cause difficulty in diagnosis. Congenital abnormalities of the vertebral bodies or the presence of a cervical rib are more common. Localized degenerative arthritis may be associated with injury, deformity or disease.

Central nervous system: Lesions of the spinal cord, e.g. syringomyelia, or of the nerve roots, e.g. herpes zoster or poliomyelitis, may give rise to diagnostic difficulties.

Cervical myelopathy and radiculopathy: As part of the gradual degenerative changes occurring in the cervical spine associated with aging there is a narrowing of the disc spaces with a bulging of disc material centrifugally. Osteophyte formation around the bulging disc may lead to significant compression of spinal nerve roots in the intervertebral foramina or lateral part of the spinal canal, or to compression of the spinal cord. This condition is really a late manifestation of cervical spondylosis. Its significance lies in the development of the most important complication – cervical myelopathy.

The symptoms and signs of cord pressure occur far less frequently than those of root pressure, since lateral protrusions from intervertebral discs are more common than posterior protrusions. When cord pressure does occur, it is usually associated with, or preceded by, symptoms of root pressure. Symptoms usually appear gradually, and a patient may complain of weakness in the legs, difficulty in walking a straight line, and pain and weakness in one or both arms. As in root pressure, the radial position of the prolapsing or bulging part of the disc determines the type of clinical picture which presents. Thus a mid-line posteriorly directed prolapse affects both pyramidal tracts, and possibly both upper and lower limbs.

The onset of cervical myelopathy is insidious, and although the patient may complain of pain and paraesthesia in the arms, these are rarely severe. The important manifestations of this condition are in the lower limbs. The patient may present with some weakness of the legs and difficulty in walking. Enquiry may reveal some paraesthesia of the lower limbs. Examination at this time usually reveals some spasticity and loss of proprioceptive sensation. It has been said that myelopathy does not develop in patients who do not have signs demonstrable at their first hospital attendance.

Treatment of cervical spondylosis

General principles

Many treatments are advocated for patients with pain in the neck and arm:

(1) Rest of the patient.
(2) Rest of the neck.
(3) Palliative physiotherapy, such as heat or ice.
(4) Collars of felt, rubber, plaster of paris, or plastic.
(5) Rest of the arm in a sling when brachialgia is severe.
(6) Traction in extension, flexion or in neutral position:
     With weights,
     By manual traction.
(7) Shoulder-raising exercises.
(8) Manipulation — with or without anaesthetic.
(9) Neck-mobilizing exercises.

There is lack of evidence to show that one treatment of pain in the neck and arm is better than any other. This lack is not a reflection on the efficacy of the forms of treatment, but merely emphasizes the need to make a pathologically based diagnosis of the precise cause of the pain in each patient, so that treatment applied may be appropriate to the underlying cause.

It is unrealistic to consider pain in the neck and arm as an entity, any more than pain in the back or pain in the abdomen can be considered a distinct symptom complex. Future research which defines accurately the source and nature of the pain throughout the course of the condition may well show the need for and the efficacy of specific treatment for each pathological situation.

The several clinical trials which have been carried out have not attempted this and have merely established that both the immediate response and the long-term follow-up are similar, whether patients are treated by the supply of a simple collar, with a time-consuming physiotherapy, or with placebo treatments. Indeed, the only factors which affect prognosis are the patient's age, the severity of the attack, the number of previous attacks and the average duration of previous attacks.

Most patients have less pain if their posture is corrected, and the majority are relieved, at least partially, by wearing an adequate collar. The disturbance of sleep can often be reduced by a collar or by instruction in the use of a 'butterfly' pillow. Many patients are greatly relieved by a frank discussion about the nature of the symptoms and, indeed, reassurance may be all that they were seeking, coupled with instruction on how to go about their daily activities in such a way as to avoid future exacerbations of their symptoms.

The basis of treatment of the symptom is rest, followed by graded activity. Rest is achieved for the neck itself by wearing a simple collar; rest for the patient by avoiding strenuous activity, and in severe cases, by rest in bed. Such rest may need to be preceded by or supplemented by traction or manipulation. Dramatic relief can certainly occur with traction or manipulation, but there is no evidence that these procedures influence the natural history of the condition as expressed by recurrences of symptoms, nor is there any guarantee that a repetition of the same procedure will successfully relieve the symptoms in successive attacks.

The clinician and therapist must therefore decide whether the use of any particular procedure is likely to produce relief from the group of symptoms present at the time of examination, and whether the symptoms and the extent of likely relief will justify the expenditure and inconvenience to the patient in attending the out-patient department for its administration.

Although it is apparent that treatment cannot be prescribed collectively but must be selected according to the physical, mental and social state of each individual patient, it is possible to generalize to a limited extent. It seems that the acute lesion with marked limitation of movement and severe pain will respond best to immobilization; the less acute lesion with restricted movement in one direction only will more appropriately be treated by mobilization techniques.

Heat and gentle mobilizing exercises during acute exacerbations of pain and stiffness in the neck usually prove helpful. If possible, heat treatment should be given daily at the physiotherapy department to relax spasm and permit exercises which involve a gradually increasing range of movements. If not, patient should be encouraged to perform their exercises at home in front of an electric fire on the days they do not attend the department.

Daily exercises to maintain the range of neck movement should be continued indefinitely, together with postural exercises and shoulder exercises, and patients should be asked to check their head and neck position in mirrors and shop windows and to correct the tendency to hold the neck protruded and the head bent forward and down.

Manual traction may relieve pain in the acute exacerbations of neck pain and stiffness, particularly if there is an associated radiculitis, with pins and needles in the hand or shooting pains to one or more fingers of that hand. While adequate for people of small and medium stature, manual traction is of little use in the case of a tall, powerfully built patient. For these patients, many physiotherapists feel that mechanical traction may be indicated. This should be applied with extreme care, under expert supervision (*see* Chapter 1).

Such traction may be effective in relieving symptoms, particularly when used in conjunction with a collar worn for the remaining part of the day and during the night as well. If not, when symptoms are severe, bed rest is necessary. A collar should be worn and only one or two soft pillows permitted. If a collar cannot be tolerated then no more than one pillow is allowed. Adequate analgesia and a nightly sedative are essential. Drugs such as diazepam and chlordiazepoxide used in conjunction with analgesics are often helpful in relieving tension and anxiety and in assisting muscular relaxation.

If the pain is severe and persists for longer than a few days despite these measures, then admission to hospital and application of sustained cervical traction may be necessary to alleviate pain. However, cervical traction is not without risk, and its use should be carefully considered. It is seldom necessary to maintain traction for more than a week, and symptoms should then continue to subside with the use of a collar, restricted exertion and daily periods of mobilizing exercises of gradually increasing range and duration.

Collars

As the pathological conditions in both the locomotor and nervous systems cannot be cured, the treatment of cervical spondylosis is a long drawn-out affair which attempts to prevent deterioration of the status quo, and to treat acute episodes of pain and dysfunction as they occur. In the acute stages of mild cases of cervical spondylosis, the symptoms usually respond rapidly to rest in an adequate collar. An 'adequate' collar is effective in preventing neck movement, and effective collars must therefore be rigid. Unfortunately, the more rigid a collar is, the more difficult it is for the therapist to apply and for the patient to tolerate. Most collars are therefore a compromise between ease of application and comfort on the one hand and rigidity and direct therapeutic value on the other. Commonly used materials are sorbo rubber, orthopaedic felt and plastazote. The collar should be worn all day and preferably all night too.

A sorbo rubber collar has one advantage because if taken off and reapplied upside down and back to front it still fits the patient, but it has virtually no mechanical ability to restrict neck movement.

A collar made from orthopaedic felt requires the concavities carved from it to admit the clavicles and to fit round the occipital protuberances and jaw. Thus, a felt collar is more restrictive than a rubber one and produces less pressure on the chin and trachea while the patient is in the horizontal position in bed.

Plastazote collars are made from expanded polystyrene, and their manufacture requires an oven for heating the sheets of material, which the physiotherapist must know how to use. The heated plastazote strip, cut in the estimated length of the collar, is moulded, while still warm, to the patient's neck and allowed to cool into the resulting shape. Its edges are then trimmed, and it is fastened by velcro tapes which may be glued or sewn on to the plastazote. It is important that the collar comes high enough up the back of the neck to cover the occipital condyles, otherwise head movement is not properly controlled nor the neck posture adequately supported. It is equally important that the neck should not be supported in hyperextension.

Once the acute symptoms are improving, the collar should be gradually discarded, the patient being advised to take it off for about an hour in the morning at first and then for an hour longer each day. If there is no discomfort, the period without the collar can be increased steadily. If discomfort is felt, the period should be decreased and then once again increased after a few days. The patient should retain the collar for some months and always wear it for car journeys and heavy work, or if he tends to get a tired, aching neck in the evening while watching television or doing any task which entails neck flexion. Many people wear their collar at night for some weeks after they have stopped wearing it during the day as they find that night posture of the head and neck is a critical factor in determining the pain level of the following day.

If symptoms respond to treatment with a collar, but are severe and likely either to recur or improve, but not completely resolve, it is advisable to try a firmer moulded collar.

Since in the acute episodes of neck pain and stiffness which occur in cervical spondylosis, the position of the neck is frequently abnormal, it is probably better, initially, to provide a collar made from orthopaedic felt as well as a plastazote collar. As pain is relieved, spasm of cervical muscles is reduced, and the head and neck resume their normal relationship with the head held erect and in neutral rotation and the neck in mild and physiological lordosis. At this stage of recovery, a plastazote collar may be worn more continuously. The advantages of the plastazote collar are that it is lighter, less bulky, less obvious, and often better tolerated. There is little difference in its heating effect on the patient. Though it is thinner than felt and may be aerated yet further by punch holes, plastazote is still a very warm material to wear and may be hard to tolerate in the summer. Many patients do not manage to wear a plastic collar at night but can tolerate the softer, felt one, retaining the more restrictive collar for day wear.

Patients with serious disorganization of the cervical spine and, in particular, patients in whom there is danger of a slip of one cervical vertebra upon another, will need immobilization in a collar giving even better support than either felt or plastazote. There are many proprietary types of rigid plastic collar, and one of these may prove particularly suitable for an individual patient.

Rigid plastic collars are of two main types.

(1) All-in-one wrap-over type, with back and side fastening.
(2) Two-piece articulated type, consisting of a front breast-plate reaching as low as the manubrium sterni and in one piece with a moulded neck and chin support, and back plate extending from scapular level to above the level of the occiput.

Many centres prefer to make their own rigid plastic collars from a cast of the patient's neck. The details of structure vary with the manufacturing centre and the patient concerned — the extent of his disability, his tolerance of a restricting support, and the degree of restriction which it is necessary to impose upon him. Thus, the depth of the collar and its height posteriorly vary considerably. The chin-piece frequently does not cover the chin, but merely provides a shelf for it to rest on. Where maximal control of neck mobility must be maintained, the collar is extended over the lower part of the prominence of the chin, cupping it and controlling its movements.

Rubber collars with parallel horizontal inflatable strips provide an alternative form of collar. Although some patients find them satisfactory, they do tend to leak and may also precipitate skin sensitivity reactions so that their abilities to support and soothe are both uncertain.

If the wearing of an adequate collar is not followed by improvement, the diagnosis should be reconsidered.

Manipulation

Cervical spondylosis may be present without symptoms, but it may so narrow the spinal canal that a sudden hyperextension or acute flexion of the cervical spine can cause a contusion of the cord, with severe neurological consequences. Despite this, millions of patients are manipulated every year by qualified and unqualified practitioners and although occasional tragedies do happen they are mercifully very rare. There is, however, little evidence that manipulation of the cervical spine has any greater long-term therapeutic effect than the conventional conservative measures used in the management of pain in the neck and arm.

The *indication* for cervical spine manipulation can be defined as pain appearing to originate in the cervical spine which is not associated with signs of cord compression, and in the presence of ligaments and vertebrae which are apparently sound.

Thus, manipulation of the cervical spine is contra-indicated in 'whiplash' injuries where there is any evidence of ligament damage or crush injury of the vertebral body; in rheumatoid arthritis which has a predilection for involving the upper cervical spine; in the presence of hypermobility of the cervical spine, or of congenital malformation or anomalies. The presence of cervical myelopathy is also a contra-indication.

Surgical intervention

Operative treatment of cervical spondylosis is indicated only when there is severe pain which has not responded to an adequate trial of conservative treatment, or when there is progressive neurological involvement. The surgery chosen can be cord decompression or cervical fusion, or a combination of these procedures.

In younger patients, the operative treatment of choice appears to be a fusion of the bodies of the vertebrae on either side of the disc protrusion, through an anterolateral approach. This permits the greater part of the disc and the cartilage plates to be removed and a cancellous bone block to be inserted into the slot cut across the front of the adjacent vertebral bodies. Trauma to the affected nerve root is reduced or prevented, and the patient is able to get up in a few days, wearing a cervical brace or collar which is discarded when a satisfactory bony union has been achieved. Further disc degeneration and osteophyte increase appear to be prevented by this measure, and it is gradually replacing the older procedure of posterior fusion.

BIBLIOGRAPHY AND REFERENCES

Brain, W.R. (1954). 'Spondylosis: the known and the unknown.' *Lancet* 1, 687
Brain, W.R., Wright, D., and Wilkinson, M. (1947). 'Spontaneous compression of both median nerves in the carpal tunnel.' *Lancet* 1, 277
British Association of Physical Medicine (1966). 'Pain in the neck and arm: a multi-centre trial of the effects of physiotherapy.' *Br. med. J.* 1, 253
Darlington, L.G. and Coombes, E.H. (1977). 'Effects of local steroid injection for supraspinatus tear.' *Rheum. and Rehab.* 16, 1972
Falconer, M.A. and Weddell, G. (1943). 'Costoclavicular compression of the subclavian artery and vein.' *Lancet* 2, 539
Hazleman, B.L. (1972). 'The painful stiff shoulder.' *Rheum. Rehab.* 2, 413
Hughes, J.T. (1966). *Pathology of the Spinal Cord*. London; Lloyd-Luke
Irvine, D.H., Forster, J.B., Newell, D.J. and Klukrim, B.N. (1965). 'Prevalence of cervical spondylosis in a general practice.' *Lancet* 1, 1089
Kellgren, J.H., Jeffrey, M.R. and Ball, J. (Eds) (1963). *Epidemiology of Chronic Rheumatism*, Vol 2. Oxford; Blackwell
Lawrence, J.S. (1963). In *Epidemiology of Chronic Rheumatism*, Vol 1, p. 100. Ed. by J.H. Kellgren, M.R. Jeffrey and J. Ball. Oxford; Blackwell
Less, F. and Turner, J.W.A. (1963). 'The natural history and prognosis of cervical spondylosis.' *Br. med. J.* 2, 1607
Lishman, W.A. and Russell, W.R. (1961). 'The brachial neuropathies.' *Lancet* 2, 941
Moseley, F.H. and Goldie, I. (1963). 'The arterial pattern of the rotator cuff of the shoulder.' *J. Bone Jt Surg.* 45B, 780
Richardson, D.T. (1975). 'The Painful Shoulder'. *Proc. Roy. Soc. Med.* 68, 731
Russell, W.R. (1956). 'Discussion on cervical spondylosis.' *Proc. R. Soc. Med.* 49, 198
Steinberg, V.L. and Mason, R.M. (1959). 'Cervical spondylosis: pilot therapeutic trial.' *Ann. phys. Med.* 5, 37
Symonds, G. (1975). 'Accurate diagnosis and treatment for painful shoulder conditions'. *J. Int. Med. Res.* 3, 261

6 Backache

INTRODUCTION

It has often been averred that backache is protean in its origins, that it is not a diagnosis, and should therefore not be dealt with as a separate condition. If this is so, a chapter on backache is superfluous in a book on rehabilitation. But rehabilitation entails the treatment of any patient and his surroundings in such a way as to restore or create for that patient a condition of optimal functional efficiency and maximal comfort, and this, in its turn, demands the relief of pain. Whatever the cause of his backache, the patient attending the Rehabilitation Department asks primarily for the relief of pain and since the measures for relieving this are applicable to the pain from a wide variety of causes, and the long-term management of backache is likewise similar in so many conditions, a chapter on backache has been included.

It is, however, important for those who treat a patient with backache to remember that when they treat the backache, they are treating a symptom; they must therefore take particular care to investigate and treat the cause of the symptom concurrently, lest by relieving the symptom, they permit the underlying pathological condition to progress undetected.

AETIOLOGY

The differential diagnoses of backache of various types are so many that to enumerate them would be to fill the pages with wearying lists. One has only to consider the anatomy of the vertebral column, the structural intricacies of its component parts, its variety of functions, and the plethora of organs to which it is related to understand that this must be so. Small wonder then that dysfunction in any system may present as backache and that the only certain deduction which can be drawn from the complaint of backache is that something is wrong somewhere. Any physiotherapeutic treatment for backache must take place concurrently with, or else follow, accurate definition of the 'something', and equally accurate delineation of the 'somewhere'.

Much has been written about backache as an expression of psychological disturbance. Perusal of the records of patients who have attended orthopaedic clinics over many years illustrates the strong tendency to consider all backache as psychological unless proved otherwise by radiological investigation. While it is undoubtedly comforting for those giving treatment to attribute the backache, which they have not cured, to psychogenic causes, it is less than comforting for the patient. Since the presence of backache is difficult to confirm, or disprove, backache has become the obvious complaint of work-shy, battle-shy or tension-shy patients who require an acceptable reason for opting out of unpleasant circumstances. The popularity of backache among malingerers has discredited its authenticity for those who really suffer from it, and this combined with failure of radiological confirmation of any underlying pathology each year puts a substantial number of patients into the 'psychogenic' category wrongly. It is chastening to recall the number of patients who develop irrefutable radiological evidence of disease some years after a diagnosis of 'psychogenic' has been affixed to their backache.

'NON-RHEUMATIC' BACKACHE

Because many pathological conditions of many systems may present as backache, treatment and rehabilitation cannot be realistic unless the underlying cause is first delineated. A detailed functional enquiry and past history are essential to the accurate diagnosis of this cause, and supplement an enquiry about appetite, bowels, micturition, menstruation and general health.

Information is elicited on:

(1) the duration, time of onset and nature of onset of symptoms;
(2) their relationship to time of day, month or year, to exercise, rest and specific activities and movements;
(3) their present location, and possible variation from their location at time of onset;
(4) their radiation and variation with posture;
(5) sources of exacerbation and relief;
(6) their response to analgesics and anti-inflammatory drugs;
(7) associated presence of pain, swelling or stiffness in any other joints, now or at any time;
(8) the presence or absence of abnormal symptoms and signs in any other system;
(9) the nature of past and present medication — type and duration with particular reference to steroids or to natural or synthetic hormones or pregnancies or abortions;
(10) past operations — with particular reference to hysterectomy and mastectomy in a woman, prostatectomy in a man, or pneumonectomy, thyroidectomy and nephrectomy in both;
(11) past or present reaction to work and leisure activities, particularly to a change or unduly long participation in either.

Such a detailed enquiry is essential in our present social structure, which necessitates a substantial number of people moving from district to district at a speed which exceeds that of their medical records, so that any doctor asked to treat them for backache may well have no information other than that obtainable from the patients themselves.

Disorders of the gastro-intestinal system, such as peptic ulcers or neoplasms situated on the posterior wall of stomach or duodeum and causing inflammatory changes on the posterior abdominal wall, may present as backache in the lower thoracic or upper lumbar region, depending on the location of the lesion. They are usually associated with poor appetite, heartburn and epigastric pain. Dysfunction of the gall bladder, such as cholecystitis, may present with acute pain between the shoulder blades, but will usually be associated with pain in the right upper quadrant of the abdomen and intolerance to fats. Pancreatitis or neoplasms of the pancreas may also be associated with back pain at the thoracolumbar level.

Disease of the genito-urinary system involving the kidney, such as pyelonephritis, may present with backache over the lower ribs and in the costovertebral angle on the affected side, and will usually be associated with frequency of micturition, haematuria and dysuria.

When the prostrate is involved, as in prostatitis or in carcinoma of the prostrate, backache is usually felt in the sacral region, although secondary deposits from prostatic carcinoma may occur anywhere in the spine, resulting in pain and tenderness in the vertebrae concerned, possibly progressing to greater tenderness and root pain if vertebral collapse ensues.

There is usually, but not always, a history of delay in starting micturition and of haematuria and dysuria. Similar symptoms arise from secondaries due to renal neoplasm, but without delay in starting micturition.

Disorders of the respiratory system involving the pleura on the posterior thoracic wall may also present as backache over the area of the pleura involved. Thus, both neoplastic and infective lesions giving rise to abscess or cavity formation may cause backache which is initially related to breathing and coughing, but may later become constant. Carcinoma of the upper-lobe bronchus frequently gives rise to backache in the subscapular region and sometimes to a painful 'frozen shoulder' as well.

The prodromal period before the eruption of the rash of herpes zoster may be evidenced by severe pain in the back along the cutaneous distribution of the nerve root affected. Persistent pain is limited to one side of the body and the single affected root and may endure for months after the rash disappears. The post-herpetic pain may respond to physical treatments such as ethylchloride spray, ice therapy or the use of a vibrator.

Muscular pain also appears as a symptom of several general diseases. Polymyositis, dermatomyositis and systemic lupus erythematosus may present with pain and muscle tenderness in the sacrospinalis, and certain infections, such as influenza and Bornholm's disease, are frequently accompanied by severe backache. This type of backache usually settles rapidly with rest and disappears as the disease process remits.

Polymyalgia rheumatica usually affects those of late middle age and the elderly and is not infrequently missed as a diagnosis. It is commoner in women than men and is characterized by severe pain and stiffness in the muscles of the shoulder and pelvic girdles. Occasionally there may be an accompanying synovitis of one or more joints, or evidence of vasculitis. Often the patients look unwell and complain of fatigue, lassitude and depression. Because of the age group affected it is usual to find accompanying radiological and clinical evidence of degenerative changes in cervical and lumbar spine. The key to diagnosis is a markedly elevated ESR (frequently values of 100 mm in the first hour (Westergren) are recorded), coupled with the complaint of incapacitating morning stiffness.

Treatment with corticosteroids is dramatic as far as symptoms are concerned, and probably shortens the course of the disease. Symptoms and the ESR are the best guides to management. This disease runs a course of 3 months to 2 years, and its severity depends upon the vasculitis (if present).

Traumatic myositis may occur after direct or indirect injury, with pain, tenderness and possibly swelling and secondary spasm of the muscles concerned. Treatment of the tenderness with ultrasonic irradiation, the application of ice, or exposure to heat, followed by mobilizing exercises all have their advocates. Occasionally, if the injury is severe, it may be necessary to restrict the mobility of the spine temporarily by the application of a plaster of paris jacket or other form of temporary corset.

Neoplasms

The presence of secondary neoplastic deposits in one or more vertebrae (or even a rib) must always be kept in mind as a possible cause of back pain at any level.

Pain frequently antedates radiological evidence of vertebral involvement, and a scan of patients with symptoms suggestive of secondary deposits in the vertebrae may be necessary to exclude this diagnosis. Local pain and tenderness over an affected vertebra may become intensified and exacerbated by root pain when vertebral collapse and root irritation supervene.

Growths of the thyroid, breast, bronchus, kidney and prostate are particularly likely to give rise to secondary deposits in the vertebrae, and involvement of these organs in any treatment — operative, radiotherapeutic or chemotherapeutic — should always be considered, together with symptoms of possible present dysfunction. Swift referral of patients with secondary deposits for radiotherapeutic or chemotherapeutic treatment is essential, as the relief of pain by appropriate treatment can be dramatic. Where fracture has occurred, or pain persists despite chemotherapy or radiotherapy, the provision of a suitable spinal brace is essential as a pain-relieving measure.

Despite the recognized danger of causing leukemia by excessive radiation, it may be essential to repeat radiographic examination of the spine from time to time if radiological evidence of the presence of a tumour is not obtained, despite clinical evidence to the contrary.

Paget's disease affecting one or more vertebrae may also cause localized pain and tenderness over the vertebrae affected. Considerable relief results from treatments with agents such as calcitonin, mithramycin, and diphosphonates.

Infections of the vertebral column often present with backache, but the more chronic the infection the more insidious the onset. Identification of the infecting organism, administration of an appropriate antibiotic and immobilization of the spine in a plaster of paris cast form the basis of treatment, with or without surgical drainage of any abscesses.

Chronic infection

Tuberculous infection can cause pain and tenderness which may vary considerably with the individual. There may be a large paravertebral abscess without pain; conversely, severe pain may precede abscess formation. Chronic infection of the vertebrae may also occur following typhoid or following a staphylococcal septicaemia when the original infection has been treated with inadequate antibiotic therapy.

Acute infection

Infections such as blastomycosis, brucellosis and tuberculosis, and infections with staphylococcus or other pyogenic organisms cause pain in the back of similar type and distribution, but the onset is swifter and the symptoms of toxicity more pronounced.

Backache may persist after the infection has been healed. Because of mechanical disruption of the normal structure, a plaster of paris jacket or spinal brace should sometimes be worn during the convalescent weight-bearing and discarded later as the vertebral bony structure is reformed.

Metabolic disorders

Demineralization of the vertebrae (osteomalacia) occurs in various metabolic disorders, with resulting vertebral compression, reduction in overall size of the patient, and a variable degree of back pain. Excessive protein withdrawal (osteoporosis) occurs after prolonged immobilization of the back, and during certain endocrine disturbances, gastro-intestinal disorders, primary or secondary malignant disease or chronic inflammatory states, and prolonged steroid administration. Osteoporosis of the vertebrae does not appear to be painful unless vertebral fracture occurs or has occurred from another cause prior to the onset of the osteoporosis. In these instances there is backache at the level of the fractured vertebra, and in the adjacent ligaments and muscles.

Gradually increasing deformity will cause further backache as other parts of the spine attempt to compensate for the collapse of the vertebra, with resulting changes in the tension of muscles, tendons and ligaments.

The aims of treatment of osteoporosis are: to prevent its continuation, to eliminate the cause where possible, to prevent or minimize deformity and to prevent or minimize pain.

The development of deformity may be minimized by a regime of graded, regularly performed exercises, designed to improve posture and reduce strain on the vertebral bodies and their ligaments by strengthening the abdominal and paraspinal musculature. At night, the patient should sleep on a firm mattress underlaid with fracture boards.

Whereas the continued performance of regular exercises is usually regarded as mandatory, there is considerable controversy about the place of a spinal brace or corset in the treatment of the pain and deformity of the osteoporotic spine. However if the pain persists and deformity increases despite strengthening exercises and night postural control, then a spinal corset is needed and should be prescribed. In prescribing a spinal corset, it is sometimes necessary to sacrifice some effiency to comfort, as most patients will discard a spinal corset if it is too restrictive. Patients wearing spinal supports should be encouraged to perform regular active and static exercises for the abdominal and paraspinal muscles within their pain tolerance.

The relief of pain in osteoporotic fractured vertebrae is attempted by the use of analgesics, combined with strengthening exercises already mentioned for the spinal and abdominal muscles.

Fractured vertebra

A fractured vertebra can often remain undiagnosed as a cause of persistent backache for some considerable time before radiography discloses its presence. Where there is a clear history of trauma, the fracture is rapidly diagnosed and treated. But in certain groups of people, such as those with metabolic disorders such as osteomalacia and osteoporosis, abnormal vertebral configuration such as Scheuermann's disease, or disease such as ankylosing spondylitis, a comparatively minor injury can cause a vertebral fracture, with resulting localized pain, tenderness and loss of function. Immobilization of the spine in a plaster of paris jacket permits the fracture to be rested and supported while ambulation continues. In this way, muscle power and bone protein and mineral content is preserved.

This immobilization should be followed by a regime of graded exercises so that muscles are strengthened to provide physiological splinting for the healed fracture. The patient is traditionally instructed to sleep on a firm mattress with the fracture site well supported, and to maintain at all times a good posture.

Gynaecological conditions

Many gynaecological conditions are associated with low lumbar and sacral backache, which usually occurs or has an exacerbation before and during the first part of the menstrual period. Uterine retroversion and prolapse, endometriosis of the recto-uterine pouch, and uterine fibroids, neoplasm or infection may all give rise to such backache in the lumbar region. Associated symptoms of heavy menstrual loss and intermenstrual bleeding help to indicate a gynaecological cause of the backache.

A large number of women complain of backache during pregnancy, and the lumbar lordosis increases to offset the weight of the protruding abdomen. The performance of regular perineal, spinal and abdominal exercises, the avoidance of lengthy standing sessions, and attention to posture while lying in bed, sitting in a chair, or standing or walking in the upright position, can do much to prevent this.

Many women complain of severe backache after childbirth, or after a gynaecological operation, in which they have remained in the lithotomy position for long periods, often in an unconscious state. There is a very real risk of muscle or ligamentous damage or of joint distraction when the lumbosacral spine is actively or passively held in prolonged flexion, and there is need for a study of the incidence of backache, correlated with the clinical and radiological findings before and after pregnancy, and before and after childbirth. Avoiding the lithotomy position during labour and operation, or else limiting its occurrence to the shortest possible time, would minimize the chance of developing this type of backache. When it has developed, palliative physiotherapy (e.g. heat) followed by gentle extension exercises may ease the pain. Injections of hydrocortisone and lignocaine into tender areas may also be helpful, and the patient should be urged to keep her weight down and to follow the usual programme of prophylactic care for the avoidance of backache.

Acute inflammatory polyarthritis

Severe backache may occur when there is sacro-iliac or intervertebral joint involvement in one of the inflammatory polyarthritides, such as idiopathic spondylitis, psoriatic arthritis and Reiter's syndrome, or in association with inflammatory bowel disease.

Treatment of these conditions is designed to control the chronic inflammatory systemic disease with adequate doses of anti-inflammatory drugs, while preserving good spinal posture by bed rest on a firm mattress and a hard-based bed. This bed rest should last as long as the pain is severe and should be followed by gradual mobilization with exercises performed up to just short of the tolerance level of pain and fatigue. Rest in bed in a position of spinal extension is particularly important in ankylosing spondylitis, in which the spine may eventually become quite rigid. Without adequate rest and therapy, the spine may fix in a flexed position. When these are available and used to best advantage, they can at least ensure that the spine stiffens with the patient able to assume an upright posture.

ANKYLOSING SPONDYLITIS

Ankylosing Spondylitis used to be regarded as a relatively uncommon condition affecting mainly young men. The discovery of the strong association between Ankylosing Spondylitis and the gene for the transplantation antigen B27 has lead to a complete revision of our knowledge.

It is now estimated that about ¾ million people in Great Britain (1.6 per cent of the population) have a well developed Ankylosing Spondylitis affecting men and women equally. Previously it was thought to run in about 0.2 per cent of men and 0.03 per cent of women.

Clearly many affected individuals will have slight or moderate symptoms only, and many will never consult a doctor. Of those that do seek help, with regular active physiotherapy and anti-inflammatory drugs most will continue their lives satisfactorily without altering the normal routine of their lives.

The classic description of a patient with a 'poker back', with radiological obliteration of the sacro-iliac joints and 'bambooing' of the lumbar spine, is true only of the late stages of the disease, in some patients. Most patients never lose a day from work, and many are only diagnosed incidentally.

In the early stages, there are three diagnostic criteria: stiffness of the lumbar spine; a raised erythrocyte sedimentation rate; radiological changes in the sacro-iliac joints.

Stiffness in the lumbar spine

Stiffness and referred pain in the low back are usually the first indications of the disease and are frequently misdiagnosed as 'growing pains' in the young and 'fibrositis' in the older age groups. A history of trauma can be obtained from most young men, and this, in patients complaining of mild low backache, may be misleading.

A common finding in the earliest stages of ankylosing spondylitis is that the patient wakes up with a slight stiffness in the back which he can 'work off'. In this so-called 'pre-spondylitic stage', the patient finds that he has to steer a careful course between insufficient exercise which makes him stiff, and excessive exercise which gives him pain.

Low backache, the commonest and main presenting symptom of ankylosing spondylitis, has certain characteristics: it is deep seated; it is worse on getting up in the morning and after prolonged periods of sitting; it often shifts from side to side; it is often referred to one or both buttocks; it tends to come and go in attacks lasting for days or weeks, with periods of freedom; it is often accompanied by mild malaise, in contradistinction to backache due to mechanical disorders of the spine, in which malaise is invariably absent.

The most important physical sign in the early stages of ankylosing spondylitis is a stiffness of the lumbar spine. This may be seen as the patient undresses and gets on the examination couch but is frequently not marked enough to be noticed in a fully-dressed patient. This stiffness also shows as limitation of forward and lateral flexion. This restriction of lateral flexion common in ankylosing spondylitis may help to distinguish the disease from chronic disc lesions.

Straight leg raising may be limited due to pain in the sacro-iliac joints, or involvement of the hip joints.

Limitation of chest expansion, which is often given as a criterion of diagnosis in ankylosing spondylitis, does not occur early in the disease process but only when involvement of the thoracic spine leads to arthritis and, later, ankylosis of the costovertebral joints.

Raised ESR
A raised ESR is an almost invariable accompaniment of the active phases of ankylosing spondylitis, but occasionally the ESR may remain within the normal limits for some months after clinical manifestations warrant the diagnosis being made. Conversely, the ESR may remain elevated for some years even though the disease is clinically in abeyance.

Radiology of the sacro-iliac joints
The radiological description of the 'bamboo spine' and the 'tramline' appearance of the lateral radiograph in ankylosing spondylitis characteristic of the established late stages are due to calcification of the intervertebral disc margins and longitudinal ligaments.

The sacro-iliac joints are usually involved early in the disease. A characteristic succession of radiological changes corresponds to progressive joint involvement:

(1) A haziness and indistinctness of outline is associated with marginal decalcification and erosion.
(2) As the erosion proceeds the joint space appears to widen.
(3) Sclerosis appears and is followed by ankylosis until the joint space is obliterated.

The posterior intervertebral joints pass through a similar series of changes, and in some patients the changes are present at a time when the radiographic signs in the sacro-iliac joints are minimal. Thus, in the presence of minimal or dubious changes in the sacro-iliac joints, oblique radiographs of the lumbar spine may confirm the diagnosis.

Difficulty of diagnosis
There is now considerable evidence that Ankylosing Spondylitis, Reiter's syndrome, acute anterior uveitis, chronic inflammatory disease of the bowel have related causes, suggesting multiple genes and environmental agents, with HLA-B27, or a susceptibility gene closely linked to it, being one of the complex factors involved. Knowledge that a patient is B27-positive will certainly help with the diagnosis, and B27 typing is useful in genetic counselling within the family of an affected person.

The greatest problem in making an early diagnosis of spondylitis is the difficulty of appreciating the significance of minor symptoms and signs. The natural history of the disease is such that suspicion of its presence is not easily aroused. It is often a slowly progressive condition with minimal symptoms and with a natural tendency to remissions. At the time when many patients first consult a doctor, their complaint is minimal and they are frequently lulled into a sense of false security by a non-specific diagnosis of 'fibrositis' or 'rheumatism', 'disc lesion' or 'postural backache' — terms which the patient knows and is willing to accept. It is only from a detailed history that suspicions may be aroused, by careful examination that the earliest signs may be found, and by full and repeated x-ray examinations that an early diagnosis can be made.

Lack of recognition of other manifestations of the condition may cause delay in diagnosis. Thus involvement of the peripheral joints may lead to a diagnosis of rheumatoid arthritis until spinal deformity supervenes, while iridocyclitis, plantar fasciitis and synovitis of the knee may be treated for a considerable time as separate conditions before the true aetiology becomes apparent.

It is well recognized that some patients are asymptomatic and that ankylosing spondylitis is only discovered as an incidental finding during examination for other reasons. Other patients experience mild symptoms only and consider them too trivial to seek medical advice. Thus the disease is frequently neither manifested nor diagnosed until affected patients reach early middle age, unless regular medical examination reveals it or the exertion of active sport or heavy work provokes further symptoms.

Treatment
The most important aspect of the general management of patients with ankylosing spondylitis is regular physiotherapy in the form of exercises to maintain and restore spinal and costovertebral mobility. Although the later changes involve fusion of the intervertebral joints, the early stages of stiffness and limitation of movement are partially preventable and even reversible. Quite marked increase in joint range and vital capacity can follow a period of intensive physical rehabilitation, and increases of chest expansion of 1–2 in (2.5–5.0 cm) are not unusual. Regular clinical review will enable the clinician to detect deterioration or relapse and will help to maintain the patient's morale and reinforce the clinician's advice to continue regular mobilizing exercises.

The patient's general health must be maintained. Dietetic advice should aim at ensuring an adequate protein intake coupled with avoidance of weight gain.

Regular breathing exercises, postural training and spinal mobility exercises, particularly hydrotherapy (exercising in a warm pool) form the basis of physical treatment. Patients are taught to lift correctly without flexing the spine, for the stiffening back is at greater risk under bending and lifting stress. Periods of intensive rehabilitation of 2 to 3 weeks' duration at about 6-month intervals are an excellent method of maintaining patients in active work. Apart from these periods, patients are encouraged to take regular exercise. Daily breathing and spinal mobilizing exercises are important. All patients are also urged to swim at least once a week. A regular game of tennis, badminton or golf is helpful. Body-contact sports and diving should be avoided as there is a real risk of severe whiplash injury to the cervical spine.

The aim of medication is to reduce pain and stiffness. Aspirin, phenylbutazone, indomethacin and naproxen all have similar effects in suppressing symptoms when given in adequate dosage. Because of problems of dyspepsia aspirin is rarely used, and although phenylbutazone has a particular specificity in ankylosing spondylitis its side effects have lead many authorities to abandon this drug. Indomethacin given as a suppository is valuable if nocturnal pain and morning stiffness are troublesome but the easiest and most effective treatment is with naproxen (500 mg daily). With adequate physiotherapy, many patients do not require analgesics, or else find that doses of these tablets can be reduced. Analgesics should be stopped as soon as the patient can manage without them.

Sleeping on a firm mattress and using a single pillow often reduces not only pain during the night, but also morning stiffness. It also eliminates a factor liable to induce spinal deformity. The use of an electric blanket prior to getting up in the morning may reduce early morning stiffness.

For some patients, a carefully moulded, adjustable spinal brace can reduce severe spinal pain and help to reduce early flexion deformity of the lumbar spine. Other braces have no part in the management of ankylosing spondylitis.

Severe cases and later manifestations
A few patients do not respond to the simple measures described and have considerable unrelenting pain. When this occurs, and the diagnosis is unequivocal, deep x-ray therapy to the painful joints will often reduce the symptoms, but there is undoubtedly an increased risk of developing leukemia as a sequel to this treatment.

Severe stiffness can often be helped considerably by a short course of steroids coupled with back-mobilizing exercises. There is, however, only one absolute indication for corticosteroids in this disease — the development of intractable uveitis. This can rapidly progress to total blindness if these drugs are withheld.

Some patients with ankylosing spondylitis have concurrent hip-joint synovitis. In a small proportion, this will lead to ankylosis and be so troublesome as to justify surgery of the hip joints. Cup arthroplasty and total hip replacement have their advocates, but the latter procedure has the advantage of early mobilization post-operatively. Pain relief can usually be provided, but increased joint mobility is not to be guaranteed, as re-ankylosis can occur after arthroplasty.

Occasionally, because of severe spinal deformity, when increasing flexion is markedly diminishing the ability of the patient to see ahead of himself, spinal osteotomy may be considered, but such surgery is acknowledged to be heroic, to carry considerable dangers, and to have rather limited success.

'SPRUNG BACK'

Soft-tissue lesions or tears of ligaments or paraspinal muscles are often diagnosed in the presence of an acute localized pain following an injury, strain or unaccustomed labour. The commonest ligamentous cause of backache is 'sprung back'. This syndrome may be summarized as follows:

(1) Low backache is felt following unaccustomed labour and is worse on slouching, lifting heavy objects with a flexed spine or standing in a poor postural position. The pain may radiate to the buttocks.
(2) Flexion of the spine and straight leg raising may be slightly limited.
(3) Tenderness is found locally over the affected posterior ligaments.
(4) The symptoms and signs are relieved temporarily by infiltration of the affected ligament with a local anaesthetic.

'Sprung back' is commoner in women and may alternatively be called the 'kitchen sink syndrome' as it particularly causes pain when the patient leans forward over washing-up or other household activities. It may also occur in women or men after athletic activity and in disabled persons with abnormal curvature of the lumbar spine.

Although the acute symptoms of 'sprung back' usually respond dramatically to infiltration of the ligaments with local anaesthetic and/or hydrocortisone, it is wise to institute more long-term measures, particularly to instil into the patient the understanding of the need to prevent unncessary straining while the spine is flexed.

Back extension exercises, postural re-education, sleeping on a firm mattress and the avoidance of lifting heavy objects with the spine flexed are the usual measures advised.

For the more severe or resistant conditions, a short period spent using a lumbar support or temporary corset may give considerable relief.

'Sprung back' may precede or accompany a prolapsed intervertebral disc. Rupture of the posterior interspinous ligaments can lead to instability and hypermobility between two lumbar vertebrae and this instability predisposes the structures holding the vertebrae together to further damage. The stress on the posterior longitudinal ligament is increased, and rupture of this ligament may occur, leading to prolapse of nucleus pulposus material.

PROLAPSED INTERVERTEBRAL DISC

During the past 40 years, an extensive literature on this subject has grown up, but there is still no universally accepted formula for the diagnosis and treatment of prolapsed intervertebral disc, and unless the patient eventually comes to operation, there is no sure means of confirming the diagnosis. A prolapsed intervertebral disc may present with severe and crippling sciatica of acute onset or as a recurrent, dull, low backache of many years' duration. The signs may vary from minimal limitation of spinal movement to an almost immobile spine accompanied by gross neurological changes in the leg.

Pathological studies indicate that loss of the normal 'turgescence of the nucleus pulposus' (which is associated with age), congenital defects of the cartilaginous end-plates of the bodies of the vertebrae, or of the annulus fibrosus, and a precipitating injury are the main factors concerned in producing a prolapse of the disc. Significant variations in the nucleus pulposus have been recorded in experimental animals in relation to stress.

Radiology of prolapsed intervertebral disc

Radiological evidence of loss of disc space only occurs after prolapse or degeneration of the nucleus pulposus has occurred. A rapid decrease in the affected disc space of some patients has been recorded after removal of the nucleus pulposus at operation, but in other patients the degree of narrowing is variable. The onset of narrowing may be delayed for months or even years after the onset of symptoms.

Radiography can indicate the level of the prolapsed intervertebral disc in approximately half of the patients diagnosed clinically as suffering from a 'prolapsed intervertebral disc' but may be negative in about one quarter of those proven by operation. In general, there is a higher incidence of radiological disc space narrowing and sciatica in the later stages of the condition, but although radiology may demonstrate an established disc lesion, it is of little value (except to exclude other conditions) in the early diagnosis of a disc lesion.

Neurological signs

Neurological signs are due to the physical involvement of the spinal cord or its nerve roots by disc prolapse. Nerve roots can slip away from any lesion which narrows the spinal canal unless that lesion is large enough to encroach significantly on the lumen. Compression, tension or angulation of a nerve root will cause symptoms; and recurrent trauma may well give rise to oedema of the nerve root, an inflammatory response, leading to organization of the oedema fluid, the formation of fibrous tissue and later to adhesions between the nerve root and the prolapse.

The mechanical factors involved are analogous to those met in certain lesions of peripheral nerves (e.g. involvement of nerve in a fracture callus; a neuroma following a peripheral nerve injury; carpal tunnel syndrome). In these conditions, continuous or intermittent mechanical involvement of the peripheral nerve may continue for weeks or months after the onset of symptoms before neurological signs can be detected. It may be assumed that similar conditions are responsible for the development of neurological signs due to prolapsed intervertebral discs, and motor weakness and muscle wasting are usually late signs in disc lesions. The time relationships for sensory changes are less clear.

The early diagnosis of prolapsed intervertebral disc

The syndrome is characterized by chronic or recurrent low backache, followed later by unilateral sciatica which is exacerbated by factors which increase intrathecal pressure. The interval between the onset of backache and sciatica is very variable, and in a few cases acute sciatica may be the first symptom.

The essential physical sign of disc prolapse is a limitation of spinal movement, with a consistent limitation of straight leg raising. Neurological and radiological evidence may confirm or exclude the diagnosis, but are not necessarily present in the early stages.

The severity, location and onset of the backache following the protrusion of the intervertebral disc varies with the size, site and rate of protrusion, and with the precipitating factors. Causing pain which varies from a dull ache to a stabbing pain radiating down the back of one or both legs, disc protrusion usually occurs at the level of L5/S1 or L4/L5 vertebral interspaces. Backache may occur without sciatic radiation, and sometimes sciatic pain without backache, although both are usually present.

Pressure from the disc protrusion may affect cord, cord and nerve roots, or nerve roots, depending on whether the protrusion is directed posteriorly, posterolaterally, or laterally. The exact relationship of the protrusion to the nerve roots crossing its interspace determines the site of the pain radiation and the associated neurological signs and symptoms. Yet due to the fact that the spinal cord ends at the level of the second lumbar vertebra and that disc protrusions may occur simultaneously at more than one intervertebral space, these signs and symptoms do not allow the deduction of the exact site of protrusion of any particular disc. (e.g. Both L5 and S1 roots cross the 4th lumbar disc; S1 root crosses the 5th lumbar disc; therefore a protrusion at the 4th lumbar disc space could press upon the L5 or S1 roots, or both; whereas a protrusion at the 5th lumbar disc space could press upon the S1 root. Thus, an irritation of the S1 root could mean a disc protrusion at *either* the 4th or 5th lumbar interspace, and an irritation of both L5 and S1 roots could mean *either* a protrustion at the 4th interspace which affected both roots, *or* two protrusions, one at the 4th and one at the 5th interspaces, pressing on L5 and S1 roots respectively.)

Treatment of prolapsed intervertebral disc lesion

Treatment of backache due to an acute protrusion of an intervertebral disc may be considered in three categories — ambulant, bed and operative. Although the initial treatment of choice is bed rest, treatment with the patient ambulant may be tried if the pain is not too severe, and the patient is a non-manual worker.

The choice of treatment of an acute prolapsed intervertebral disc must depend upon the physical and mental conditions of each individual patient and upon his work and home conditions.

The choice lies among four basic treatments, which may be used singly or in conjunction with each other: (1) rest in bed; (2) immobilization; (3) manipulation; or (4) traction.

Rest in bed

Most patients with severe backache are best treated in the initial stages by rest in bed and adequate analgesics. Not only the rest, but the position of the spine during that rest is important. To avoid the spinal flexion induced by a sagging mattress, patients are instructed to use a firm mattress laid over fracture boards, planks or a door.

Absolute rest is attempted with the patient in the position of maximal comfort. This he usually finds to be the supine position, with the affected leg flexed at hip and knee, and with only one pillow under his head. Analgesics or anti-inflammatory tablets are given for day or night use, and a night sedative supplied.

It is important to control the pain of prolapsed intervertebral disc adequately, since otherwise muscle spasm will continue and a self-perpetuating cycle of pain and spasm will result. When it is necessary to use the more potent analgesics initially, these should be used with caution and tailed off rapidly.

A gentle bulk laxative should be started immediately so as to avoid constipation and straining at stool. Bowel action should be into bedpan, commode or lavatory pedestal, according to the capability and inclination of the patient.

The patient should be encouraged to micturate into a urinal. Male and female urinals made of plastic are now readily available from all large chemists, and their use obviates the need for frequent painful sessions on bedpan, commode or lavatory seat.

Most patients with acute prolapsed intervertebral disc are nursed at home. Severe pain unrelieved by the above measures, or the presence of increasing paraesthesia or of neurological signs in the legs are indications for admission to hospital. Here a patient may be put into a plaster of paris jacket and discharged home if the symptoms and signs are controlled thereby or else treated by bed rest with continuous lumbar traction. Weights of up to 20 lb (9 kg) are gradually suspended from the legs by skin traction, 8—10 lb (3·6—4·5 kg) for each leg. The use of traction for a patient nursed at home is not practical unless continuous care is available.

While traction is applied to the legs, the foot of the bed is raised on blocks and, once again, the patient is nursed on a hard-based bed and firm mattress, using one or no pillows. Traction is maintained for about 3 weeks, depending upon the improvement or otherwise of the back pain. Static exercises are performed frequently and regularly for the muscles of the trunk and lower limbs throughout the period of traction and active exercises for trunk and upper limbs. When pain permits, and the traction is discontinued, graduated active exercises are urged and weight-bearing gradually resumed.

If pain has resolved completely, patients are discharged home without any spinal support and then have a period of regular out-patient physiotherapy, but if there is still unresolved pain, a period in a plaster of paris jacket may be tried, followed in some instances by a surgical corset.

In those few cases when conservative treatment has been tried and has failed, surgical intervention is called for.

Immobilization

Immobilization in a lumbar corset is used particularly for those patients whose financial straits or domestic and work commitments demand that they continue ambulant without repeated attendances for treatment at a physiotherapy department.

For these patients, long-term immobilization in purpose-designed, individually tailored, surgical corsets may provide effective pain relief. When measurements have been taken for these corsets, patients are temporarily immobilized in plaster of paris jackets, in instant corsets made of plaster of paris slabs applied to a tubigrip corset, or else in belts from the store of spinal supports which are stocked in many orthopaedic hospitals. This temporary form of immobilization is worn in each case until it can be exchanged for the finished, made-to-measure corset.

Whichever form of spinal support is worn, it should be kept on at night as well as by day, until the back pain has been relieved. Once this has occurred, and the straight leg raising is almost normal, the spinal support may be left off during the night but worn consistently by day for a further few weeks or even months, depending upon the occupation of the individual patient. Many people discard their supports before they should do because of the discomfort of wearing them. This is reduced considerably if the support is put on while the patient is supine.

As soon as the pain permits, static and then active exercises are introduced for the spinal and abdominal muscles. It is urged upon the patient that a surgical belt is not a substitute for efficient muscular action, and that the strength of the trunk musculature must be maintained throughout the entire period of immobilization. A twice-daily exercise routine before the corset is put on and after it is taken off, together with a further interval of static exercises which can be performed with the corset in situ should prevent the spine from stiffening and the muscles from losing bulk and strength. The exercises should be graduated in intensity and duration, so that by the time the surgical corset is discarded they have increased sufficiently to produce normal or near-normal muscle function.

The corset should be kept available for use when particularly hard physical work, likely to predispose to further disc protrusion, must be undertaken. When it is possible to avoid such work, patients should be urged to do so. Unfortunately, it is not easy to find or pay people to do the manual work attached to the care of the house or the garden, and many people are forced by circumstances to cope with tasks much better avoided.

Manipulation
The following are indications for manipulation.

(1) A thorough clinical examination has excluded the presence of abnormal neurological signs indicative of root pressure or of pressure on the cord.
(2) A radiological examination has excluded the presence of a neoplastic or infective lesion in the vertebrae, or of any indication of vertebral disease or frailty.
(3) A detailed history and thorough clinical examination has excluded lesions in other systems as causes of the backache, and it has been definitely established that the pain arises from the musculoskeletal system.

Even when these conditions have been satisfied, manipulation is by no means universally indicated, or invariably effective. First or recurrent attacks of backache of sudden onset may respond dramatically to a single manipulation. In the management of chronic low back pain, intermittent manipulation may also be useful.

The object of manipulation is to impart involuntary movement to the intervertebral joint from which the disc protrusion has occurred, so to allow the protrusion to be 'reduced' between the momentarily distracted joint surfaces by the tension of the surrounding muscles. When sufficient relaxation cannot be obtained with the patient conscious, manipulation under anaesthesia is sometimes performed. The danger of causing further damage to the patient is greater when he is manipulated in an unconscious state, and special care must be taken to ensure that no greater force is used than that for the conscious patient. Whenever possible, manipulation under anaesthesia should be avoided.

Manipulative treatment must be followed up by a regime of exercises, performed both in the physiotherapy department and at home. These should be initially static or isometric exercises for the erectores spinae and the anterior and lateral abdominal muscles, progressing, as pain permits, to graded active exercises for these muscles.

Contra-indications for manipulation are:
(1) Pregnancy.
(2) Significant root pain in one or both legs.
(3) Marked deviation of the lumbar spine from the vertical when standing as erect as possible, i.e. sciatic scoliosis.
(4) Straight leg raising reduced to 30 degrees on either side.
(5) Continuous paraesthesia in one leg, or paraesthesia induced by standing.
(6) Disturbances of micturition apparently associated with this episode of backache.
(7) Neurological signs associated with the backache and sciatica, e.g. abnormal reflexes.
(8) Sensory loss.
(9) Significant weakness or wasting.
(10) Clinical evidence of sacro-ilitis.
(11) Significant osteoporosis of one or both hips.

(12) Radiological evidence of osteoporosis, spondylosis, spondylolisthesis, hemivertebra, local bone disease, and vertebral anomalies associated with systemic disease.

Intermittent lumbar traction is another active technique which theoretically attempts to reduce the size of the intervertebral protusion. There are various forms of equipment designed to exert traction on the lumbar spine while patients lie on specially designed traction tables. The efficacy of these is unproven, and a number of patients are in more pain after treatment than before it.

Operative treatment of prolapsed intervertebral disc
The criteria which induce surgeons to undertake operative treatment may be summarised as follows.

(1) Persistent or recurrent low backache.
(2) Limitation of movements of the lumbar spine.
(3) Radiological evidence of loss of disc space.
(4) Persistent sciatica.
(5) Persistent neurological signs.
  (a) Limitation of straight leg raising.
  (b) Muscle weakness.
  (c) Loss of tendon reflexes.

Since the relief of pain following operative treatment of a prolapsed intervertebral disc is not absolutely certain, operation should not be undertaken unless the medical and physical treatment given has been adequate and prolonged. When pain persists and is severe, when neurological signs have developed and are increasing, or when pain recurs in frequent and distressing bouts, operation should be considered. It becomes essential only when paraplegia develops from compression of the cauda equina by a prolapsed intervertebral disc.

Post-operative care depends upon the extent of the surgery. If it has been necessary to remove the lamina then rehabilitation is slower than if the operation was carried out through a laminotomy.

Although post-operative bed rest for up to 2 weeks has been advocated, many surgeons prefer to get their patients out of bed after 2 or 3 days. Static exercises for the trunk are commenced immediately post-operatively, and graduated exercises are increasingly added until there is full recovery of muscle strength.

Post-operative care involves instilling a regimen of 'back care' while encouraging the patient to return to normal activities as soon as possible. Avoidance of prolonged stooping and lifting and carrying of heavy objects with the spine in a position of mechanical disadvantage (i.e. flexed instead of extended), the practice of regular strengthening exercises for the spine, the use of a firm bed and mattress and a well-upholstered easy chair with adequate lumbar support are simple measures which are easily incorporated into the pattern of life for most people.

This attitude of sensible prophylactic care for the back should be encouraged in all patients who have back pain from any cause. Far from preventing them from living active lives, it permits the maximal possible participation in all activities, other than those especially conducive to back pain, by producing and maintaining optimal functional efficiency in the spine and its musculature. The prevention of pain by active conditioning of the affected part rather than by passive abstention from activity constitutes a mode of existence which some patients find hard to understand and harder still to follow. The medical and paramedical staff giving treatment need to emphasize and re-emphasize the necessity of continuing active prophylactic self-care throughout life.

OSTEO–ARTHROSIS OF THE LUMBAR SPINE

A prolapsed intervertebral disc acts as a major aetiological factor in the onset of degenerative changes in the lumbar spine (lumbar spondylosis or lumbar osteo-arthrosis).

It is the gradual transition from acute prolapsed intervertebral disc into general lumbar osteo-arthrosis over a period of years which gives rise to such a broad spectrum of clinical presentation and paradoxical response to therapy. During this process patients with similar symptoms and signs may respond to very different treatments, and one particular patient may respond differently as he gets older.

As prolapse of the intervertebral disc inevitably leads to narrowing of the intervertebral disc space, it also inevitably leads to subluxation of the posterior intervertebral joints. As these joints are synovial, such a mechanical disruption will inevitably lead to osteo-arthrosis. The narrowing of the intervertebral disc will also lead to osteophytosis of the lumbar spine.

Much confusion seems to have arisen from lack of differentiation between true oesteo-arthrosis (of the posterior intervertebral joints) and osteophytosis or spondylosis of the vertebral bodies of the lumbar spine.

The diagnosis of osteo-arthrosis of the lumbar spine will depend on the radiological demonstration of generalized changes in the posterior intervertebral joints of the lumbar spine, usually in the middle-aged or elderly patient.

CONGENITAL ABNORMALITIES OF THE LUMBAR SPINE

Congenital deformities of the lumbar spine depend on radiography for their diagnosis. Those which can be associated with low back pain are:

(1) Spondylolisthesis.
(2) Spondylolysis.
(3) Abnormalities in the number of mobile lumbar vertebrae.
(4) Transitional vertebrae.
(5) Spinous process impingement.
(6) Spina bifida.
(7) Abnormalities of the posterior articular facets.

The incidence of congenital defects has been estimated variously as 0.5–27 per cent in patients with backache and 2–7 per cent in controls. The clinical significance of the defects is thus far from clear.

It is likely that congenital deformities of the lumbar spine are significant mainly because they represent a mechanical defect and, as such, are a contributory factor to the development of degenerative changes in the inter-vertebral joints.

'POSTURAL DEFECTS'

'Postural defects' have been variously recorded as being present in from 5 to 50 per cent of patients with backache, the incidence depending upon the patient group surveyed and the reporter's interests. These variations are partly due to selection of cases, and partly to the diagnostic criteria applied (which are seldom defined). All 'postural defects' are variations from the accepted 'normal' posture which can be corrected by the active effort of the patient. It is seldom that one part of the body alone is involved, and usually the entire posture is at fault. The main source of difference of opinion is the definition of 'normal posture'.

The 'postural defects' commonly met may be classified into three types, depending on the primary defect:

(1) Anterior-posterior curves of the spine.
(2) Lateral curves of the spine.
(3) Foot defects.

A few patients with 'postural defects' present with backache; many others present with foot defects; others are asymptomatic. As far as treatment is concerned, general postural re-education is more important than treatment of the feet alone.

'SHORT LEG' SYNDROME

The incidence of differences in leg lengths will depend upon the method of length assessment and upon the criteria by which patients are selected for leg measurement. The smaller the unit of measurement, the greater will be the incidence of length difference, and the larger the unit of measurement, the greater will be the agreement between observers.

The amount of leg difference which is clinically significant has been assessed at figures varying from $\frac{1}{4}$ in (0·625 cm) to $\frac{5}{6}$ in (2·10 cm). Differences of this magnitude demand considerable accuracy in measurement, which is difficult to ensure when it is generally accepted that it is impossible for one person to measure leg length more accurately than to within $\frac{1}{2}$ in (1·25 cm), and when there is considerable variation among individual observers. Until the technique of measurement can be standardized and its degree of accuracy improved, it is not possible to estimate the magnitude of the clinical problem attributed to difference in leg length.

Significant differences in leg length have been recorded in association with chronic infection of one joint (e.g. TB hip); local hypertrophy (e.g. angiectatic hypertrophy); haemangioma or lymphangioma; neurofibromatosis; injury; muscle disease (e.g. poliomyelitis) and congenital malformities; but the commonest form of leg length difference appears to be idiopathic.

Differences in leg lengths of less than $\frac{1}{2}$ in (1·25 cm) have little clinical significance, and there is an incidence of asymptomatic leg length difference of $\frac{1}{2}$ in (1·25 cm) or more in 7 per cent of the general population. The association between leg length differences and low back pain is emphasized by the fact that among patients with this type of pain such a difference in leg length occurs 3 times more commonly than it does among members of the population as a whole.

The clinical diagnosis of 'short leg' has been defined as depending on the presence of $\frac{1}{2}$ in (1·25 cm) leg length differences or more. The clinical diagnosis of 'short leg' syndrome assumes the presence of 'short leg' with associated symptoms.

'Short leg' syndrome is a condition commonly presenting as low backache of gradual onset, but occasionally as low backache of sudden onset, or pains in the legs, in which the only physical findings are those directly related to a leg length difference of $\frac{1}{2}$ in or more.

Although the symptoms are usually of gradual onset, they may sometimes be precipitated by minor trauma. In either case they are made worse by standing and activity, and relieved both by rest and by correction of the deformity (providing structural changes do not prevent the correction).

When associated with postural or congenital defects of the lumbar spine, however, the symptoms are not relieved by correction of the difference in leg length. 'Short leg' syndrome may prelude the development of a prolapsed intervertebral disc and may contibute to the aetiology of this condition. 'Short leg' may also be associated with idiopathic structural scoliosis.

Post-traumatic 'short leg' may interfere with functional recovery from the causative injury; this is a short-term effect of leg length discrepancy. The more serious effect is the long-term resulting degenerative disease which may develop in the weight-bearing joints of both shortened and normal limb, when excessive changes occur in the mechanical stresses to which they are subjected.

This relationship between 'short-leg' and low backache resembles that between congenital defects of the lumbar spine and backache. Both defects may or may not cause symptoms in their own right. Both probably predispose to the development of ligamentous strains and consequent discomfort.

Although it has been estimated that 'short leg' occurs in approximately 7 per cent of the population without giving rise to symptoms, it would seem desirable to correct any inequality in leg lengths of more than half an inch, whether or not it is currently asymptomatic. Long-standing deformities need to be corrected in stages, but length discrepancies of short duration (e.g. post-traumatic 'short leg') may be corrected by a single procedure. In all instances, correction may be made simply by raising one heel and/or lowering the other to produce an adjustment of up to 1 in (2·5 cm). Raises of more than $\frac{1}{2}$ in (1·25 cm) in one heel should be accompanied by some thickening of the sole of the shoe.

CORSETS AND SPINAL SUPPORTS

The advisability of prescribing corsets or spinal supports is a matter about which there is a considerable difference of opinion. Some doctors prescribe a corset, or a support, almost routinely for any patients with recurrent backache; others refuse to prescribe either. It is interesting that such an 'all or none' attitude is adopted by many advocates of either policy, when the analogous prescription of a collar for pain in the neck is more laissez-faire. It has been adequately shown that consistent external support is beneficial for attacks of acute neckache, but as symptoms decrease, most doctors introduce a period of 'weaning off', allowing the collar to be removed for an increasing number of short intervals, and then for increasingly longer intervals.

A spinal support of some kind is appropriate for the patient with acute backache:

(1) Who needs or wants to remain ambulant but for whom manipulation is

not indicated and physical measures such as heat or lumbar traction are insufficient to effect prolonged pain relief.

(2) Who has tried bed rest at home and had found it ineffective in controlling symptoms, but is not sufficiently inconvenienced to need hospitalization for continuous lumbar traction or for surgical intervention.

(3) Who has recurrent attacks of backache, despite an adequate programme of prophylactic exercises and strict attention to back care in all activities of daily living.

When back pain is acute the need for back support is equally acute and can be fulfilled by the provision of:

(1) A plaster of paris spinal jacket.

(2) A spinal jacket made of thermoplastic material (e.g. expanded polystyrene – plastazote).

(3) A standard surgical corset, ready-made in a range of different sizes and available 'off the shelf'.

(4) An 'instant corset' made from tubular elastic bandage strengthened in the back with slabs of plaster of paris bandage or of thermoplastic or orthopaedic felt.

The disadvantages of the plaster of paris jacket are that it is heavy, does not allow for adjustment, and often produces a condition of unbearable claustrophobia. Its main advantage is that it does provide a very real restriction of all spinal movements. Less effective in producing such restrictions are the 'ready-made' surgical corset, the 'thermoplastic' corset and the 'instant corset'. All these forms of support, however, act as deterrents from attempts at flexion, lateral flexion and rotation of the spine, as well as reminders that patients must keep within their range of pain-free movements.

Application of a temporary back support during an acute episode of back pain should be preceded by the measurement of the patient for a more permanent form of corset. Both made-to-measure corsets of cotton material reinforced with steel strips, and the more complex spinal supports take several weeks, with one or more fittings to be made satisfactory. The temporary, or 'instant', corset attempts to keep the patient's back relatively immobile until the definitive brace or corset is completed. Often the patient becomes symptom-free before the permanent corset arrives. In this case the corset is retained and kept for use during long car journeys, heavy work (when unavoidable), prolonged activities which tend to cause backache, recurrences of back pain, and periods of malaise or fatigue. Prophylactic use of a corset can be very helpful in preventing the occurrence of severe back and sciatic pain. If the patient is *not* pain free when the definitive corset or support is ready, it should be worn until freedom from pain has lasted for several weeks, and then should be very gradually discarded.

The more rigid surgical braces are usually reserved for conditions more serious than prolapsed intervertebral disc or idiopathic low back pain. Whichever type of spinal corset, brace, belt or support is worn, it is important that static exercises should be carried out for the spinal extensor and abdominal muscles as a part of the regime involved with its use.

GENERAL MANAGEMENT OF PATIENTS WITH BACKACHE

Although the treatment of backache in its acute stages must necessarily vary with the causative lesion, the management of a patient who has backache or recurrent backache, or who is likely to have backache, has many constant features. Such management attempts to achieve a balance between the demands of family, work and environment upon the patient's back, and his functional capacity to fulfil those demands. It seeks to enable him to enjoy the fullest possible life without precipitating further attacks of pain.

The clinician and physiotherapist combine in advising regular exercises for spinal and abdominal muscles, weight control and the correct position of the spine during daily living activities. The occupational therapist advises how such activities may themselves be modified in order to avoid the fatigue or strain which may lead to further backache.

Prolonged standing, standing with the weight mainly on one leg and standing in a slumped or stooping posture should be avoided. A standing patient should never attempt to pick up heavy objects while his knees are extended but should squat down to grasp them and should lift by straightening his legs.

Prolonged sitting without adequate lumbar support should also be avoided. Drivers may need a small firm cushion, a backrest or one of the speciallly designed seats for drivers with painful backs. Patients who work in the sitting position for most of the day should avoid using stools or uncomfortable chairs. The use of an upright chair is best, with a seat of such a height that the patient can sit comfortably with thighs horizontal, both feet flat on the ground and the lumbar spine well supported. Such a chair is appropriate also for the housewife with backache, so that she may sit to iron, wash up and do as much of her kitchen work as possible. In an easy chair, patients are advised to avoid sitting with knees crossed or with their feet tucked under them and to place a firm cushion behind their backs. Prolonged stooping almost invariably precipitates backache. To avoid this patients are asked to sit or kneel whenever possible for tasks which otherwise require a stooping posture. Alternatively, the heights of working surfaces, sink, ironing board etc. can be lowered to enable patients to sit at them comfortably.

Lifting or carrying heavy objects should be left to others, but if it is unavoidable, the patient can protect her back by balancing the load on her hip or abdomen.

Prophylactic organization of housework, shopping and gardening for the patient with backache is based on similar principles to those established for the patient with cervical spondylosis. This is particularly important when the two conditions occur in the same patient, as they frequently do.

Leisure activities should not include sporting activities which involve heavy lifting and pulling. During sedentary activities such as reading, writing, painting, sewing, knitting and crocheting, the patient with backache needs to sit in the type of chair already described.

Insufficient care is at present given to the design of chairs for children at school, young people working in lecture rooms, classrooms and libraries, and adults who follow sedentary occupations. Backache is not as infrequent among the young as it should be, which is not surprising when 2 hours at a stretch are often spent sitting on a high stool during double science periods and when there is no choice of seat heights available. It seems ludicrous that a tall and a short child must sit on chairs of the same height and lean over horizontal tables of constant height. A return to the sloping working surfaces of earlier school desks and a realistic approach to the need to relate the seat height to the height of the working surface for each child could do much to improve matters. The spines of the young are resilient, but when children are subjected to unnatural conditions and prolonged sitting they need the assistance of a well-positioned chairback constructed to provide lumbar support; equally they need to have their feet firmly on the ground – to assist a good spinal posture, to enable them to change position easily in the chair and to provide some weight relief to their buttocks.

BACKACHE AND THE DISABLED

Here it is appropriate to consider, in particular, the parent, spouse or child who cares for a disabled relative. The incidence of prolapsed intervertebral disc and consequent back pain among such patients is high, and as both patient and helper become older and less resilient, and the disabled person becomes heavier, the strain on the helper's back increases. The provision of adequate aids in the home to prevent the onset of back pain of such intensity as to necessitate bed rest for the helper, with consequent breakdown of the home situation, becomes a matter of urgency. Unfortunately, many people are reluctant to accept help until such a crisis has been precipitated. Once it has occurred and its consequences become apparent, the affected helper can usually be persuaded to wear a supporting corset, to follow a definite regime of prophylactic self-care, and to pay proper attention to the maintenance of the strength of spinal and abdominal musculature, while avoiding further provocation of disc prolapse by using a hoist for transfers and encouraging the disabled patient to lose weight.

The general practitioners who treat disabled patients have particular need to anticipate the onset of serious back trouble in those giving the most care. They can ensure the early provision of a hoist through the local social services and a visit by an experienced domiciliary occupational therapist to advise both patient and helper on possible problems associated with activities of daily living.

If difficulty is experienced in providing a hoist suitable for patient, helper and the home in which they live, referral of patient and helper to a disabled living centre or rehabilitation unit is indicated, where accurate assessment and prescription of the most suitable type of hoist can be made.

The cost of installing an electric hoist with an overhead track or of rehousing a family in a house where a portable hoist can be effectively used is insignificant compared with the cost of accommodating a disabled person permanently in an institution, simply because the relative giving care has also become disabled with back pain.

AGE GROUPS AT PARTICULAR RISK

When examining patients who present with backache, it is important to recall that backache from certain causes is particularly likely to occur in different age groups, and to be vigilant in excluding these causes.

Young people
In young people complaining of backache, symptoms may arise from:
    Scoliosis (1) idiopathic or primary; (2) secondary to (a) vertebral anomaly; (b) paraspinal neuromuscular dysfunction.

Kyphosis secondary to bony abnormalities such as Scheuermann's disease.
Infection such as vertebral abscess or osteomyelitis from TB, staphylococcal or typhoid infection.
Injury such as crush fracture following accidents at sport and work or on the road.
Involvement of the posterior vertebral joints in one of the acute arthritides (including ankylosing spondylitis).

Young women
In young women complaining of backache, in addition to the causes listed above:
Structural or functional abnormality in the genital system must be excluded.
Backache of locomotor origin is especially likely to occur during pregnancy, after labour and after gynaecological operations.

Middle-aged patients
In such patients more frequent causes of backache presenting for the first time are:
Degenerative joint disease.
Vertebral metastatic involvement.

Older people
In older people likely causes are:
Osteoporosis.
Degenerative joint disease.

SUMMARY

The structure of the lumbosacral spine predisposes to mechanical problems, and it is not in the least surprising that low back pain is so common. Indeed, mechanical causes are responsible for most cases.

Identification of cause entails a detailed examination of the patient and careful attention to his history. Appropriate treatment demands not only the elimination of serious and removable causes of pain, but also the reassurance of the patient, an adequate explanation of his symptoms and advice on future care relative to work, leisure and daily living activities.

Certainly, if the patient has an acute disc lesion, with persistent neurological signs, there is good reason to consider surgical removal of the offending disc. If bony inadequacy is present (e.g. spondylolisthesis) or persistent pain associated with other congenital deformities, there is a good case for considering spinal fusion. Polymyalgia rheumatica, osteoporosis, neoplasm, myelomatosis, tuberculosis, ankylosing spondylitis or fracture call for special care and treatment.

The majority of cases of backache are associated with minor strains with or without associated degenerative changes. The patients are often reassured by old-fashioned non-specific terms – 'lumbago' is often more acceptable and sounds less disabling than a slipped disc or 'arthritis', which are emotive terms with serious connotations.

At some stage, most of these cases of low back pain respond to:

(1) Palliative heat.
(2) Rest on a firm bed.

(3) Restriction of movement by a corset.

(4) Active mobilization by exercises, preferably in warm water (hydrotherapy).

In the majority of cases, the natural history is one of progressive radiological changes of osteo-arthrosis and osteophytosis (spondylosis) and progressive loss of joint range, associated with intermittent symptoms of backache with or without referred pain in the buttocks or legs. The more acute the symptoms, the more restrictive and intensive should be the treatment prescribed.

Acute, severe, disabling pain warrants immediate radiological examination, whether or not there is a history of trauma, and in the absence of serious causes, the best treatment is rest in bed with a firm mattress. Chronic recurrent low backache responds well to palliative physiotherapy.

In both types, the immediate acute phase, the exacerbation and the recurrence will respond to total rest. The period of immobility should be followed by a period of back-strengthening (extension) exercises and then mobilizing exercises.

Pain is the guide. Exercises and other activities that cause pain should be avoided. Static exercises of the extensors are rarely painful and more active mobilizing exercises including extension, flexion, rotation etc. can be introduced when they can be performed without pain.

The indication for rest in bed or rest in a spinal support will be determined by the severity of the backache experienced by the particular patient and by his physical, psychological and social state.

When loss of movement is a significant feature, stretching and manipulative techniques may achieve dramatic results.

At all times, postural re-education and strengthening exercises are essential except when they themselves precipitate severe pain, when treatment by further rest is indicated.

There are a number of serious conditions which may present as low back pain, with or without sciatica, and these must always be excluded. Haemoglobin estimation, ESR and appropriate radiographs are mandatory investigations supplementing full clinical examination.

Backache tends to be a recurring symptom, for the sufferers are notoriously reluctant to abide by the advice given them. They will not exercise to strengthen their spinal musculature, lose weight, limit their activity to a level below the threshold of pain onset, abstain from precipitating activities, limit the duration of their activities, limit the time for which they take up any particular spinal posture or organize their leisure/work/household activities to avoid exacerbations of their pain. They persist in 'finishing the job' instead of changing from task to task to avoid becoming fatigued. They refuse to cut down their arduous physical activities and supplement them with mechanical aids or to acknowledge the passage of time. They will not accept that the older a man is the shorter the time for which he can hold any particular trunk posture without causing muscular pain. Above all they refuse to recognize the particular precipitating cause of their backache and are therefore unable to effect its removal, or else, recognizing it, do not, or cannot, choose to remove it.

BIBLIOGRAPHY AND REFERENCES

Barnes, C.G. (1971). 'The differential diagnosis of backache.' *Br. J. Hosp. Med.* 5, 219
Brain, W.R. (1954), 'Spondylosis: the known and the unknown.' *Lancet* 1, 687

Brav, E.A. (1942). 'Diagnosis of low back pain of orthopaedic origin: analysis of 62 cases.'
   Am. J. Surg. 55, 57
Brewerton, D.A. (1976). HLA—B27 and the inheritance of susceptibility to rheumatic
   disease.' Arthritis and Rheumatism 4, 656
Brewerton, D.A., Caffrey, M., Hart, F.D., James, D.C.O., Nicholls, A., and Sturrock, R.D.
   (1973). 'Ankylosing spondylitis and HL—A27.' Lancet, 1, 7809, 904
Charnley, J. (1951). 'Orthopaedic signs in the diagnosis of disc protrusion.' Lancet 1, 186
Clymer, G., Mixter, W.J. and Mella, H. (1921). 'Experience with spinal cord tumours during
   the past 10 years.' J. nerv. ment. Dis. 53, 229
Falconer, M.A., McGeorge, M. and Begg, A.C. (1948). 'Observations on the cause and
   mechanism of symptom-production in sciatica and low back pain.' J. Neurol. Neurosurg.
   Psychiat. 11, 13
Floyd, W.F. and Silver, P.H.S. (1951). 'Function of erectores spinae in flexion of the trunk'.
   Lancet, 1, 133
Hart, F.D., Robinson, K.C., Allchin, F.M. and MacLagan, N.F. (1949). 'Ankylosing spondy-
   litis.' Q. Jl Med. 18, 217
Hurst, A. (1943). 'Treatment of sciatica: essay in debuning.' Br. med. J. 2, 773
Jayson, M.I.V. (1970). 'The problem of backache.' Practitioner 205, 615—21
Jayson, M.I.V. (Ed.) (1976). 'The lumbar spine and back pain.' Sector Pub. Ltd.
Kellgren, J.H. (1939). 'On distribution of pain arising from deep somatic structures with
   charts of segmental pain area.' Clin. Sci. 4, 35
Kellgren, J.H. (1941). 'Sciatica.' Lancet 240, 561
Mixter, W.J. and Barr, J.S. (1934). 'Rupture of intervertebral disc with involvement of
   spinal cord.' New Engl. J. Med. 211, 210
Mowat, A.G. and Camp, A.V. (1971). 'Polymyalgia rheumatica.' J. Bone Jt. Surg. 53B, 701
Newman, P.H. (1952). 'Sprung back.' J. Bone Jt. Surg. 34B, 30
Nichols, P.J.R. (1960). 'Short leg syndrome.' Br. med. J. 1, 1863
Pearce, J. and Moll, J.H.M. (1967). 'Conservative treatment and natural history of acute
   lumbar disc lesions.' J. Neurol. Neurosurg. Psychiat. 30, 13
Rush, W.A. and Steiner, H.A. (1946). 'Study of lower extremity length inequality.' Am. J.
   Roentg. Rad. Ther. 56, 616
Tegner, W.S. (1954). 'Physical medicine.' Proc. R. Soc. Med. 47, 389
Van Leuven, R.M. and Troup, J.D.G. (1969). 'The "instant" lumbar corset.' Physiotherapy
   55, 499
Wright, V. and Moll, J.M.H. (1973). 'Ankylosing spondylitis.' Br. J. Hosp. Med. 9, 331
Wright, V. and Moll, J.M.H. (1976). 'Seronegative Polyarthritis.' North Holland Publishing
   Co., Amsterdam
Wyke, B.D. (1967). 'The neurology of joints.' Ann. R. Coll. Surg. 41, 25
Wyke, B.D. (1970). 'The neurological basis of thoracic spinal pain.' Rheum. phys. Med. 10,
   356

7 Osteo-arthrosis

INTRODUCTION

Changes in connective tissue not only affect its mechanical properties but also the metabolic behaviour of the cells within it.

Furthermore the articular cartilage of different individuals varies considerably in the distribution of collagen, chondroitin sulphate and sceratan sulphate, in a manner characteristic of the individual, irrespective of age and sex. There is likely to be a genetically determined factor predisposing some people to develop osteoarthrosis.

Osteo-arthrosis is a pathological condition of a synovial joint, which though occurring spontaneously in the middle-aged and elderly, may also be precipitated by injury, disease or deformity. Osteo-arthrosis in its initial stage appears to invoke profound changes in the metabolism of cartilage cells set in train by increased hydration of the tissues. Later, in the advanced stages, the changes become degenerative. The diagnosis of osteoarthritis may only be made at a later stage when radiological changes have developed. It is a progressive condition involving the destruction of hyaline cartilage and ultimately involving all the structures of the joint in changes which are mainly degenerative. In generalized osteo-arthrosis there is asymmetrical involvement characteristically of the terminal phalangeal, first metacarpophalangeal, first metatarsophalangeal, the apophyseal joints of the spine, the knees and the acromioclavicular joints. It occurs most commonly in women and constitutes a familial tendency.

Secondary osteo-arthrosis usually follows some mechanical, occupational or traumatic factor and tends to affect single joints, or a few joints asymmetrically.

Heberden's nodes are common, affecting any or all of the distal interphalangeal joints. They may become red, hot, swollen and tender. They are of no clinical significance, but may be a nuisance because of pain, their size or their appearance. Clinically, there may be crepitus on movement, restriction of the range of motion and effusion into the joint cavity with enlargement or alteration of the joint contours. The diagnosis is established by the occurrence of the characteristic radiological changes of narrowing of joint space, subchondral sclerosis and cyst formation, and osteophytosis. Such a joint has become worn and mechanically defective, and is more prone to mechanical strains. Clinically the condition may be symptomless, and the severity of the symptoms is rarely related to the severity of the radiographic changes. Symptoms are more frequently associated with trauma and are thus often more significant in the weight-bearing joints of lower limb and spine than in the upper limb joints.

As the condition progresses, joint range becomes increasingly restricted, often reducing the severity of the symptoms. However, osteo-arthrosis in a weight-bearing joint, such as a hip or knee, associated with a mechanical abnormality due to old injury or disease, can progress with considerable speed and rapidly lead to painful joint destruction.

SYMPTOMS

It is helpful to review the symptoms associated with osteo-arthrosis, as they are usually a guide to treatment. Patients with osteo-arthrosis commonly complain of pain, stiffness and reduced range of movement. In addition, they may complain of intermittent swelling, due to effusion, or to permanent increase and change in size, due to bony enlargement. Joint laxity, locking or grating may also be presenting symptoms.

Pain

The pain is often worst after prolonged exercise, though it may be relieved by exercise once the initial stiffness on commencing movement has worn off. Depending upon the nature, severity and location of joint involvement, bed rest may relieve or exacerbate it: frequently, osteo-arthritic pain will light up as the muscles relax after the patient has been in bed a short time and will disturb sleep. Persistent maintenance of any one body posture also tends to bring on pain.

Most patients assert that as long as they can 'keep going', 'chop and change' and 'take their own time' about their various tasks they can also reduce their pain. For every arthritic joint there will usually be one 'position of ease' in which maximal relief of pain for long periods is experienced. The pain from osteo-arthrosis is not constant but varies with position, activity and weather. Although it is not accompanied by the systemic upsets of rheumatoid arthritis, it is nevertheless distressing, and has a 'wearing' quality remarked upon by the majority of those who suffer from it; and under certain circumstances it can be intensely painful.

Stiffness

Unlike that of rheumatoid arthritis, the stiffness of osteo-arthrosis is not necessarily worst in the mornings. It may be evident at any time of the day in which a posture is held constantly for a long time. A patient with osteo-arthrosis of the knees and spine may complain of the need to assist himself out of an easy chair either by pushing on the arms of the chair or else by rocking himself in increasing arcs until he manages to stand at the end of the forward rock.

Some stiffness is muscular in origin, and some of it may be due to a permanently diminished range of movement due to alteration in joint structure. Stiffness of the former variety wears off with exercise and is minimized by frequent changes of posture. Conversely, it is exacerbated by prolonged exercise. As with the pain of osteo-arthritic joints, this muscular stiffness is less when patients are able to change often from task to task, so varying their patterns of movement.

Diminished range of movement

In the early stages of osteo-arthrosis, restriction of joint movement may be partly due to a voluntary decision to avoid pain, and partly to the involuntary spasm of the muscles to which pain is referred from the inflamed joint structures. In the later stages, in which cartilage destruction and bony overgrowth have occurred, this restriction follows the actual mechanical block to joint movement which such overgrowth can produce. Pain may be felt while some movement remains in the joint.

Swelling

The swelling complained of may be due to bony overgrowth or to an effusion or it may be due to inflammation in the periarticular tissues, as in the Heberden's nodes of the interphalangeal joints. Occasionally swelling may be apparently extra-articular and yet derive from the joint itself, as in the case of cystic swelling, particularly of the knee and elbow.

'Locking' or 'giving way'

'Locking' or 'giving way' of weight-bearing joints are occasional symptoms usually associated with an effusion in the joint. The knee joint is particularly prone to these symptoms which are probably due to detached fragments of osteophytes, cartilage or menisci lodging momentarily between opposing joint surfaces.

MEDICATION

Either simple analgesics or non-steroidal anti-inflammatory drugs are given in sufficient doses to eliminate pain or reduce it to a reasonable level. There is a great deal of individual variation in the responses of different patients to these various drugs.

Side-effects are frequent, and are most commonly upsets of the digestive tract. Care is needed when salicylates or indomethacin are given to patients with past history of indigestion or peptic ulceration. Whenever possible soluble or enteric-coated tablets should be used, and administered during meals. Persistent indigestion is an indication for stopping any particular type of tablet, as haematemesis or melaena may result if this symptom is ignored. Sometimes a reduction in dosage level, the use of the same medicament in an enteric-coated capsule, or the addition of an antacid permits medication to be continued.

More recently, ibuprofen, aclofenac and benorylate have been added to the armamentarium of drugs for the treatment of osteo-arthritis. Their long-term effects have not yet been fully evaluated and therefore they should be reserved for patients who are intolerant of, or unhelped by, the longer established preparations.

Many patients with osteo-arthrosis have acute inflammatory episodes of affected joints related to appearance of hydroxyapatite or calcium pyrophosphate crystals in the joints. On these occasions the use of anti-inflammatory drugs is particularly recommended. The *long term* use of non-steroidal anti-inflammatory drugs is considered by some authorities to be contraindicated.

The establishment of a satisfactory drug regime presents a very real difficulty in a large number of patients. In effective doses, many of the drugs commonly used have untoward side-effects which outweigh their usefulness as analgesics.

Apart from the tendency of the salicylates, phenylbutazone and indomethacin to cause gastro-intestinal pain and bleeding, phenylbutazone and indomethacin may both cause fluid retention and indomethacin may produce insomnia and depress normal intellectual function. Many patients need to strike a balance between an effective and a tolerable level of medication.

When sleep is regularly disturbed by a serious joint pain, and operative corrective treatment for the joint concerned is not feasible, a stronger analgesic may need to be given at night in addition to the sedative.

It is important that patients with osteo-arthrosis who are on a regular drug regime should be instructed how to prevent constipation, both by dietary means and by taking regular doses of bulk laxatives such as bran or mucilaginous preparations.

PHYSIOTHERAPY

Physiotherapy can be a great help in osteo-arthrosis. The procedures employed must naturally depend upon the particular joint or joints involved and also on the amount of articular and periarticular damage which is present. The patient's pain threshold, his degree of functional disability and his commitments both at home and at work must be taken into consideration.

Physiotherapeutic treatment is usually combined with medication, and with advice by the medical adviser and the occupational therapist on the day-to-day management of the patient as a whole.

The aims of the physiotherapeutic treatment of osteo-arthrosis are:

(1) Pain relief.
(2) Restoration of function.
(3) Prevention of further deformity.
(4) Stabilization of unstable joints.
(5) Enforced rest by splintage or bracing.

When, despite adequate medication and physiotherapy, it is not possible to prevent progressive joint destruction, or to achieve adequate pain relief, surgical treatment must be considered.

Symptomatic treatment

Osteo-arthrosis manifests itself clinically as a painful, swollen joint with some restriction in joint range and with associated muscle wasting and weakness.

Passive palliative physiotherapy in the form of heat (wet or dry) can be very soothing and pleasant for the patient. Such treatment forms an excellent way for the therapist to establish rapport with the patient, and to pave the way for the acceptance of other treatment, whether this be advice or active strenuous exercise.

Radiant heat, infra-red heat, short-wave diathermy, ultrasonics, hot packs, hot-water sprays, hydrotherapy or wax are all methods of applying heat, and there is no convincing evidence that there is any physiological reason for selecting one rather than another. The choice should be left to the physiotherapist and will depend on the availability of the apparatus, the time available for treatment and the personal predilections of the therapist and the patient.

Muscle power and joint effusion

It is universally accepted that the quadriceps muscle is the guardian of the knee joint. When an acute effusion of the knee joint occurs, whether due to minor trauma, surgery or an exacerbation of arthritis, the quadriceps muscle shows a tendency to waste. This wasting appears to be a prelude to an exacerbation of arthritis, and thus a vicious circle of events is initiated to perpetuate a progressive disorganization of the joint.

There is some evidence that the quadriceps wasting is associated with an inhibition of its normal contraction; increasing the tension within the knee joints by intra-articular injection has been shown to induce temporary inhibition of voluntary contraction of the quadriceps. Certainly from the clinical stand-point, acute effusion of any aetiology is often associated with difficulty in obtaining active quadriceps contraction and leads to marked wasting. The condition can be helped by active stimulation of the quadriceps muscle with electrical impulses. Usually three or four treatment sessions over 2–3 days is enough to re-establish voluntary contractions.

This vicious cycle can be broken by a combination of intensive non-weight-bearing quadriceps exercises and passive splinting and support of the knee during essential weight-bearing. A simple back-splint of plaster of paris, plastic, or other available materials may be adequate.

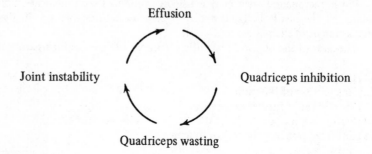

Effusion

Joint instability

Quadriceps inhibition

Quadriceps wasting

A plaster of paris cylinder is sometimes necessary. For more chronic and severe conditions, weight-relieving calipers are useful.

It may be that other muscles or muscle grousp are the 'key' muscles for various other joints and of the same importance to their ability as the quadriceps is to the knee. Certainly abduction of the hip is often weak and painful during an exacerbation of symptoms due to osteo-arthrosis of the hip, and intensive non-weight-bearing abduction exercises of the hip are often followed by a reduction in pain. Perhaps the gluteus medius is inhibited by effusion in the hip joint. Similarly, the calf muscles are often slow to repond to strengthening exercises in the presence of ankle injuries.

Obesity

The part that obesity has to play in the aetiology of osteo-arthrosis may be subject to discussion, but the reduction of obesity in the presence of symptomatic osteo-arthrosis of weight-bearing joints is universally recommended. Indeed, the loss of surplus weight in the presence of osteo-arthrosis of hips, knees, ankles and spine should be a primary aim. There are many who will refuse to introduce other forms of treatment until weight has been reduced to 'normal'.

The process is often difficult for patients in active employment or in the lower income groups, and for some a short period of hospitalization and the administration of a low (800 calories per day) diet may be the only way of initiating weight reduction. For most patients a sympathetic dietician, and membership of a group of 'weight-watchers' are successful once they understand the real need for reducing their weight.

GENERAL ADVICE

Living with osteo-arthrosis is an exercise in invention, substitution, compromise and, above all, organization. When a doctor says to a patient 'You have wear-and-tear arthritis. We can help you a great deal, but we cannot actually undo the damage which has been done − you will have to learn to live with it', this should not be seen as a negative attitude, and it does not call for passive acceptance on the part of the patient.

Where osteo-arthritis follows direct trauma or infection, one joint only may be involved, but in the older patients, osteo-arthrosis seldom strikes at a single joint. Several joints are usually affected, albeit to varying degrees. The patient who could cope well with the vicissitudes of one abnormal joint is faced with the knowledge that to do so would be to precipitate pain in several others. He lives therefore in a state of perpetual compromise, where the joint or joints giving most discomfort at any one time are managed with concessions consistent with the optimal good of the body as a whole.

The essence of living fully and successfully with osteo-arthrosis is the mutual acknowledgement by doctor and patient that osteo-arthrosis may have repercussions affecting every aspect of life, and the recognition of the importance of managing the life of the patient in such a way that these repercussions are minimized. This can only be achieved by a broad outlook on the work and leisure activities of the patient.

Probably the most important contribution that can be made to the management of osteo-arthrosis in a rehabilitation department is the dispensation of reassurance and good general advice. The confident reassurance that the symptoms do not herald a serious, progressive, crippling disorder is based upon accurate diagnosis. The patient should be given a clear and simple explanation of the pathology, the likely prognosis, the alternatives of long-term and short-term treatment available and a rational explanation of the reasons for choosing or changing a particular treatment regimen. The importance of preventing obesity and other forms of excessive strain and of maintaining general physical fitness and local muscular strength must be stressed.

Emphasis must be placed on the need to rest during a period of acute joint pain while yet avoiding prolonged inactivity during quiescent phases. The difference between non-weight-bearing exercises and free activity must also be clearly demonstrated and the necessity of avoiding undue stress and trauma to the affected joints explained. Such advice may range from discussion concerning the patient's work (particularly for those in heavy industry) to the problems of inadequate or unsuitable housing. It may also include instruction on the use of a simple appliance such as knee bandage or wrist support whilst undertaking certain tasks.

The dispensation of useful advice is a time-consuming activity if it is to be relevant and meaningful. Unfortunately, it is not always possible for the doctor to spend as much time as is really necessary in explanation. In these circumstances, it is incumbent upon the clinician to ensure that someone else is given the time to accomplish this most important part of the patient's care. Much of this important work properly falls to the physiotherapists and occupational therapists. For many patients, the doctor's reassurance is the most important part of the treatment, but the majority will benefit from more general advice and direction from the therapists.

DETAILED ADVICE

Detailed advice may with advantage be the combined responsibility of the physiotherapist and occupational therapist attending the clinic or concerned in treatment. It is well recognized that patients do not remember clearly the instructions and advice given by doctors. Repeated reiteration of this advice during treatment sessions or follow-up clinics is often better remembered and therefore of greater use. Thus, the more relaxed interview with the therapist following that at which the doctor has made his enquiry, examination and prescription for investigation and treatment, is often the more important for the patient's rehabilitation.

The therapist translates the doctor's advice into domestic terms. She enquires further into difficulties with activities of daily living and gives detailed advice on how to minimize pain and exertion. In addition, she suggests alternative methods of arranging domestic routines and ways of rearranging furniture and household fixtures, and she will also supply essential aids, or arrange for them to be supplied. Although it is traditionally the occupational therapist who does this, ideally this aspect of management should be the combined responsibility of physiotherapist and occupational therapist working together. The physiotherapist supplements the necessary knowledge of the home situation from further information which she gathers during treatment sessions. Under the warmth of the heat lamp, relaxed and confident, because the fear of being left with pain has been removed, a patient will often reveal details which have been concealed from the doctor. Some aggravating factor at work or home is described which has precipitated or contributed to the present state. This may be a financial difficulty, a marital problem or a work situation, a clinical fear or some domestic or social stress.

When a patient has pain and dysfunction from osteo-arthrosis, the discovery of predisposing factors in the history is of considerable importance. Since the condition cannot be cured, it must be managed, and the more detailed the knowledge of a patient's pain, the more likely it is that the pain can be reduced to a minimum. As in so many other fields of rehabilitation, the wiser the therapist, the less therapy she will need to dispense. Counselling pays better dividends than empirical physical therapy.

Many of the key factors in a particular patient's pain pattern can be quickly elicited. Others can only be discovered by detailed questioning. One of the greatest values of a period of palliative physiotherapy is that it provides time for the patient to relax and establish a rapport with the therapist. During these periods much essential and therapeutic discussion can take place.

If the patient is not clearly and authoritatively informed about his symptoms and their prevention, he will acquire a great deal of uninformed folklore or invent concepts for himself. Thus, an adequate explanation to the patient of the natural history of the disease, so that he understands the part which he can play in influencing its progress, is the corner-stone of his management.

Work

The elimination or reduction of predisposing factors which cause exacerbations of the patient's symptoms necessitates a frequent reassessment of their relationship to his work, transport, home, leisure activities and personal care. Some of the most important advice to be sought and given relates to a man's work. To give sensible and relevant advice, considerable information is needed. Careful enquiry is needed about his postures and movement during work, and their duration, repetition and capacity to cause pain or stiffness. It is helpful to the doctor and therapists if the patient is able to describe in mime the sequence of movements which make up the basic pattern of his day's work so that the causes of the pain can be made apparent.

Gratuitous advice to 'take it easy' or to 'find a light job' may precipitate a sequence of events leading to permanent unnecessary unemployment. Detailed advice regarding work activities should only be given when an accurate prognosis can be matched with a detailed knowledge of the type of employment. Preferably such advice should be constructive, indicating capability and not negatively restricting activity. Many patients have lost their jobs through ill-considered advice. Many others have kept them in relative comfort following suitable alterations to equipment, working surfaces, seating heights, or the method in which they use these.

Transport

Here, too, pertinent questioning often reveals a host of precipitating factors leading to pain and dysfunction in affected joints. Such questions include:

(1) Does the patient drive a car — what make is it?
(2) Does it cause any discomfort?
(3) Does the seat cause backache?
(4) Do the controls cause wrist, elbow or shoulder discomfort?
(5) Are the door handles stiff and do they cause pain in the wrists or hands?
(6) Is there an awkward stretch to reach the handle or lock on the back door?
(7) Does he get pain when he looks around to reverse?
(8) Does he get pain when he brakes suddenly?
(9) Does he do minor car maintenance and repair jobs himself?
(10) Does he wear a seat belt?
(11) Has he a well-designed headrest?
(12) Does he ride a bicycle?
(13) Can he dismount easily?
(14) Can he mount it easily or must this be done from a kerb?
(15) Can he pedal it easily?
(16) Does he travel by bus or train?
(17) If so, does he fall asleep while travelling?
(18) Does he strap-hang for long intervals, and must he stand frequently?

Home

Enquiries about a patient's home establish:

(1) Does he have a warm house?

(2) What is his usual chair like, and does sitting cause pain?

(3) Does he fall asleep often in his chair?

(4) Has he difficulty in getting up and down from the toilet, or climbing up and down stairs?

(5) What is his bed like, and does he get pain at night?

(6) What is the layout of his house, and does any of the work in the house cause particular pain?

Housework and leisure activities

Everyday activities at home are often a potent source of pain. A patient should therefore be questioned about his home, hobbies or other household commitments.

Leisure activities are particularly important and become increasingly so in the older age groups. Relevant questions to a patient include:

(1) In general:
   (a) What are his hobbies?
   (b) Does he do a lot of gardening?
   (c) Does he do a lot of decorating and do-it-yourself work, or participate in a competitive or exacting sport?

(2) If a housewife:
   (a) Does the patient clean, cook or polish excessively?
   (b) Has she a part-time job? If so, what?

(3) Family commitments:
   (a) Are there children? How many and how dependent?
   (b) Are there lodgers? How many and how dependent?
   (c) Is there family or outside help for domestic work?
   (d) Is there difficulty or pain with personal care — washing, dressing, grooming and toiletting?

For patients in hospital, such assessment is the province of the occupational therapist and indirectly of the physiotherapist, but for patients seen in the GP's surgery, out-patient departments or their own homes, it is the GP or consultant who needs to initiate the assessment. Though time-consuming, it is an essential preliminary to the correct management of osteo-arthrosis and indicates in which of the many aspects of daily activity help is required.

With the wide range of assistance from the Department of Health and Social Security now available, it is usually possible to provide considerable help for patients in need, but the provision of the right help at the right time, and in an acceptable form, is difficult; without accurate functional assessment it is impossible.

SUMMARY OF POSSIBLE TREATMENT IN OSTEO-ARTHROSIS

These are the essential parts of the *management* of all patients with osteo-arthrosis:

(1) An adequate explanation of the natural history of the disease and of the part which the patient can play in influencing its progress.

(2) Instruction in activities of daily living so that he avoids fatigue and pain whenever possible.
(3) Initial instruction and advice by the doctor caring for him, confirmed and re-enforced by the therapists who treat him.
(4) Instruction in the importance of maintaining optimal general physical fitness and correct body weight.
(5) Organization of house and garden to minimize effort, fatigue and pain during their maintenance.
(6) Organization of working conditions to ease or avoid discomfort — if necessary by changing occupation.
(7) Assessment of transport, hobbies and leisure activities. Reorganization to avoid pain and effort.

Some, or all of the forms of *treatment* listed below need to be incorporated in the overall management of the condition:

(1) Medication by means of analgesic drugs, night sedatives and laxatives.
(2) Injection of hydrocortisone with or without local anaesthetic, into and around joints, bursae, tendons and muscles.
(3) Support or stabilization in the form of splints and calipers to prevent the exacerbation of pain caused by movements of painful joints and by excessive mobility in unstable joints. This includes, collars, spinal braces and corsets.
(4) Intermittent attendance at the rehabilitation department for appropriate palliative treatment, general assessment and advice.
(5) Surgical intervention to alter the stresses on a joint by means of an osteotomy, to fix a joint in one position by means of an arthrodesis, or to change its internal structure by means of excision, interposition or replacement arthroplasty.
(6) The issue of aids and appliances to enable a patient to compensate for the grossly restricted or absent function of lower limb joints, whether this stems from pain, stiffness, weakness or a combination of all of these symptoms. Such aids are those offering weight-relief or stabilization to joints of the lower limbs: e.g. weight relieving calipers; sticks, quadruped sticks, crutches or walking frames; wheelchairs; and outdoor transport.
(7) The issue of aids and devices to improve function and reduce stress for upper limbs. Such devices increase the range of upper limb movement (e.g. lazy tongs, helping-hand aids, curtain-pulling stick, stocking aids) and decrease the effort needed to manipulate household fixtures or equipment (e.g. tap turner, padded glove).

BIBLIOGRAPHY AND REFERENCES

Dixon, A. St. J. (Ed.) (1965). *Progress in Clinical Rheumatology*. London; J. & A. Churchill
Golding, D.N. (1969). 'General management of osteo-arthrosis.' *Br. med. J.* 3, 575
Law, W.A. (1967). 'Surgery in the treatment of osteo-arthrosis.' *Hosp. Med.* 1, 612–616
Licht, S. (Ed.) (1969). *Arthritis and Physical Medicine*. U.S.A.; E. Litcht
Muir, H. (1977). 'Molecular approach to the understanding of osteo-arthrosis Heberden Oration 1976.' *Ann. Rheum: Dis.* 36, 199

8 Fractures, Dislocations and Other Injuries

INTRODUCTION

The rehabilitation of a patient with a fracture should start as soon as the fracture is reduced and the reduction has been firmly held. Indeed, the most important factor in determining the end result and therefore in determining the need for rehabilitation is the quality of the treatment of the fracture and the associated soft-tissue injury.

For each fracture there is an ideal rehabilitative routine which falls into several sections:

(1) The routine followed during the period the fracture is consolidating:
  (a) In hospital, whether as an in-patient or out-patient.
  (b) At home.

(2) The routine followed when the fractured bone ends have joined in a well-consolidated union.
  (a) In hospital, whether as an in-patient or out-patient.
  (b) At home.

(3) The issue of appropriate aids to assist the function of the fractured part and the patient as a whole.
(4) Training and advice on personal care and daily living activities during the period of fracture consolidation and the ensuing one of patient mobilization.

Throughout the entire period of rehabilitation it is essential that five separate aspects of the healing of the injured part should be considered concurrently: bone healing; soft-tissue conservation; joint mobility; maintenance of muscle strength and co-ordination; total patient health.

Bone healing
The prime object of the treatment of a fractured bone is to cause the two ends to unite in a firmly consolidated union in the optimal functional position.

Soft-tissue conservation
Soft-tissue conservation encourages the repair and resumption of the normal functional interrelationship of the various soft-tissue components – muscle, nerve, blood vessels, lymphatics, connective tissue and skin.

128

Maintenance of joint mobility and muscle strength

The maintenance of joint mobility seeks to retain a full range of motion for the unimpeded joints of the whole body and to regain the maximal possible amount of movement for any joints immobilized during the period of fracture consolidation. The regular performance of active exercises throughout the period of fracture consolidation is the key-stone to the total rehabilitative treatment of the patient. Such activity:

(1) Assists the preservation of the mobility of the joints of the fractured limb.
(2) Promotes the circulation of blood, lymph and tissue fluid.
(3) Prevents disuse osteoporosis in the bones of the fractured limb.
(4) Minimizes adhesion formation.
(5) Preserves muscle power, tone and co-ordination.

Total patient health

Total patient health may well be inadvertently allowed to deteriorate while the fracture site is receiving maximal attention during the early stages of fracture healing, particularly if the patient is confined to bed or chair during a prolonged period of non-weight-bearing. The rehabilitative treatment for the whole patient should be started when the fracture has been reduced and continued throughout the period of immobilization required for bone healing. A programme of planned, graduated activity should be supplemented by mobility and independence training when the healing of the fracture permits, and is completed only when optimal functional efficiency has been restored to the injured part and the patient as a whole.

The rehabilitation of a patient with a fracture varies so much with the type of fracture that it may conveniently be considered in four sections:

$$
\text{Rehabilitation of } \begin{cases} \text{Upper limb fractures} \\ \text{Lower limb fractures} \\ \text{Spine and pelvic fractures} \\ \text{Fractures associated with} \\ \quad \text{multiple injuries} \end{cases}
$$

The differences in the problems presented by the rehabilitation of fractures of these various types relate to:

(1) The relative independence of people with upper limb fractures from the time the fracture is reduced.
(2) The need to avoid weight-bearing and to protect lower limb fractures during the healing phase.
(3) The difficulties of combining the needs of adequate nursing with adequate measures to ensure the achievement of maximal power and mobility in spinal and multiple injuries.

In each case rehabilitation presents problems of specific and general management. The specific problems relate to the maintenance of muscle power in the injured part during the period of fracture healing and to the re-establishment of maximal mobility and power when movement of the part is introduced.

The general management is concerned with the maintenance of general physical fitness, morale and motivation during prolonged immobilization of the injured part which may possibly involve immobilization and hospitalization of the patient. It is concerned also with the assessment of the probable outcome of injury and the preparation for work resettlement. This may entail return to the patient's original work, initiation into a different but more suitable type of employment, or preparation for prolonged or permanent disability of a minor or major degree.

As far as the rehabilitation of adults is concerned, the primary responsibility of rehabilitation personnel is first, to minimize or prevent residual disability, and secondly, to utilize normal daily and work activities to maintain or regain physical function and to re-establish a patient's confidence in his physical capability.

Frequently patients remain away from work or fail to return to full normal activities. This is commonly due to lack of authoritative guidance on the therapeutic advantages of rapid return to those everyday activities within their capabilities. Some patients who have severe multiple injuries or special injuries such as crush injuries of the hand, or who are engaged in particularly heavy physical labour or competitive sport may need special intensive rehabilitation.

The rehabilitation of children with limb fractures rarely presents problems. Most children need to be restrained from over-exertion rather than encouraged to exercise. Indeed, adequate immobilization is usually the only post-reduction therapy which is required. Some instruction in the importance of preventing plaster becoming immersed in water, together with some instruction in the use of crutches or similar appliances is often all that the physiotherapist is called upon to do.

LINES OF COMMUNICATION

Communication with the patient
When patients are treated as out-patients following fractures or dislocations, it is often difficult to ensure that they supplement exercise sessions at the physiotherapy department by regular sessions in their own homes. This is partly because they do not understand that they are expected to do so. It is also partly because they do not appreciate the benefits which can accrue from muscular exercise nor the damage that may result from inactivity.

Reiteration of the need and reason for frequent exercise sessions should be started by the doctor supervising rehabilitation, and followed by the physiotherapists, nurses and occupational therapists who combine to give their care. Even with such repeated explanation, it is advisable to present patients with a small information card, detailing the type and timing of exercises which they should perform, what signs of improvement can be looked for, what to do if their condition deteriorates and whom to consult when they are worried. These cards should also carry the telephone numbers of the hospital and the GP and the time of the next appointment.

Communication with the general practitioner
A brief notification should be despatched to the general practitioner from the consultant at the Fracture Clinic or Accident Service, before or at the time of departure of the patient for home. Ideally, this should be backed by a telephone call to the surgery or health centre attended by the patient. Such liaison enables

the general practitioner and his team of ancillary staff to take over smoothly their task of supporting the patient in the immediate post-fracture period. This may involve the supply of analgesics or hypnotics, nursing care or domestic help. It will also consist of checking the circulation in a plastered limb, and, if local facilities are available, initiating physiotherapy so that long ambulance journeys are not needed.

Communication with social services
Patients with fractures or dislocations who are not independent personally, domestically and socially, should not be sent home from hospital until the presence of adequate family or social service backing has been confirmed. This is often best done by direct contact between the medical social worker or ward sister and the family or area social services concerned. It is not enough to ask the patient about this. Many old people are confused and often imply that their home situations are as they would like them to be rather than as they are. Others are simply too proud to accept what they consider as 'charity'.

Those living alone, particularly when elderly, may find themselves unable to manage at home without assistance during the period of rehabilitation following a fracture or dislocation. The ideal solution will often be transfer to a local community hospital. They will be near friends, and the GP and his staff will be able to carry on with their care. If this is not possible, the local health visitor, social worker or domiciliary occupational therapist may be able to visit and give care at home. However, many old or solitary people strongly resent what they consider to be an intrusion on their privacy by unasked visitors, and refuse the help which they need. It is wise therefore to make a routine referral via the hospital social work department to the social services so that a direct check can be made on the real needs at home. Through such a referral the following help can be provided:

The district nurse may make a regular visit to help with personal care activities and any dressings or slings, and to assist with the weekly bath.

The domiciliary occupational therapist will check on the need for help in all activities of daily living (washing, dressing, toilet, cooking, housework), and supply necessary aids.

The home help may be particularly concerned in managing some of the heavier housework (cleaning the grate, laying the fire, shopping, collecting the pension, and doing the washing). Once it is safe to attempt them, these domestic activities provide an excellent form of rehabilitative exercise for fractured limbs, and patients should be encouraged to reassume them at the earliest opportunity.

FRACTURES AND DISLOCATIONS IN THE UPPER LIMB

Fractures and dislocations in the shoulder region
Since the immobilized, traumatized shoulder joint readily stiffens, treatment of injuries in the shoulder region aims at the minimal period of immobilization for the glenohumeral joint. This must be consistent with the stable union or reduction of the fracture or dislocation concerned, and must aim to produce optimal conditions for the maintenance of joint function during this period and throughout the period of remobilization.

Four principles of rehabilitative treatment of shoulder injuries therefore emerge as being applicable for fractures of the upper end of the humerus, or of the scapula and for dislocations of the glenohumeral joint.

(1) If reduction is unnecessary or impossible, treatment is concentrated on regaining shoulder movement, and the fracture or dislocation is largely disregarded.
(2) If the reduction is necessary and possible, it may need to be held, and shoulder movements must then be regained by active exercise as soon as possible.
(3) Whether or not reduction is effected and whatever treatment is given, in all shoulder injuries the elbow, wrist, thumb and fingers must be kept freely mobile from the start.
(4) Active use of the hand for personal and domestic tasks is encouraged even while the shoulder is supported by a sling or plaster.

In the later stages of rehabilitation progressive active exercises for the shoulder are introduced early and practised assiduously to re-establish the range and power of shoulder movement. But the timing and degree of such exercises must vary with the type of fracture or dislocation under treatment, the age and general condition of the patient, and the nature and severity of any associated lesions in the shoulder region.

Diagnosis of these associated lesions at time of injury may be difficult or impossible and the anticipation of their occurrence and recognition of their presence during rehabilitative treatment is therefore vital. Thus, whereas shoulder stiffness may well be due to neglect, fear or prolonged immobilization, it may also be due to:

(1) Damage to the rotator cuff, which may be clearly localized (e.g. supra-spinatus rupture) or less well defined (e.g. capsulitis or 'frozen shoulder').
(2) Nerve damage. The circumflex nerve is particularly at risk and more severe injuries may damage the brachial plexus.
(3) Damage to the articular surfaces of the glenohumeral joint.
(4) Unrecognized associated fracture.
(5) Detachment of the greater tuberosity or fracture of the humeral neck. These may accompany other injuries around the shoulder and may not be apparent until delayed recovery of function suggests the need for further investigation.

Some shoulder stiffness is likely to follow the period of immobilization of the arm in the sling, which forms an essential part of the treatment of so many shoulder injuries. Necessarily, the glenohumeral joint is internally rotated and adducted while held in the sling position, and in this position damaged muscle and capsule soon lose the ability to stretch. Loss of external rotation and limitation of abduction ensue. For this reason the period of immobilization of the glenohumeral joint following shoulder injuries is the minimal one consistent with stable reduction and is always followed by early active movements. Active exercises may prevent stiffness and can usually cure it. Passive exercises are usually contra-indicated, but the shoulder is the one joint which may respond to passive movements or mobilization techniques when recovery of joint movement ceases to improve with active exercises. Such techniques are contra-indicated when the joint shows evidence of active synovitis and should be used with the utmost care in elderly people.

The painful stiff shoulder can be a very disabling complication. It may respond to ice packs or to applications of heat. Active exercises for the shoulder and entire arm in a warm pool are often beneficial, and this form of therapy can be introduced early even before consolidation has occurred, while the arm is still supported in a sling between hydrotherapy treatments.

Purposeful occupational therapy provides active exercises to overcome shoulder stiffness in the early stages of active mobilization. It is important that the activities should be chosen and adapted for each patient so that elevation of the shoulder should be required in doing them. In the early stages, traditional craft activities have their value. Later, heavier activities such as carpentry and gardening can be introduced, progressing to log-splitting, cement-mixing and heavy digging, to build up muscle bulk and strength. The harder tasks of housework such as window cleaning, furniture and floor polishing, and eventually interior decorating, provide the same power-building exercise for women.

Fracture of the humerus

Whether the fracture is of the neck of the humerus or of the shaft, transverse or spiral, union is usually rapid and rehabilitation relatively straightforward. Immobilization may be accomplished by a simple sling or 'U'-shaped plaster. In all instances finger and hand movements are essential from the outset. 'Pendulum' exercises (practised with the patient leaning forward while the arm hangs supported by plaster or sling) for the shoulder joint can usually be introduced early, but abduction exercises are avoided until there is evidence of consolidation.

Radial-nerve damage requires special treatment with the early use of a simple lively 'radial-nerve' splint. Such a splint should not impede the active use of the finger and hand during the recovery phase.

Fracture of the elbow

Fractures in the region of the elbow are notorious for producing some loss of range in all planes of movement — flexion, extension, pronation and supination. The combination of these movements is of paramount importance in placing the hand at the appropriate distance from the trunk and face. Thus, in the majority of daily living activities and in all those movements involved in personal care, elbow movement plays an essential part, and marked restriction of elbow range may lead to a significant loss of independence.

Because of its tendency to become stiff after injury, the elbow joint should only be immobilized for the minimal time consistent with a stable reduction of the fracture or dislocation concerned.

Except in a supracondylar fracture with forward displacement of the lower fragment in children, the elbow is immobilized in flexion rather than extension. Should elbow stiffness follow immobilization, whatever range of movement is recoverable is of far more use from a position of 90 degrees of flexion than from a position of full extension.

Closed reduction of fractures and dislocations in the elbow region is preferred, and open reduction and internal fixation are only employed when it is necessary to hold the fractured fragments in the reduced position.

Whenever possible, reduction of an elbow fracture is maintained by gravity traction, and the forearm is held in a collar and cuff sling with or without a supporting backslab. Simple sling immobilization is usually needed for 3 weeks only, but when a backslab is used the sling is usually retained for up to 3 weeks after the slab has been removed.

Active finger movements are practised immediately following reduction and are maintained assiduously throughout the period of elbow immobilization. Active shoulder and wrist movements are added when fracture healing permits. Their early institution is particularly important in adults in whom a 'frozen shoulder' may easily follow sling treatment of elbow injury.

Elbow movement is regained when the period of elbow immobilization has been completed by means of active non-resisted exercises, but some limitation of extension is almost inevitable following severe elbow fracture. Formal physio-therapeutic treatment seldom needs to be prolonged since normal use of the injured arm at home or at work will encourage recovery of movement over a period of at least 6 months.

Passive elbow movement must be avoided at all times, and elbow manipulation by physiotherapists, relatives and patient is *absolutely* contra-indicated. So is 'therapeutic stretching' by carrying heavy shopping bags and suitcases.

Apart from complications, which may accompany fractures or dislocations in the elbow region, further injury to the upper limb may occur during the actual treatment of these conditions. Volkmann's ischaemia and myositis ossificans are the two most serious sequelae which may occur, and these must be diagnosed early and treated promptly unless serious functional loss is to result.

Forearm fractures

In the treatment of fractures of the radius and ulna, perfect apposition of the fractured bones is necessary to avoid a rotation deficit. Thus, although closed reduction of such fractures is usually initially attempted, unless this reduction can be held by an above-elbow plaster, open reduction and plating of the bones is indicated.

In all cases, shoulder and finger exercises are practised regularly and frequently from the start, and elbow flexion/extension and forearm pronation/supination are regained by progressive active exercises when the plaster is removed. As with fractures around the elbow, elbow and forearm movement must never be forced or assisted, and the elbow must not be passively manipulated.

Non-union, mal-union, joint stiffness and ischaemia of the hand are possible complications to be avoided by careful reduction and immobilization.

The commonest fracture of the wrist, a Colles' fracture of the lower end of the radius, is treated by closed reduction and a below-elbow plaster slab which extends to the metacarpal heads. Swelling of the hand and fingers frequently occurs shortly after reduction and any medical or paramedical personnel treating a patient who has developed blue, swollen or painful fingers needs to split the bandage holding the slab immediately. The development of oedema is discouraged by the elevation of the arm at night and its support by day in a sling for the first few days after fracture. Active shoulder and finger exercises are prescribed, and the use of the hand for light tasks is encouraged. The sling should be withdrawn within a few days so that secondary capsulitis of the shoulder due to immobilization may not develop.

Shoulder stiffness should be preventable and is certainly treatable either by ice and active exercises, or heat and active exercises. Finger stiffness may arise from disuse. Repeated explanation and demonstration of finger exercises may be needed to convince elderly patients that they are not doing irreparable damage by moving their fingers. Rarely, stiffness of the fingers is persistent and arises from Sudeck's atrophy, in which pain and stiffness of the fingers with puffiness, patchy discoloration and moist hyperaesthetic skin come on a few weeks after injury. Regular, persevering physiotherapy assists recovery over many months, and with heat, elevation and progressive exercises, the fingers gradually approach normality.

Severe and persistent stiffness of the wrist seldom follows a simple Colles' but is more likely to occur when the fracture line involves the joint or when there has been associated dislocation of one or more carpal bones. Mobilization of such stiff, weak wrists by progressively active exercises preceded by heat or ice is greatly assisted by appropriate occupational therapy.

Rehabilitative treatment of other fractures of the lower end of the radius is similar to that following a Colles' fracture. Out-patients are able to follow recommended occupational therapy in their own homes in household and do-it-yourself activities.

Fractures and dislocations of the carpal bones
Following reduction of fractures or dislocated carpal bones, the forearm and hand are immobilized in plaster. Finger movement is encouraged by directing the patient to undertake as many normal activities as possible, consistent with preserving the plaster's integrity. Only when this advice is not followed, or cannot be followed, should it be necessary to institute regular sessions of formal physiotherapy and to instruct the patient in active exercises for the fingers in the hospital rehabilitation department.

Scaphoid fractures are usually treated by 8 weeks in plaster. If union has occurred and the fingers have been actively exercised throughout the period of immobilization, rapid recovery of wrist movement and power follow plaster removal. Non-union of the fracture and possible avascular necrosis of the proximal fragment may occur, and a weak and painful wrist results. Should this be so the wrist is immobilized for a further 3 weeks after the customary 2 months in plaster. If this fails to relieve the pain and weakness, excision of the radial styloid and the removal of the necrotic segment of the scaphoid may be considered. Wrist function is regained by active exercises post-operatively, and by an early return to normal activities.

When osteo-arthritis results from non-union of the scaphoid fragments, provision of a plastic wrist-splint and possible intra-articular steroid injections at weekly intervals for 3 weeks may be sufficient to ensure comfort, but arthrodesis may become necessary to produce a pain-free stable wrist.

Lunate dislocations may occur separately or in association with a fracture of the scaphoid. Simple dislocations are treated by closed reduction and held by a plaster of paris slab, while active exercises for shoulder, elbow and fingers are started at once. Damage to the arterial supply of the lunate may follow dislocation, and avascular necrosis may develop. Operative removal of the bone becomes necessary, and permanent stiffness of the wrist is likely to result. This is treated in the same way as the wrist stiffness following injury to the scaphoid bone.

Fractures and dislocations in the hand
Fractures in the hand almost always unite, and immobilized fingers almost

invariably stiffen. The treatment of fractures and dislocations in the hand therefore aims at the minimal period of finger immobilization and at the restoration of maximal functional efficiency rather than exact anatomical outline.

Constant factors of management therefore involve:

Control of swelling: By elevation of the hand and early active exercises for the fingers.

Minimal splintage: Only the finger which is injured should be splinted, either individually, or else by a narrow garter attachment to an adjacent finger. The functional position of partial flexion is adopted for fractures of any digit other than the thumb under certain conditions. When external splintage would immobilize several fingers unnecessarily, internal wire fixation is used instead.

Skin care: When skin damage accompanies bone injury, treatment of the skin takes precedence over treatment of fracture.

Maintenance of finger movement: During the period of immobilization of the fractured bones, use of the remaining fingers is encouraged and the arm as a whole is used and exercised regularly. Following the removal of the splintage, finger movement is regained by active exercises. Playing a musical instrument is excellent occupational therapy, and craftwork and housework are also helpful in restoring co-ordinated finger movement.

During the period of remobilization after removal of the supporting splintage, home physiotherapy in which both hands are exercised several times daily, supplements, or follows, the more sophisticated treatment offered in the physiotherapy department. Specific regimes involving, for example, the immersion of the hand in warm water, help to impress the habit of regular exercise upon the patient.

Patients with severe hand injuries in which, in addition to bone fracture, there has been much soft-tissue damage and subsequent fibrous contracture, need admission to hospital for specialized intensive care. To correct the contractures, warm-oil massage and gentle, gradual stretching are repeated for short intervals several times daily, and the correction is maintained by applications of a light plaster splint, renewed daily in the early stages and at longer intervals later, according to response to treatment. Manipulation and sudden stretching are absolutely contra-indicated. Specially programmed occupational therapy assists in the structural and functional recovery of the fingers and hand and their reintegration into the body image.

Crush injuries of the hand are relatively common in heavy industry and frequently lead to considerable time off work and loss of earning power. Intensive rehabilitation in the purposive atmosphere of an active rehabilitation unit can reduce morbidity and improve the end results of treatment. When nerves are involved in the injury, careful, detailed supervision of the rehabilitation is even more important, and close collaboration between the orthopaedic surgeon or plastic surgeon and the rehabilitation team is of the highest importance.

INJURIES OF THE SPINE

General

The immediate and rehabilitative treatment of fractures of the spine vary according to the stability or instability of the fracture and the actual or potential cord damage involved. This chapter is not concerned with the management of paraplegia and tetraplegia associated with spinal injury but only with the rehabilitation of patients without cord injury.

Cervical spine
The reduction of fractures of the cervical spine is followed by a period of immobilization in which the fracture is held reduced by traction, plaster or internal fixation.

After the period of continuous immobilization, a polythene collar is usually prescribed and worn for some weeks. The patient should be instructed to take this off for gradually lengthening periods each day, and the physiotherapist teaches him to perform gentle strengthening exercises for practice during the unsupported intervals. Manipulation and passive movements are contra-indicated. Prolonged attendance for out-patient physiotherapy is common but usually unrewarding. Movements return with natural usage when the immobilization is discarded.

Fractures of the thoracic and lumbar spine
The treatment of spinal fractures uncomplicated by neurological deficit may be divided into two distinct groups:

(1) Patients with potentially unstable fractures who are treated by strict immobilization. They progress through a sequence of bed rest, with or without traction, plaster of paris immobilization, spinal brace and then spinal corset.
(2) Patients with more stable fractures, who may progress directly from a period of best rest to a spinal brace or corset. A few of these patients may return immediately to full activity.

In all cases the rehabilitation programme is concerned with:

(1) Maintaining the power and volume of the paraspinal musculature and the function of all other muscle groups.
(2) Instilling into the patient the concept of maintaining the optimal position of the spinal column while undertaking many activities.
(3) Teaching the patient to lift by using the power of his legs while his back is held straight.
(4) Graduating and increasing the general activity and physical fitness of the patient and strengthening his trunk musculature proportionally.
(5) Preventing unnecessary fear and inactivity by active demonstration of the progressive increase in functional capability.

In such a programme, the rehabilitative activity is always in parallel with the progress of the clinical and radiological stabilization and eventual consolidation of the fractured vertebrae.

In the past, many injuries of the spine from industrial accidents have been associated with unnecessarily prolonged immobilization. In recent years, it has been clearly demonstrated by the routine treatment of personnel injured in the armed services, that with careful and understanding rehabilitation, such injuries need cause no more than a few months relative inconvenience preceding a return to full activity.

Fractures of the pelvis

Following simple, isolated fractures of the pelvic ring, bed rest without reduction is advised until the patient is comfortable. He is then gradually mobilized, first standing and then walking with whichever walking aid gives him greatest confidence and stability.

Following pelvic-ring disruption in which the ring is fractured in two places and displacement and complications are common, immediate and rehabilitative treatment varies with the type of disruption produced. As a general principle, however, non-weight-bearing exercise in bed will maintain muscle power, and when the fractures are united, increasing weight-bearing activities can be introduced. Exercise in the swimming pool is particularly valuable in this type of injury as it enables the physiotherapist to introduce a wide range of activity before weight-bearing is allowed.

FRACTURES AND DISLOCATIONS OF THE LOWER LIMB

General

The management of all fractures falls into four phases which follow the natural history of bone healing:

(1) Fracture reduction and holding.
(2) Union.
(3) Consolidation.
(4) Remodelling.

But the treatment of fractures of the lower limb differs from that of those of the upper limb in the longer periods which must elapse before full function may be restored. This is directly related to the need for a healed fracture of a lower limb to be able to bear weight.

To reduce the long period of immobilization in bed which adequate fracture healing might otherwise necessitate, whenever possible, a lower limb fracture is protected from abnormal lateral and rotation stress by internal or external fixation, weight relief is provided by a caliper or crutches, and preconsolidation ambulation is encouraged. Despite this technique of fracture treatment which permits early protected walking, most lower limb fractures entail some period of bed rest since during the immediate post-reduction stage the swelling consequent on soft-tissue damage necessitates elevation.

During the intervals between the different stages of healing, physiotherapeutic treatment consisting of bed rest, assisted ambulation and protected and unprotected activity is essential. The overall rehabilitative programme following a lower limb fracture involves:

(1) Exercise in bed following reduction and immobilization, usually restricted to static exercises only for muscles acting over the fracture line and immobilized joints. Active exercises for all movable joints of all four limbs and trunk.
(2) Early mobilization during the interval from reduction to union, with supervision of non-weight-bearing activities and introduction of partial weight-bearing for the injured limb; continuance of progressive exercises to maintain strength and mobility of all four limbs and trunk.

(3) Later mobilization during the interval from union to consolidation, with supervision of the gradual resumption of full weight-bearing and the maintenance of regular exercise sessions while fracture protection is being maintained.

(4) Final rehabilitation following fracture consolidation and removal of external plaster protection when muscle power and co-ordination and joint range are developed; retraining for work, sport and full activity may now occur.

Early phases of treatment

Patients with upper limb injuries can get up, walk about and become independent using one hand, and thus, almost inadvertently, accomplish their own rehabilitation and resettlement as the injury recovers. They usually only require instruction and encouragement. Patients with lower limb injuries, however, present a very different problem. Both during the initial period of bed rest and during the ensuing period of active rehabilitation to achieve walking, they may need considerable support, training and active encouragement from experienced staff. Elderly and fragile people are at severe risk while recumbent in bed, and the secondary effects of immobilization − pressure sores, chest infection, osteoporosis, and sheer inanition − may often be more disabling than the original injury. Thus, the early part of the period of mobilization is often critical and is a period in which not only physical improvement in muscle power, joint mobility and stamina are to be achieved, but considerable psychological barriers may have to be overcome, such as fear of further injury, fear of the future, anxiety about family, compensation and loss of work. Much of the routine suggested is directed towards the patient's general rehabilitation as well as to specific recovery from lower limb injury.

During the initial stage of physiotherapeutic management of the lower limb fracture, reduction has been effected, union is awaited, and it is essential to ensure that fracture immobilization is not synonymous with patient immobilization. Whether internal fixation, traction or plaster of paris is being used to hold reduction while the patient is at bed rest with his leg elevated, his exercise regime is designed to promote rapid removal of oedema fluid from the fractured limb. The patient must safeguard muscle action and joint mobility by static contractions of the muscles spanning the fracture and the joints immobilized in its treatment, and by active exercises for all the mobile joints in all four limbs and trunk.

A specific exercise programme is devised, taught and rehearsed with each patient at least twice daily by the therapist giving treatment. In addition, a group or class section can be held for the ward each day in which static exercises for gluteal, quadriceps and calf muscles can be taught and practised together with breathing exercises and exercises for upper limbs and trunk. More active exercises can be introduced on an individual basis and graded by the use of springs and slings attached to an overhead beam or to the foot of the bed.

Bed rest may be of short duration, merely until the swelling disperses in fractures which involve the distal part of the limb and are simple in nature and uncomplicated in mode of reduction. It may be prolonged for weeks or months following fractures which involve the proximal part of the lower limb, or which form part of a multiple injury complex with associated damage to the brain or cord. However severe the total clinical picture may be, regular physiotherapeutic treatment should be started as soon as it is medically allowed and pursued energetically throughout the period of recumbence.

Nursing and physiotherapeutic care overlap each other considerably during this initial post-reduction phase. Seriously injured, frail, elderly or relatively immobile patients need to be nursed on firm-based beds in which the heights of both ends are adjustable and on mattresses which both support the spine and protect the skin. Often a firm sponge-rubber mattress is adequate, but when skin ulceration is a possibility, the use of a sheepskin, a ripple mattress, or a 'cubex' mattress may be indicated. (The 'cubex' mattress consists of aerated polystyrene granules compartmentalized into various patterns to make a firm whole.) Alternatively, large foam blocks may be used to make a composite surface from which removal of appropriate blocks allows toiletting, washing or the easier performance of exercises. When skin health is severely threatened, a water mattress or 'flotation bed' is occasionally indicated.

For a female patient especially, the early days following reduction and fixation of a fractured femur can be fraught with unnecessary additional pain. Use of a bedpan for micturition, particularly when only one nurse is available to assist the patient on and off, is intensely painful. The alternative use of one of the many plastic female urinals which are now obtainable could minimize the discomfort for the patient and the work for the nursing staff. A bedpan should be reserved for defaecation only and it should be mandatory that two nurses should be present to administer and remove it. The use of a bedside commode should be introduced as soon as it is possible.

Physiotherapists attend each patient only twice or thrice daily, while nurses are in the ward throughout the day and night. With collaboration between the physiotherapist and the nursing staff, an extended supervision of the patient's exercise regime becomes possible. Particularly when backed by a written exercise chart, explanation by the physiotherapist to the nurse of her requirements can ensure that the requisite exercises are performed more regularly because they are monitored and encouraged by the nurses giving care.

Routine use of a physiotherapy chart, kept at the foot of the patient's bed with other charts and medical notes, not only facilitates closer supervision by the nursing staff, but also enables all staff to make detailed enquiries and observations of a patient's rehabilitative progress.

Early mobilization

In the absence of associated injuries, unless maintenance of fracture reduction demands external traction, once swelling has been reduced patients with lower limb fractures are allowed up. Periods of dependence of the limb, during which exercises are performed within the plaster cast, are then alternated with periods of elevation, when the limb is elevated on chair, stool or the elevating leg rest of a wheelchair.

Sitting with the foot dependent and inactive should be forbidden as this quickly leads to hypostatic oedema, swollen toes and all the discomforts of an overtight plaster. A dependent foot must be an active foot. Toe-wriggling and static contractions of muscles controlling immobilized joints should be regularly and frequently practised.

Non-weight-bearing is taught at this stage, using elbow crutches initially, and progressing to sticks if and when fracture stability permits. Accurate adjustment of the height of the handrests of the crutches and sticks is essential so that this corresponds with the level of the tip of the greater trochanter when the patient is standing in a shoe.

Occasional walking is not enough in itself to ensure the steady functional gain required of the patient as a whole and the injured limb in particular. It is still necessary to continue with regular exercise sessions for all four limbs and trunk several times daily.

There are many theoretical and practical advantages and disadvantages of allowing early weight-bearing, and each fracture must be considered individually. Decision will depend upon the position and stage of healing of the fracture itself, the amount of soft-tissue injury, whether internal fixation has been used, and the general state of the patient. The after-care of fractures of the lower limb calls for the utilization of much of the art and skill of clinical practice, and critical decisions taken by the orthopaedic surgeon will often depend upon the calibre of the rehabilitation services available to him.

During the first few days after removal of plaster or caliper, walking is supervised closely. Initially the patient reverts to the use of crutches and partial weight-bearing, gradually increasing the weight taken by the fractured limb until full weight-bearing has been achieved.

Control of weight-bearing

Unless some disability prevents their use, standard elbow crutches are used to teach crutch walking. The length of the crutch upright from handgrip to tip is adjusted for each patient, the presence of an adequately grooved ferrule is checked, and handgrips and forearm grips are tested for comfort. In many cases this entails winding plastic foam round the rigid plastic from which the grips are made and then covering the padding with chamois leather or rexine.

Once weight-bearing begins, the patient is encouraged to take steps of equal length and to swing the injured leg in the natural rhythm of walking. Walking sticks are later substituted for the crutches and are retained until normal balance and a limp-free walk have been re-established. Regular class work in the gymnasium at this stage is designed particularly to improve the power and co-ordination of the calf muscles and so to promote a springy step, preparing the way to running, jumping and sporting activities as rehabilitation proceeds. For this reason also it is important to use two sticks and not one, when crutches are eventually discarded, since two sticks permit a more symmetrical walking pattern. They should be retained until rehabilitative treatment is completed and weight relief is no longer needed.

Assisted walking with crutches gives considerable weight relief to the fractured limb, but involves extra work for the other lower and both upper limbs. The performance of regular exercises for all four limbs and trunk throughout the period of patient immobilization and the gradual introduction of longer intervals of crutch walking interspersed with intervals of rest and elevation of both lower limbs are essential if discomfort and oedema are to be avoided.

Plaster walking

Efficient walking with a limb encased in plaster of paris involves the provision of a walking plaster which not only protects the fracture from stress, but also permits as normal a gait as possible. While the strength of the plaster protects the fracture, its shape and size influence gait. For ease of walking and to prevent unnecessary strain on other joints, the foot of the plastered limb needs to be in the plantigrade position (i.e. the neutral position) and not in the 10 degrees of flexion which is commonly advocated.

A rocker may be incorporated into the plaster sole and the patient is taught to walk by rocking himself vertically over the rocker which he uses as a fulcrum, assisting the following swing-through of the plastered limb by a pelvic 'hitch' from the quadratus lumborum, and using gluteal action to level the pelvis during the action of the rocking. The spring of the uninjured leg and the upward thrust from the crutch handles provide additional propulsion and lift for the plastered leg and help to prevent external rotation while pivoting on the rocker, and also circumduction during the swing-through phase.

An alternative to a rocker incorporated in the plaster sole is the use of an overboot with a rocker-type sole, which is worn over a walking plaster. This has many advantages, not the least being the greater ease with which a normal heel-toe gait may be acquired during its use. It protects the toes from trauma and cold and the plaster from rain. It facilitates the active participation of the long toe muscles during walking and the performance of exercises for the intrinsic muscles of the feet while at rest.

In patients who are frail or elderly or have a disability of the uninjured leg, a raise fitted to the shoe of the non-plastered leg may be needed to facilitate a more normal swing-through action of the plastered one.

Walking in calipers
The reduction of certain lower limb fractures is held by means of traction. This is maintained until the fracture has united, and the patient is then mobilized in a weight-bearing caliper. A simple half-ring caliper, ischial-bearing and of adjustable length, permits partial weight-bearing with fracture protection until consolidation has occurred. Use of such a caliper reduces the long period of bed rest otherwise necessitated by the treatment of some inherently unstable fractures and allows muscle strength and joint range to be built up by the greater range of exercises which ambulation makes possible. The caliper is removed for non-weight-bearing mobilizing exercises during the regular sessions of physiotherapy in the gymnasium and warm pool which are incorporated into the daily routine of the ambulant patient. Repeated instruction and possible adjustment of the caliper is essential to ensure that it is fully weight-relieving and is providing adequate protection against stress for the fracture concerned.

Walking without protection
When fracture consolidation has been confirmed by radiological and clinical examination, full weight-bearing without fracture protection becomes permissible, and caliper and plaster alike are discarded.

The success and comfort of the ensuing period of rehabilitation depend upon the extent to which the patient has carried out his earlier exercise programme of muscle exercise and joint movement, the efficiency with which hypostatic oedema of his fractured leg can be controlled, and his total motivation to regain normal function.

The time at which protection is removed varies with the type of fracture, the blood supply to the fractured limb, and the age, constitution and associated injuries of each patient. Allowing for these variable factors, it is nevertheless possible to make an approximate forecast of the probable times at which union and consolidation are likely to occur in any particular type of fracture.

Cast bracing

Non-operative management of fractures of the long bones of the leg imposes a relatively long period of immobilization and consequently a long period of remobilization and rehabilitation. Internal fixation permits early mobilization and thus early restoration of function. Consequently open reduction and internal fixation, particularly intramedullary fixation, has found considerable favour. Recently a cast-brace device has been introduced which allows weight-bearing with joint movement some 6 − 8 weeks after fracture. The technique is particularly suitable for supracondylar and the more comminuted fractures of the femoral shaft which are least amenable to internal fixation.

The fractures are treated by reduction or skeletal traction. As soon as the patient's condition allows (one to three weeks after injury) the cast-brace is applied. In essence, the device consists of an above and below knee cast with a caliper-type knee joint. The casts are carefully moulded to the patient and the knee joints (often polycentric) are carefully fitted with a special zip and incorporated into the above and below knee casts.

BIBLIOGRAPHY AND REFERENCES

Apley, G.A. (1968). *A System of Orthopaedics and Fractures* (3rd edn). London; Butterworths

Connolly, J.F., and King, P. (1973). 'Closed reduction and early cast brace ambulation in the treatment of femoral fracture. Pt. 1.' *J. Bone and Jt. Surg.* 55A, 1559

Connolly, J.F., Dehne, E., and Larollette, B. (1973), 'Closed reduction and early cast brace ambulation in the treatment of femoral fracture. Pt 2.' *J. Bone and Jt. Surg.* 55A, 1581

Gardner, D.C., Goodwill, C.J. and Bridges, P.K. (1968a). 'Absence from work after fracture of the wrist and hand.' *J. occup. Med.* 10, 114

Gardner, D.C., Goodwill, C.J. and Bridges, P.K. (1968b). 'Cost of incapacity due to fractures of the wrist and hand.' *J. occup. Med.* 10, 118

Nichols, P.J.R. (1963). 'Rehabilitation after fracture of the shaft of the femur.' *J. Bone Jt. Surg.* 45B, 1, 96–102

Nichols, P.J.R. and Parish, J.G. (1959a). 'Rehbilitation after fractures of the tibia and fibula.' *Ann. phys. Med.* 5, 3, 73–87

Nichols, P.J.R. and Parish, J.G. (1959b). 'Rehabilitation of malleolar fractures of the tibia and fibula.' *Ann. phys. Med.* 5, 128–40

Nichols, P.J.R. and Wynn Parry, C.B. (1958). 'Rehabilitation after reconstruction of the shoulder for recurrent forward dislocation.' *Ann. phys. Med.* 4, 8, 281–7

Sarmiento, A. (1967). 'A functional below knee cast for tibial fracture.' *J. Bone and Jt. Surg.* 49A, 855

Watson-Jones, Sir R. (1955). *Fracture and Joint Injuries* (4th edn.). London; Livingstone

Wynn Parry, C.B. and Nichols, P.J.R. (1966). 'Rehabilitation.' *Clin. Surg.* 12, 236–64

Wynn Parry, C.B., Nichols, P.J.R. and Lewis, R.N. (1958). 'Meniscectomy, a review of 1723 cases.' *Ann. phys. Med.*, 4, 6, 201–15

Wynn Parry, C.B. (1973). *Rehabilitation of the Hand* (3rd edn). London; Butterworths

9 Disorders of Peripheral Nerves

CHRISTOPHER WYNN PARRY

A wide variety of conditions can affect the peripheral nerves. They all cause the same clinical disorders – wasting and weakness of muscles, sensory loss and paraesthaesiae, the brunt usually falling on the distal part of the limbs. Some aetiological agents favour motor rather than sensory nerves, some sensory rather than motor, and in a few diseases the clinical pattern is specific enough to be almost diagnostic as in, for example, diabetic neuropathy and porphyria. In a few conditions the face is also affected – such as sarcoid, and the Guillain Barré neuropathy.

But in the majority of clinical conditions it is with sensory-motor problems in the hands and feet that patients present.

It is not far from the truth to say that if the presenting cause of a peripheral neuropathy is not obvious clinically, or is not made clear by the routine screening tests, a definitive cause is unlikely to be found in over half the cases, despite exhaustive investigations. Clearly remediable causes must be sought, and the common conditions that are treatable always kept in mind when diagnosis is being considered.

The following are common causes:

(1) *Trauma*
   (a) Direct violence, such as putting the hand through a window or falling on glass and severing the median and ulnar nerves at the wrist.
   (b) entrapment, such as compression of the median nerve in the carpal tunnel or the ulnar nerve at the elbow.
(2) *Infections*   Leprosy is by far the single commonest cause of neuropathies in the world. With travel so widespread, it must constantly be kept in mind. Sarcoid. Tuberculosis.
(3) *Metabolic*   Diabetes, uraemia.
(4) *Deficiency diseases*   Particularly the B vitamins – Beri Beri, subacute combined degeneration of the cord.
(5) *Alcoholism*   Both direct poisoning of the nerve and due to vitamin deficiencies as a result of too liquid a diet.
(6) *Guillain Barré syndrome*   Probably an autoimmune response to a virus.
(7) *Carcinomatous neuropathy*   This refers to a group of neurological disorders associated with a small primary carcinoma and due to some abnormal reaction (whether metabolic or immunological is not known). Often they

144

precede the demonstration of the primary by months or years and the peripheral nerve disorder may be the first sign of malignancy. The common manifestations are a proximal myopathy, a mixed sensory-motor neuropathy, a myaesthenic syndrome, a cerebellar picture, or dementia.

(8) *Poisons*   Such as organic phosphorus compounds in weedkillers and oils, lead, arsenic.

(9) *Collagen diseases*   Rheumatoid arthritis can affect the nerves in a variety of ways. Pressure of Rheumatoid Synovitis on the flexor tendons can compress the median nerve in the carpal tunnel, or a large effusion in the elbow joint compress the ulnar nerve. There is a specific affection of the digital nerves giving patchy sensory loss – carrying a good prognosis. Rheumatoid vasculitis can affect one or more nerves, and there is finally the diffuse symmetrical polyneuropathy, usually associated with a high titre of rheumatoid factor and a poor prognosis. Other causes are amyloid infiltration and generalized amyloidosis.

(10) *Drugs*   Phenytoin, isoniazid, thalidomide.

(11) *Hereditary neuropathies*   Hereditary motor sensory neuropathies recently classified by Thomas, Dyck and Lambert (1975).

Peripheral neuropathies can be classified by cause, by clinical presentation, or by pathology. Thus one speaks of mononeuritis simplex (a single nerve e.g. an isolated foot drop), mononeuritis multiplex (two or more nerves affected), and diffuse symmetrical polyneuropathy.

Pathologically there are two major disorders depending on whether the disease process involves primarily the axis cylinder or the myelin sheath. Toxins and poisons tend to affect the axis cylinder, whereas the rheumatological and malignant disorders affect the myelin sheath, causing segmental demyelination. These two varieties can be distinguished by electrical studies, for conduction is markedly slowed in the demyelinating neuropathies. The prognosis tends to be better in these, for the myelin can reform whereas any degree of axis cylinder disease usually leads to permanent weakness. In some neuropathies there are elements of both.

In myelopathies the disease process affects the anterior horn cells, such as poliomyelitis, syringomyelia, and motor neurone disease. In some neurological diseases such as Charcot-Marie-Tooth disease there is a mixed neuropathy and myelopathy. Whatever the cause the clinical picture is similar.

Motor involvement causes weakness, wasting and contractures if not prevented. Sensory involvement has two effects: loss or diminution of sensation, i.e. touch, pain, temperature, pressure sense; and paraesthesiae, i.e. tinglings, pins and needles, electric shocks in the distribution of the nerve affected, commonly being most pronounced in the terminal parts – fingers and toes. Affection of the automatic system causes stagnation of the circulation with colour changes – blue in cold weather, red in hot weather. These are excessive reactions to heat and cold, and they may cause severe burning pain which is worst at night, driving patients to all sorts of manoeuvres to gain relief, e.g. placing electric fans by the feet, or sleeping with the feet in cold water. Trophic lesions can easily develop from lack of care in anaesthetic areas – cold burns from the refrigerator, cigarette burns, burns from inadvertently leaning the anaesthetic hand on a hot radiator.

ASSESSMENT

Whenever possible it is desirable to record function quantitatively so as to judge the progress of the disorder and the value of treatment.

Motor function

Muscle bulk can be measured and the quality of the reflexes recorded. The MRC grading of power 0—5 is universally used. Often a more subtle grading is required and use of dynamometers to measure power grip, and strain-gauges to measure individual muscles such as the first dorsal interosseus or pinch grip, are valuable.

Sensory function

Classically the response to touch using the Von Frey hair and the response to pain with a pin are used. Two point discrimination (2PD) measures fibre density not function, for it is well established that sensory function after nerve repair can be good but two point discrimination is almost invariably poor, being 15 mm or more (Wynn Parry, 1976: Javely, 1976). 2PD is useful to assess severity of disease and progress but not as a yardstick of function.

We have for many years included in our routine sensory testing, the ability of the blindfold patient to recognize objects and textures and to localize a touch. These seem to us realities of sensation.

Autonomic function

Temperature is recorded, presence or absence of sweating, trophic lesions and the atrophy of the fingers and toes.

Trick movements can deceive the uninitiated into thinking muscles are working when they are not. The classic example is the ability of patients to extend the interphalangeal joint of the thumb in a complete radial nerve palsy through the action of the short abductor and flexor of the thumb which have an insertion into the extensor expansion. The trick is soon spotted if the patient is prevented from abducting the thumb. The long extensor tendons can imitate abduction of the fingers in ulnar nerve paralysis. If the hand is laid flat on the table and the middle finger raised in the air attempts to abduct will fail and a characteristic movement of the palm and wrist from side to side is seen, the fingers remaining still, the extensor tendon being prevented from abducting as it is fully occupied in maintaining the finger raised (Wynn Parry, 1973). In a complete foot drop it can seem as if the tibialis anterior is working, for a strong movement of plantar flexion followed by relaxation causes a rebound and the ankle dorsiflexes slightly. The tendon must always be felt as well or the muscle watched in order not to be misled by these trick actions.

In circumflex nerve lesions the deltoid is paralysed, but full abduction and elevation is often possible (and can almost always be taught). The infraspinatus externally rotates the humerus and this allows the clavicular fibres of pectoralis major and the long heads of the biceps and triceps to act as elevators. The brachioradialis can provide very strong elbow flexion in paralysis of the biceps.

Functional assessment

What, of course, really matters to the patients is what functional disability does the neuropathy cause. It is essential to record a realistic functional profile. In lower limb disorders, how far can the patient walk? How many stairs? What aids are required? In upper limb disorders, what are the problems of dressing, feeding, toilet, writing, work, hobbies? There is no universally accepted method of assessment, so much depends on the use to which the patient puts his limbs. An assessment for a labourer is quite different from a watchmaker, and the assessment for a patient with rheumatoid disease different from a patient with hemiplegia.

Two useful indices are the Northwick Park assessment scheme (Sheik *et al.*, 1974) and the Barthel Index (Mahoney and Baning, 1965). Both attempt to quantify function and thus allow comparison of ability and disability over a period of time. Often an individual assessment scheme has to be drawn up for each patient and repeated testing will show alterations. Accuracy, and time taken to complete a set task in the workshops are measured. Many of the tests to measure hand function require a combination of motor and sensory skills, and it is not possible to dissociate the two. One must be absolutely clear as to what one is testing – motor power, sensation – or co-ordination, a combination of the two.

ELECTRODIAGNOSIS

Electrical investigations in peripheral nerve disorders are of great value in diagnosis and assessment of progress.

Diagnosis

In cases where doubt exists as to whether the lesion is in the peripheral nerve, muscle or anterior horn cell, electromyography will help to localize the lesion.

In muscle disease voluntary effort is accompanied by a full pattern of units on the oscilloscope screen but the units are low in amplitude and of short duration – muscle fibres are lost but the number of motor units is not diminished. In myelopathies the number of units is reduced as the disease attacks anterior horn cells. Many of the units will be of much larger amplitude than normal, because neighbouring normal axons send sprouts to incorporate denervated fibres within their territory – the so called giant units. As the surviving motor units are normal, motor conduction velocity will be normal or only slightly reduced – measurement of the amplitude of the response of the muscle using surface electrodes to supra maximal stimulation will be reduced in proportion to the loss of motor units and serial studies are a guide to progress of the disease.

In neuropathies the findings depend on whether the disease attacks mainly the myelin or the axis cylinder.

In myelin disorders conduction velocity is considerably reduced, for the speed and conduction along the axon depends on the intact myelin sheath – so called saltatory conduction. In extreme cases, when almost all myelin has atrophied, conduction is by transmission along the axis cylinder itself and no longer jumps from one node of Ranvier to another – speeds as low as 10 metres per second are recorded compared with the normal of 50 metres per second or greater. Sensory conduction is often reduced earlier than motor conduction and it is not uncommon to be unable to detect sensory action potentials in the fingers or along the sural nerve when motor conduction is normal and even when sensory symptoms are minimal. If there is localized pressure over a nerve, as in the entrapment neuropathies, there is slowing of motor and sensory conduction at that level. In an ulnar neuritis at the elbow for example, sensory action potentials will be reduced or absent from little finger to wrist and from wrist to elbow, but will be normal from above elbow to axilla. Motor conduction velocity will be normal in the upper arm and forearm but slowed across the elbow: amplitudes recorded over the abductor digiti minimi will be normal when stimulating at the wrist but reduced when the ulnar nerve is stimulated above the elbow. These objective measurements allow a precise localization of the level of compression and serial studies will show if the lesion is deteriorating or recovering after surgical transposition. Such studies are invaluable in distinguishing if symptoms of paraesthesiae in the median nerve distribution are due to pressure in the carpal tunnel – when sensory and motor conduction will be normal in the forearm but slowed at the wrist – and cervical spondylosis when they will be normal.

In the Guillain Barré syndrome serial electrical studies are of the greatest help in prognosis. As the disease process recedes so the amplitudes of the sensory and motor unit action potentials will steadily increase and conduction velocity becomes faster.

In some cases of the Guillain Barré disorder the brunt of the disease falls on the axis cylinder when denervation as shown by fibrillation will be pronounced, whereas in others the disorder is primarily one of segmental demyelination when fibrillation will be scanty and the predominant finding is gross slowing of conduction.

In lesions of the brachial plexus, it is important to establish whether the roots are avulsed from the spinal cord, in which case recovery is impossible, or if there is a lesion in continuity, when some spontaneous recovery can be expected, or a rupture of a root distal to the intervertebral foramen which is amenable to nerve grafting.

The demonstration of sensory action potentials in the presence of anaesthesia must mean that the lesion is proximal to the posterior root ganglion. Demonstration of fibrillation potentials only and no units on effort indicate a complete lesion – in the case of the posterior spinal muscles this again implies a preganglionic lesion, and in the rhomboids a very high lesion with a poor prognosis.

There are a number of factors that help to distinguish these three types of lesion. The more associated injuries, the higher the speed of impact, the more likely is a rupture or avulsion. The presence of severe burning pain in the hand and a Horner's syndrome and meningoceles on myelography indicate avulsion of T1 at least.

The implications for treatment are these: if the lesion is an avulsion then the possibility of neurotization, rerouting the accessory nerve or the intercostals into the musculocutaneous or median nerves, arises in order to restore some proximal function – elbow flexion, adduction of the arm and possibly finger flexion.

If there is a strong painful Tinel Sign in the neck referred to the root dermatome then a rupture can be suspected and grafting undertaken. It has repeatedly been shown that traction lesions in continuity have a reasonable prognosis and it is the concensus of opinion among the experts in this field that resection of fibrotic sections of nerve is unjustified and only neurolysis should be attempted.

Thus electromyography in conjunction with history and clinical signs will materially help in deciding the rehabilitation of these tragic injuries. Electromyography is of great help in assessing the success of nerve suture, sometimes recovery is delayed and the detection of polyphasic recovery potentials will reassure the surgeon that all is well. Serial recordings of motor unit action potentials will show if reinnervation is progressing and will help to decide if re-exploration is needed.

In all peripheral neuropathies these tests help to establish the degree and extent of nerve involvement, the preponderance of motor or sensory affection, and the rate and degree of recovery or deterioration, and should be a routine aid in their management.

MANAGEMENT

The specific treatment of neuropathies of course is determined by the aetiology — stabilization of diabetes, control of the rheumatoid process, removal of poisons or drugs, vitamin replacements, dapsone therapy and removal of malignant tumours.

In traumatic lesions of nerves, definitive repair is required if the nerve sheath has been divided (neurotomosis). Primary suture is indicated if the patient is seen within 6 hours, the wound is clean, and an experienced hand surgeon available; otherwise suture is delayed by 3 weeks or more when the extent of the damage can be more accurately assessed. Controversy is raging at present between the orthodox technique of repairing the epineurium or putting in interfascicular grafts. Millessi (1972) has reviewed this subject and it is clear that indications exist for each procedure.

The key to success lies not so much on accurate approximation of nerve ends in the hope of routing axons down their pre-existing channels for the work of Sunderland (1968) has shown that fascicles rotate, cross and interconnect at all levels and the architecture of the nerve is entirely different at a difference of 2 cm. Moreover a high proportion of axons never reach the periphery even in near perfect sutures (Wall, 1979). Tension of the suture line is perhaps the most important factor. To avoid this the nerve is mobilized and the joints flexed to facilitate approximation, or grafts are used, but here two suture lines have to be crossed. Among key factors in the overall result are careful *preoperative preparation* of the limb, restoration of full passive movements to joints, correction of deformity by intensive oil massage, slow stretches and serial plasters, and encouragement of maximal muscle power. The patient then understands what will be required of him when rehabilitation starts.

Management in the paralysed stage, whether one is dealing with wasting and sensory loss after a neuropathic disorder or after nerve suture, requires that paralysed joints must be kept mobile and deformities prevented by correct splinting. In the acute stage of a generalized neuropathy, e.g. Guillain Barré, the body must be kept in the position of function, the shoulders kept by pillows in 45° abduction, 30° forward flexion and neutral rotation, the elbow at 90° and neutral rotation, the wrist in 10° dorsiflexion, the fingers flexed at 45° and the MP joints and the thumb in half opposition. The back is supported by a rest, the hips in neutral rotation and no more than 10° flexion. the knees *never* in more than 10° flexion, the ankles at 90° and neither inverted or everted. Light plaster or plastazote splints are the most convenient. If the muscles are acutely tender, hot packs are helpful and the joints put through a gentle range twice daily once pain has subsided. In severe Guillain Barré disease tracheostomy and assisted respiration are necessary and because of advances in intensive care, few such patients perish. Once the acute phase has passed, oedema must be prevented by elevation of the foot of the bed and massage and bandaging, and restoration of mobility and sensory function can start.

In paralysis of the shoulder muscles abduction splints are no longer used. In intrinsic paralysis it may be necessary to prevent the deforming action of unopposed antagonists.

The claw hand in ulnar paralysis can be corrected by a lively splint that prevents hyperextension at the MP joints and by virtue of a helical spring of piano wire at the MP joint allows active use of the hand. The 'monkey hand' of median paralysis can be treated by a splint which supports the thumb in palmar abduction, thus preventing the long thumb extensor stretching the paralysed thenar muscles and allows, by its spring, the long flexor to oppose the thumb to the fingers. In combined median and ulnar paralysis the two splints are combined.

Wrist drop is treated by a wrist support which by virtue of a spring at the wrist allows active movements. Perspex spider attachments sometimes help achieve finger extension.

Foot drop is most conveniently treated by an ortholene orthosis worn in the shoe. The material has enough spring to allow some active dorsiflexion. A special use of functional splinting can be seen in lesions of the brachial plexus.

In total elbow paralysis with sparing of the hand (C5–6 Palsy) an elbow lock splint allows the patient to position his elbow in one of four positions and this gives him stability for using his wrist and hand. If there is also a wrist drop, a wrist support can be added. If the whole arm is paralysed (C5–T1 lesion) patients often find the flail arm splint valuable. This consists of a supportive shoulder cap to counteract subluxation of the joint, the elbow lock as described and a forearm platform into which the terminal appliances of the standard artificial limb can be inserted and powered by a cable on the opposite shoulder.

To date we have supplied 50 patients with total plexus lesions with these splints and at one year follow-up 70 per cent were using them functionally at work or hobbies. Almost all found the basic splint valuable as a support, preferring it to a sling. It allows some function as a prop or support for tools, or stabilizing paper when writing, and many of our patients have helped in devising specific appliances for their individual jobs, e.g. gardening, engineering, model making. Moreover, the use of the splint keeps the paralysed arm in the body image and makes it much more likely that the patient will use his hand when reinnervation starts, either from surgery or spontaneously.

In the rare cases of femoral neuropathy (usually traumatic) paralysis of the quadriceps can be treated by a full caliper with knee stop, the Stanmore cosmetic caliper is light and efficient.

As recovery in the muscles progresses so the classical range of physiotherapy techniques are deployed, starting with gravity-eliminated active supported exercises in the pool or on a board, progressing to sling suspension and then to exercises against graduated resistance using the physiotherapist's hands, water and weights.

Proprioceptive neuromuscular techniques are invaluable. Interspersed with sessions in the physiotherapy department and in the pool, will be periods in occupational therapy in realistic crafts — metal work, carpentry etc. and later, periods in the swimming pool, general games in the gymnasium, walks, and cycle rides. A total integrated progressive programme is essential. Periodic quantitative assessment by muscle charting, dynamometers, amplitudes and velocities with electromyography and ratings of stamina in occupational therapy are helpful both to the therapist and patient. It is our practice to keep regular charts and patients are enormously encouraged to see progress when it may seem slow.

Biofeedback is helpful if patients have lost the idea of mucle action, which is often the case when nerves have been blocked for some time.

CASE HISTORY: MANAGEMENT OF A CASE OF ACUTE GUILLAIN BARRÉ POLYNEURITIS
V. Frampton MCSP, Senior Physiotherapist, Royal National Orthopaedic Hospital, Stanmore

Onset: 22.12.77
Admitted to hospital abroad. Within 24 hours of onset of flu-like illness he had virtual total paralysis of all limbs and impaired respiratory function – he first noticed weakness in his wrists, as he could not use his cigarette lighter. During the day he had increased difficulty in walking and by the evening he was virtually unable to walk, could not climb stairs, could not get up from sitting and was unable to undress or dress himself. He was admitted to hospital the following morning. Although his lung function was severely impaired he was never on a respirator. Despite prophylactic chest care he developed pneumonia which responded to antibiotics and physiotherapy.

Means of treatment in early stages:

(1) *Breathing exercises*   Diaphragmatic and intercostal breathing. Bird respirator three hourly (during period of pneumonia).
(2) *Passive movements to all limbs*
(3) *Splintage*   To rest ankles in dorsiflexion to prevent shortening of the tendo Achilles.
(4) *Positioning*   By the use of pillows and splints to support arms, wrists, fingers, hips and knees, and so preventing contractures and joint damage during period of muscle inactivity.

Aims of treatment – early stages:

(1) To maintain a clear chest.
(2) To prevent contractures.
(3) To maintain elasticity and extensibility of muscles.
(4) To prevent trophic skin lesions.

Recovery:
Recovery started four to six weeks following onset. First active movement noticed in his fingers.

Assessments were carried out as follows:

(1) Measurement of passive movements of all joints and recorded on muscle chart.
(2) Muscle charting of shoulder girdle. All muscles MRC Scale. Repeated at

six-weekly intervals. As new muscles showed contraction they were charted serially.

(3) Locomotor ability was charted, e.g. rolling to right and left, bridging, sitting to lying, sitting to standing, kneeling, standing and walking.

(4) Functional assessment. Activities of daily living by occupational therapists. Functional hand assessment.

(6) Video — a film was taken showing his locomotor ability, transfers from bed to chair, chair to standing, management of wheelchair, walking, stairs and hand activities. The video was repeated periodically to show patient and treatment staff his progress.

Aims of treatment at later stage:

(1) To maintain full range of movement in all joints.
(2) To re-educate and improve general locomotor mobility.
(3) Strengthen recovering muscles.
(4) Functional splinting; drop foot appliances.
(5) To restore hand function.
(6) Restore balance and co-ordination.

Means:

(1) Passive movements.
(2) Mat work — rolling, bridging, trunk strengthening, incorporating PNF patterns to shoulder and pelvic girdles, sit-ups — commencing with an incline of 45 degrees, gradually reducing this until he was able to sit up from lying flat and then from sitting up holding a weight.

Although he at no time had cutaneous sensory loss, his proprioceptive function was impaired and therefore he needed his own visual aid. This was helped by the use of mirrors during balancing exercises which included rhythmic stabilizations in all positions, i.e. long sitting, high sitting, prone kneeling, half kneeling, high kneeling, and throwing and catching a ball in these positions and also crawling, resisted crawling and co-ordination exercises, e.g. alternate elbow and knee flexion and extension to command.

Pool therapy including hydrotherapy and swimming in large indoor pool with the aid of rings.

Owing to muscle imbalance he had very poor hip control and this was a great hindrance in walking and transference from sitting to standing.

Gait re-education:

Walking with elbow crutches held on with tubigrip (because of loss of strength in grip of hand), transfers using crutches as a lever to get up, firstly from sitting on a high plinth and then gradually increasing until he was able to stand up from his chair. Because of his very weak quadriceps (Grade 2) and weak glutei (Grade 2) as well as hamstrings and ankle dorsiflexors he walked by hyperextending his knees; by increased lordosis he stabilized his hips. The use of ortholene splints corrected his foot drop and thus he managed 4 point gait with crutches.

Facilitatory techniques: (upper limb)

(1) PNF patterns   active assisted/active movements to arms, slow reversals, repeated contractions, static holds. To encourage overflow into wrist extensors and flexors.
(2) Re-education board for wrist and elbow flexors and extensors, gravity counteracted using quick stretch and active assisted movements.
(3) Brisk stroking and 'slapping' to biceps, triceps, wrist flexors and extensors. These exercises were made more difficult as strength increased by use of increased force of gravity by increasing incline of the re-education board until he was able to resist gravity (Grade 3). Having reached this stage he progressed on to intermediate stage exercise as follows:
(4) Push-ups on pummels, press-ups for latissimus dorsi, serratus anterior, etc.
(5) PNF   Bent and straight arm patterns, active resisted movements, bilateral arm patterns, repeated contractions, static holds, slow reversals with quick change from strong pattern into weak pattern.
(6) In later stage the use of Westminster pulleys, poundage being regularly increased.

Facilitatory techniques: (upper limb)

(1) Active assisted hip and knee flexions by use of re-education board and springs, also by using spring in this position enabled active resisted knee and hip extension was encouraged.
(2) Brisk stroking and 'slapping' to quadriceps, anterior tibial group, and hamstrings, incorporating quick stretching and static holds. Owing to proprioceptive loss re-education of hamstrings in prone lying was not effective but use of PNF in high sitting was more effective when augmented by visual aid.
(3) Hip abduction and adduction — gravity eliminated re-education board — progressing to gravity resisted side lying, progressing onto intermediate exercises.
(4) Quadriceps exercises — knee extension over low edge, progressing to lifting weights.
(5) Graded resisted strengthening exercises to hip flexors, extensors, abductors, and adductors.
(6) PNF patterns resisted bent and straight leg patterns, bilateral leg patterns.

Walking:
Early stage: Walking with two crutches, 4-point gait.
Intermediate stage: Two sticks 4-point gait progressing to 2-point gait.
On discharge: Was able to walk unaided but used one stick out of doors.
   In the early stages of recovery intrinsic function was poor and his power grip too weak to grip crutches or bannisters. This was aided by the use of a non-slip leather hand grip, worn like a mitten and fastened with velcro. He managed to continue to use the hand although thumb abduction and opposition was virtually lost, by using trick movements and he did not use any splintage on the hand with the exception of Futura wrist splints which he used for some activities requiring more strength.

Treatment of the hand in the early stage was by:

(1) Passive movements to all joints, also stretching of the thumb web.
(2) Hand games (occupational therapy) to improve precision grip, power grip, activities in the workshop (making a backgammon board).

Towards discharge, he began a programme of walking around the grounds, encountering different surfaces, steps and slopes, and on discharge was walking distances of ¾ − 1 mile.

SENSORY RE-EDUCATION

During the paralysed stage trophic lesions must be prevented by constant education of the patient to avoid hot and cold to the skin. Gloves should be worn in any but the mildest weather, and care taken of the nails. Once sensation returns to the finger tips and fingers, it has been found most valuable to start formal sensory re-education. Theoretically, it should not be necessary to re-educate neuropathies for the correct axons should reach their receptors. In practice this is not always so − reinnervation may exceed the period of nine months, by which time receptors have atrophied (Wyke, 1979) and re-education will help in their reformation. After neurotmesis re-education is essential.

It used to be thought that the inevitable cross innervation after nerve suture made stereognosis impossible, if a fibre distined for a pressure corpuscle innervated a touch receptor then false information would be transmitted centrally. The poor 2PD after nerve suture reinforced the view that sensory function must be poor.

We now know that receptor specificity is much less clearcut than classical teaching has led us to believe. Receptors are organized in units that have a specially low threshold to one specific modality but fire off with almost any type of stimulus, and it is not so much the actual receptor that determines the sensation felt centrally but the spatial and temporal patterns along groups of nerve fibres.

To recognize an object we instinctively rub it between fingers and thumb to produce a series of impulses both spatially and temporally orientated. We cannot recognize an object if it is placed statically on a finger tip and so 2PD is not a measure of function.

We have shown that sensory training can restore a high degree of stereognosis and that recognition of objects and textures can be not far short of normal yet 2PD is as Onne (1962) correctly stated, very poor (Wynn Parry and Salter, 1976). Patients have been able to take up needlework again and play keyboard instruments.

Training is started as soon as sensation returns to the finger tips. In a lesion at the wrist this will usually be between 6 and 9 months. The patient is blindfold, or if co-operative, shuts his eyes, and a number of different blocks of wood of various shapes and weights are presented to him. He is asked to feel round them and describe their shape − oblong, square, round; note if the surfaces are all identical and to put them in order of weight. The rationale is to introduce him to the basic parameters of sensation − texture, shape, density, temperature. If he fails he then opens his eyes and relates what he feels to what he sees. The tests are repeated, the time for recognition taken and numbers of correct answers are recorded. Once he becomes adept at this procedure, large familiar objects are used, then textures, and finally small objects. Variations are introduced as, for example, asking the patient to find a named object in a bowl of sand, to put different shaped pieces into their correct place in a cut-out board, or to spell words using wooden letters. The therapist encourages the patient to describe out loud the various parameters and to build them up into a meaningful image. Thus, for example, in feeling a key he will describe its texture, its temperature, its shape, and work out what it must be by its particular configurations. Short sessions of 10 minutes repeated 2-3 times a day have been found to yield the best results. Patients get easily tired and frustrated if sessions are prolonged. At monthly intervals tests are carried out with different objects from those used in the training, and the number correctly identified, and the time taken is recorded. If he cannot identify the nature of the object within 60 seconds a failure is recorded. At no time is the patient told if he is right or wrong in the test situation in order to minimize a training effect.

Localization is always disturbed after nerve lesions and correct localization is therefore taught also. The patient is blindfolded and asked to indicate where he is being touched. The site indicated is recorded on a chart and if incorrect, the patient opens his eyes and relates what he feels to what he sees. The therapist then gives systematic training, starting proximally and progressing distally. Within 5 weeks it is usually possible to restore almost perfect localization.

PAIN

In the early stages of neuropathy pain can be a prominent and distressing feature. The severe burning pain in diabetic autonomic neuropathy prevents sleep and has been known to lead to suicide. Unfortunately even careful control of the diabetes is not necessarily successful and drugs are not often helpful. Large doses of intravenous vitamins are always worth trying and transcutaneous electrical stimulation is sometimes dramatic. Richardson and Akil (1974) implanted a cerebral stimulator in a patient with a diabetic neuropathy and intractable pain with dramatic success — minutes of stimulation gave hours of relief.

The painful neuromas are not uncommon after nerve suture and often do not respond to repeated surgery even with meticulous fascicular suture under microscopic control.

Surgeons specializing in peripheral nerve lesions are only too familiar with the patient who has had two or even three attempts at suture without relief of pain and patients with amputation stumps of fingers who suffer severe paraesthesiae and burning pains that prevent function and make life a misery. Causalgia refers to the burning pain in the territory of a partially damaged nerve so graphically described by Weir Mitchell (Melzack 1973) which renders the patient a nervous wreck, prey to even the mildest external stimulus that exacerbates his pain.

Recent advances in neurophysiology have partly lifted the veil of this mysterious realm. We now know that damage to peripheral nerves leads to spontaneous discharges of small diameter unmyelinated fibres which are supersensitive to noradrenalin (Wall and Gutnick, 1974; Wall and Scadding, 1979), and that sympathetic blocking by guanethedine or other anti-sympathetic drugs can successfully abolish or modify this pain.

Wall has pointed out that when peripheral nerves are damaged there are central effects also. Any degree of deafferentation is likely to release spontaneously firing neurones in the dorsal horn which is construed as pain. The extreme example is the continuous burning pain of the plexus avulsion, unaffected by any external stimuli, electrical stimulation or drugs, the experimental counterpart of which is beautifully shown by Loeser and Ward (1967). Wall and Gutnick (1974) showed that the spontaneous firing of painful neuromas could be inhibited by electrical stimulation. Electrical stimulation (TES) has proved its value in such patients and we routinely treat such patients with prolonged spells of stimulation.

The precise positioning of the electrodes and the parameters of pulse duration, frequency, and amplitude of current are a matter of trial and error. It is important to apply this treatment for prolonged periods — 2 hours, 2 or 3 times daily is far more successful than short spells, and it is this that has led to disappointing reports from some centres.

It is likely that TES works both distally by preventing the discharges of small fibres and centrally by selectively stimulating the large diameter fibres which it is known inhibit the activity of cells in laminas I and V to which the nociceptive fibres relay (Cervero, 1976). There is no doubt that TES is a major breakthrough in these painful neurological conditions. Being non-invasive and non-painful it is always worth a trial (Wynn Parry, 1979).

CASE HISTORY

On November 30th Mrs. E.K. fell while carrying a milk bottle and sustained lacerations of the palm of the left hand leading to loss of feeling in the thumb and index finger. The median nerve was repaired on the same day.

Thereafter she complained of increasing pain in the thumb and index fingers. In January 1977 the median nerve was explored and found to be densely scarred. It was freed and silastic was wrapped around the nerve. This in no way relieved her pain. When seen in September she could not use the thumb, index or middle fingers. There was marked hyperpathia and much spontaneous paraesthesiae and burning pain. It was aggravated by cold, touch and vibration. Striking improvement followed two weeks of TES 2 hours twice a day combined with intensive exercises and occupational therapy. She could hold cups, and knit for the first time in 4 years.

All went well until February 1978 when the symptoms returned, for no obvious reasons.

In May she had another operation. The silastic was removed and the median was grafted to the radial digital nerve, using 6 cm sural graft. The pain recurred in June but rapidly responded to the same regime of TES and activity as before. In December she was using the hand normally, had virtually no pain, and used the stimulator occasionally if the pain threatened to recur.

RECONSTRUCTIVE SURGERY

There are occasions when recovery does not occur or is insufficient for adequate function. In severe axis cylinder neuropathies there may be permanent paralysis of the intrinsics so that fine hand function is poor, or foot drop prevents a normal gait. In plexus lesions there may be permanent elbow paralysis (C5—6) or permanent wrist drop (C7). The following reconstructive procedures are available.

Shoulder paralysis: It is impossible to restore elevation of the shoulder by dynamic muscle transfers. Occasionally transfer of latissimus dorsi and teres major to the rotator cuff can allow external rotation and if pectorals are working some abduction. More often shoulder stability is given by arthrodesis.

Elbow paralysis: Three procedures are available. The Steindler operation in which the original common flexor and extensor origins are moved further up the humerus. Elbow flexion for the first year after operation is perforce accompanied by flexion of the fingers.

The pectoralis major can be inserted into the biceps but it is often necessary to perform an external rotation osteotomy of the humerus to prevent the excessive adduction of the arm in elbow flexion.

Recently whole muscle transfer of the latissimus dorsi has been used to replace the biceps and this bids fair to be a highly successful procedure, having neither of the drawbacks of the other two operations.

Wrist drop: Radial palsy or C7 lesion. The standard tendon transfers here are flexor carpi ulnaris into extensor communis and extensor pollicis longus and pronator teres into extensor carpi radials brevis and palmaris longus, if present, into abductor pollicis longus. If insufficient tendons are available for transfer arthrodesis of the wrist allows the use of a flexor to give finger extension.

Median paralysis: Opposition can be restored by transferring flexor sublimus of the ring finger into the first metacarpal and extensor expansion.

Ulnar paralysis: Often no surgery is needed but if pinch grip is poor, extensor pollicis brevis is put into the first dorsal interosseus. Clawing can be controlled by Zancolli's procedure of plicating the volar plate and tightening the structures in front of the MP joint.

Foot drop: Tibialis posterior can be put into tibialis anterior. Arthrodesis of the ankle is sometimes helpful.

Muscles must be at least MRC grade 4 as they lose one grade on transfer. When muscles are not available for transfer functional splints can be worn permanently and we have five patients with plexus lesions who have been wearing elbow splints and wrist drop attachment for skilled work for several years.

CASE HISTORY

Mr. A. had an obscure heredo-familial neuropathy which gave him a bilaterial foot drop and inability to extend his wrist and fingers. Unfortunately he sustained a complete left-side brachial plexus avulsion and he was greatly dependent on his right hand. The condition had been static for some years, so the classical radial tendon transfers were carried out which improved his function in eating, dressing, and writing. His bilateral foot drops were controlled with ortholene supports.

CONCLUSION

The causes of neuropathies are legion but all present the same problem in management. Accurate diagnosis leading to definitive treatment, whether of disease or injury, maintenance of joint range and prevention of deformity when paralysed, restoration of motor and sensory function when reinnervation takes place, and provision of appropriate splinting to encourage function and return to work early.

Finally, surgical reconstruction has much to offer when paralysis is permanent.

BIBLIOGRAPHY AND REFERENCES

Bradley, W.G. (1974). *Disorders of peripheral nerves.* Oxford; Blackwells

Cervero, F. and Ogawa, M. (1976). 'Nociceptor driven dorsal horn neurones in the lumbar spinal cord of the cat.' *Pain* 2, 5–24

Hall, M.R.P. (1970). 'The assessment of disability in geriatric patients.' *Rheum. U Rehab.* 15, 59

Javely, M.E., Burne, J.E., Oncutt, B.S., and Bryant, W.M. (1976). 'Comparison of histologic and functional recovery after peripheral nerve repair.' *J. Hand. Surg.* 2, 119–138

Loeser, J.D. and Ward, A.A. (1967). 'Some effects of deafferentation on neurons of the cat spinal cord.' *Arch. Neurol. (Chic.)* 17, 629–36

Mahoney, Fl. and Barthel, D.W. (1965). 'Functional evaluation. The Barthel Index.' *Maryland Med. J.* 14, 61

Melzack, R. (1973). *The Puzzle of Pain.* Penguin Books

Melzack, R. and Wall, P.D. (1965). 'Pain mechanisms. A new theory.' *Science* 150, 971–9

Millessi, M., Meissl, G. and Berger, A. (1972). 'The interfascicular nerve grafting of the median and ulnar nerves.' *J. Bone Jt. Surg.* 54A, 727–750

Richardson, D.E. and Akil, H. (1974). 'Electrical, surgical and pharmacological management of pain.' *Proc. Neuolect. Soc.* p. 50

Sheikh, D.S., Meade, T.W., Goldenberg, E., Brennan, P.J. and Kinsella, G. (1979). 'Repeatability and validity of a modified acitivites of daily living (ADL) index in studies of chronic disability.' *Int. Rehab. Med.* 1, 2, 51

Sunderland, S. (1968). *Nerves and Nerve Injuries.* Edinburgh and London; Livingstone

Thomas, P.K., Dyck, P.J., and Lambert, E.H. (1975). *Peripheral Neuropathies.* W.B. Saunders

Wall, P.D. and Gutnick, M. (1974). 'Properties of afferent nerve impulses originating from a neuroma.' *Nature* 248, 740–3

Wall, P.D. and Scadding, J. (In press)

Wall, P.D. (1979). Personal communication.

Wyke, B. (1979). Personal communication.

Wynn Parry, C.B. (1973). *Rehabilitation of the Hand.* Butterworths

Wynn Parry, C.B. and Salter, M. (1976). 'Sensory re-education after median nerve lesions.' *The Hand* 8, 250–7

Wynn Parry, C.B. (1979). 'Management of peripheral nerve injuries and traction lesions of the brachial plexus.' *Int. Rehab. Med. Assoc.* 1, 9–20

10 Strokes

THE NATURE AND SIZE OF THE PROBLEM

There are probably at present about half a million patients in the United Kingdom suffering from hemiplegia following a cardiovascular accident. Hemiplegia is therefore one of the most commonly occurring physical disabilities. The severity of the disability in any one hemiplegic patient depends on the density of the initial ischaemia, the adequacy of collateral circulation and the severity of the residual brain damage; these in turn vary with the type of acute lesion with which circulatory dysfunction presents.

Cerebral thrombosis associated with hypertension and arteriosclerosis, intracerebral haemorrhage, subarachnoid haemorrhage and cerebral embolism are the four main cerebrovascular lesions which may result in hemiplegia. Prognosis and the delineation of a programme of rehabilitation depend on a knowledge of the natural history of each condition. Unfortunately, it is often only possible to establish the diagnosis accurately at autopsy, since the presentation of all four lesions during life may be remarkably similar. Despite the difficulty of making an early differential diagnosis of the causative lesion, various general characteristics of the patient assist in prognostication of life expectancy and rehabilitation potential.

Mortality
Life expectancy varies inversely with age, severity of preceding hypertension, severity of accompanying cardiac dysfunction, and duration and depth of initial unconsciousness. As far as *cerebral embolism* is concerned, about 1 in 3 patients die within 3 months of the initial episode and a further one third die within 3 years. Thus two thirds die within 3 years, and the average survival period is 2 years. *Cerebral infarction* carries a slightly better prognosis, since only 1 in 4 patients with this condition dies within 3 months and another quarter die within 3 years. Only half are therefore dead in 3 years and the average survival time is 3 or 4 years.

Morbidity
The delineation of a realistic rehabilitation programme following stroke entails accurate and repeated assessments of the residual disability and functional capacity of any one patient. An early single assessment is often of little value,

since the patterns of recovery from stroke are so variable, and the earlier the assessment is made the less likely it is to give an accurate prognosis. Yet some initial tentative prognosis is urgently needed, so that the type of long-term care required may be given the earliest possible consideration, and an approximate plan of management formulated. Patient, relatives and remedial staff need information on the rate and extent of probable recovery, the ability to return home, and the care which will be needed either in the home itself or, alternatively, in a residential institution should return home prove impossible.

Such information requires not only an assessment of the patient's physical and mental condition both before and after the stroke, but also a knowledge of his premorbid education, training and skill, and an assessment of his home and social conditions.

Assessment of the clinical condition after a stroke embraces that selection of particular signs and symptoms, variable in number, association and degree, which follow a stroke in any one patient. These signs and symptoms are:

(1) Loss of motor power.
(2) Loss of sensation.
(3) Hemianopia.
(4) Aphasia.
(5) Apraxia.
(6) Dementia.
(7) Incontinence of urine.

In addition to the characteristics of the stroke itself, assessment of the clinical condition of a patient must take into account any associated disabilities which may be present.

Seventy-five per cent of the patients with stroke are over 60 years of age, and of those referred for rehabilitation to a hospital or a rehabilitation unit, 70 per cent are over 50 years and 25 per cent are over 60 years. Commonly associated disabilities in stroke patients are, therefore, arteriosclerosis, hypertension, diabetes mellitus, cardiac insufficiency, osteo-arthrosis, visual defects, hearing defects and the general frailties of the elderly.

The onset and the pattern of recovery from stroke is itself of prognostic value. The onset may be sudden or insidious; a gradually extending paralysis and prolonged, deepening unconsciousness indicate a bad prognosis. Usually the initial paralysis which develops is flaccid with absent tendon reflexes, becoming gradually hypertonic with exaggerated reflexes during the course of the first few days; persistence of flaccidity seems to carry a poor prognosis, and so, too, does intense hypertonicity. Spontaneous recovery starts soon after the initial episode and continues for many months, but usually the greatest degree of recovery is seen in the first few months and often in the first 6 to 8 weeks. Subsequent recovery is slower and correspondingly less likely to affect ultimate functional capacity; thus a patient who has not regained much of his personal independence and some ability to walk within 3 months of the onset of the stroke is unlikely to do so at a later date.

The rehabilitation potential of young hemiplegic patients naturally differs from that of patients in the older age group. Their functional recovery is likely to be swifter, and the prognosis is often less gloomy. Management is correspondingly different in detail, and rehabilitation should be planned on a more energetic basis.

REHABILITATION IN THE EARLY STAGES

General care

The immediate care of the patient with stroke depends on the severity of the cardiovascular accident and its effect on his condition, and is initially concerned with the maintenance of the life processes, the diagnosis of the causative lesion and its treatment, and the prevention of deterioration in the locomotor system while its control is no longer properly co-ordinated.

During the acute phase, physiotherapy is directed towards:

(1) Passive movements of all limb joints of the affected side to prevent contractures.
(2) Prevention of deformity by the use of a bed cage, foot-boards, axillary pillow, palmar wrist-splint.

While the patient is in bed, whether during the period of unconsciousness or during the early recovery stage, a foot-board to discourage foot drop and a bed cradle to remove the weight of the bed-clothes from the legs should always be used. During the early comatose phases, a pillow in the axilla may help to prevent a fixed adduction of the shoulder. These passive preventive measures are used to supplement more active measures to maintain joint range and prevent contracture. These will consist of putting all affected joints through the full range of movement several times each day. If the patient is unconscious, then the movement of the shoulders in particular, and all joints of both arms and legs should be carried out at regular nursing sessions. During these sessions the patient is turned, washed and cleaned; pressure areas are attended to, oral hygiene is carried out, and catheterization is undertaken when necessary.

During the initial phase of the acute post-stroke stage, the hemiplegia is usually flaccid and passive movements are relatively easily elicited. Great care and gentleness are required to prevent overstretching of muscles and ligaments and consequent soft-tissue damage. As spasticity supervenes, there is a continuing need for skill and experience if soft-tissue injury is to be avoided. The risks of a musculotendinous tear which later becomes calcified cannot be overemphasized. If the patient is dying, then unwarranted disturbance should be avoided, but if there is a reasonable chance of recovery, it is essential to avoid delay in active prevention of unnecessary stiffness and deformity.

The length of time the patient needs to be kept strictly bedridden will vary with the cause and severity of the lesion but should be minimal. As soon as possible, sitting and bed-edge activity are introduced (sitting, leaning and balancing exercises). At this stage, physical treatment is directed towards:

(1) Prevention of chest complications — breathing exercises, postural drainage (particularly for patients with a history of bronchitis).
(2) Continued mobilization of joints (particularly shoulder).
(3) Prevention of contractures of hip, knee and foot.
(4) Retraining in balance and postural control.

A stiff, painful shoulder may well permanently complicate the weakness and spasticity of the upper limb of the hemiplegic patient, unless the physiotherapist has been gentle in her handling of the arm and the nursing staff have refrained from pulling on the paralysed arm during nursing, toiletting and bed-making. A hemiplegic patient should *never* be moved by *one* member of the nursing staff unaided during the acute stage of stroke, but always by *two* nurses using a grip which obviates the need for traction on the paralysed arm.

Between sessions of exercises with the physiotherapist, the patient should lie on alternate sides when unconscious and should alternate between side and back when consciousness returns. When side-lying, the pelvis should be positioned so that the underlying half is displaced backwards, the legs should be partly flexed, and the hemiplegic arm supported on one pillow and held in partial abduction by another. If the paralysed hand tends to become swollen, the arm may be elevated and supported by a forearm cuff-sling from an upright stand beside or attached to the bed.

Speech disorders are common and in the very early stages may cause the patient considerable distress and frustration. It is often very worthwhile providing a simple communication board with appropriate pictures and words so that the patient can make known his requirements.

Early mobilization

As recovery begins, active rehabilitation is introduced. Standing, walking and arm mobilizing exercises, supplemented by passive movements of those joints which the patient cannot move himself, form the basis of early active treatment. The importance of regular exercise sessions on the bed cannot be over-emphasized and should be started as soon as the patient can be mobilized. Achieving the sitting or standing position is often complicated by defective balance and an apparent increase of spasticity when changing from the horizontal to the vertical position. However difficult they may be, voluntary movements of trunk and limb muscles and active attempts to sit and stand several times daily should be encouraged. Standing up and sitting down independently may be practised in the ward (or bedroom) if a stable 'geriatric' chair is placed facing the foot of the bed. The patient then grasps the bed-end and assists himself out of bed and into this chair. It is usually necessary to fix a foot-stop between the legs of the bed to prevent the patient's feet from sliding away from him while he practises these movements.

As soon as the patient is able to sit up and stand, his paralysed arm should be supported in a suitable sling. There are various designs which are suitable, their common features being that they give some support to the arm at or under the elbow to prevent glenohumeral subluxation and that they support the hand at such a level over the opposite breast that they prevent oedema of the hand and fingers. The common slings are the 'double loop' sling (with a loop over the hand and a loop over the upper forearm) and the 'trough sling'. Although the use of one of these slings prevents swelling of the hand and distraction of the shoulder, it may also predispose to stiffness of the shoulder and elbow unless the arm is removed from it frequently. Regular exercise sessions for the arm are particularly important for the patient who wears a sling.

The early walking training of a patient with a stroke is a time-consuming activity. At first it is necessary for the physioptherapist to have a colleague or a helper so that the first stages of standing and walking are controlled by two people, one on either side of the patient. While the leg is flaccid, a temporary back-splint made from plastic or plaster of paris may be helpful to prevent the leg 'giving way'. As spasticity supervenes, temporary drop-foot springs, slings, or even simple bandages may be used to help the patient through the swing phase of movement of the hemiplegic leg. Progression to walking bars, walking frames, quadruped sticks and walking sticks depends upon the patient's general rate of recovery.

After the first few weeks, rehabilitation can be directed towards functional activity, and it is at this stage that the complications and associated disorders which may accompany strokes play a dominant part in determining the rate of progress in the pattern of achievement.

Incontinence

While the patient is unconscious, catheterization may become necessary. Unless a highly efficient team is present to ensure regular aseptic, intermittent catheterization at frequent intervals, it is better to use an indwelling catheter, changing it weekly or fortnightly.

When consciousness returns, the patient may recover his ability to control micturition. The return of this ability may be indicated when the spigotted catheter is released at 2-hourly intervals and the patient attempts to micturate. The catheter is then removed, the patient is given a bottle or bedpan at frequent intervals, and, if co-operative, instructed how to assist micturition by tapping, pressing, squeezing or rubbing the abdominal wall overlying the bladder. Particular care is needed during this period with aphasic, demented, hemiplegic patients, as well as patients with sensory loss, since incontinence may be suspected merely because of urine spilt from receptacles which cannot be properly supported or utilized.

Most patients affected by incontinence regain some degree of control. If a normal micturition pattern does not return, it is possible to build up in many patients the ability to stay dry by frequent visits to the lavatory, regulated drinking of moderate quantities of fluid, and timed stimulation of the bladder to contract by manual stimulation of the abdominal wall, assisted by forward flexion of the abdomen and contraction of the abdominal muscles.

Some patients will remain incontinent, and no recovery of control of micturition of any sort can be taught them. The use of an indwelling catheter then becomes necessary as a permanent measure to keep female patients comfortable and socially acceptable. With the plastic disposable bag now available for catheter attachment, it is possible to fasten this around the thigh and so to retain some personal dignity. Women patients need to be persuaded into wearing longer skirts or else trouser suits if they are to wear the urinals inconspicuously. Small taps are fitted to the lower end of the plastic bags to enable them to be emptied. Male patients can more easily be fitted with satisfactory drainage appliances, and they have their trousers to conceal these urinals.

Particular care should be taken by all those giving care to a hemiplegic patient to ensure that these urinals are emptied regularly and remain concealed as much as possible. A burst, detached or leaking urinal may cause great distress to the fastidious patient for whom the idea of catheterization is often extremely distasteful.

Relationship of clinical findings and rehabilitation

Early assessment of the long-term prognosis is very difficult, but is all-important if realistic decisions and plans are to be made. The characteristics of strokes which bear most relevance in the long-term rehabilitation are: loss of motor power; disturbances of sensation, including perception of body image and visual field defects; spasticity; impairment of speech; impairment of mental status.

Motor problems

Loss of muscle power, muscle control and muscle tone all contribute to the disability, but motor defect alone is seldom a real bar to functional recovery. A patient with hemiparesis from polio may have complete independence, and a patient with an arm and a leg amputated on one side, although clearly handicapped, can achieve considerable functional skill. It is the disturbance of muscular tone inherent in stroke which has such a profoundly disabling effect. Not only must the patient who is hemiplegic from stroke compensate for the weakness due to loss of motor power, but he must also overcome the spasm of the affected muscles when he attempts voluntary movement of the hemiplegic side. This spasm is often cumulative in effect – a man who can walk two steps easily, may be forced to a halt after 20 because of inability to move his spastic limbs.

Sensory defects

A variable amount of sensory defect may accompany the unilateral loss of power and occurs in about 10–15 per cent of strokes. These are most frequently defects of superficial sensation (e.g. touch and temperature), but may involve cortical sensation (e.g. loss of joint position sense, spatial orientation or object recognition – astereognosis). A patient with defects of position-sense or astereognosis, or disturbance of spatial orientation and perception, is unable to respond to a training programme requiring the redevelopment of many functional activities. Thus, the failure of a patient to perform and improve as well as might be expected may well derive from sensory disturbance. Among those who care for hemiplegics, there is therefore a need for greater awareness of the possibility that such sensory disturbances may co-exist with the spastic hemiparesis. In their presence, the conventional rehabilitation programme and the expected standard of achievement may need considerable modification.

Sensory inattention (anoscognosia) is the denial of the true-self-image and occurs when a patient is either completely unaware of the hemiplegic side or refuses to admit that it is an integral part of himself. It usually involves touch or pain, but may involve hearing aversion. It may not be noticed by an observer unless specifically looked for. It is associated with right (non-dominant) hemisphere lesions, and although the clinical picture may improve slowly over many months, recovery is seldom significant. The condition indicates a poor prognosis for functional recovery. Such a patient may initially be thought unco-operative until anoscognosia is recognized. He is not, however, failing to co-operate, but is failing to achieve what is required of him because he is not properly aware of the presence and activity of affected parts of his body.

Any disturbance of body image leads to a sensation of instability associated with a fear of failling, which is quite distinct from the disturbances of balance which may occur through involvement of the vestibulocerebellar system or through impairment of visuospacial perception.

Impairment of perception of the body image interferes with activities such as dressing and walking. Persistent attempts to achieve these activities may be doomed to failure unless the patient can be taught to recognize, understand and compensate for his disturbed body image. A simple test is to ask the patient to draw a clock, a star or even himself. A characteristically distorted drawing is a clear indication that the patient is likely to have difficulty in activities requiring an awareness of the paralysed side.

Apraxia is the inability to perform previously learned, skilled tasks and can be demonstrated by the patient's inability to copy simple drawings of various designs. It should be distinguished from *ataxia* which is muscular inco-ordination. *Agnosia* means loss of ability to recognize the impact of sensory stimuli, and results in an inability to understand the function of the articles although the patient can clearly describe them. *Perseveration* is a response which is more appropriate to previous instructions than current ones and can be applied to speech and thought as well as action.

The disturbances of co-ordination of muscular action which result from such disturbances of sensation provide early indications that conventional physical therapy and rehabilitation regimes are likely to be unavailing. At best, their achievements will be minimal and will be accomplished only with great effort by the therapists concerned over long periods. Some units are now developing programmes of perceptual and behaviour training which may prove more rewarding.

Spasticity
The intensity of spasticity demonstrable in a hemiplegic patient is variable, and depends upon both cerebral and non-cerebral factors.

It is the extent and location of the cerebral damage which primarily determines the degree of spasticity or flaccidity of the affected muscles. Many non-cerebral factors exert a secondary affect upon the muscle tone, and it is important that those giving care should recognize these factors and enhance or counteract them to increase the patient's mobility.

Particularly important is the influence which body posture has on spasticity. A patient whose arm is semi-fixed in the typical hemiplegic position when the body is erect will often be able to move the arm through a wide range of movements when his body is supine. It is therefore incumbent on the physiotherapist to instruct the patient to exercise his hemiplegic limbs night and morning while lying on the bed, so that joint movement may be better maintained.

Intense or noxious stimuli of many kinds may provoke increased spasticity, particularly when due to infection, injury or increased mechanical tension. Thus, pressure sores, bladder distension, bladder infection or paronychia of the toes may be provocative. General cold also increases spasm, and spastic limbs need to be warmly clad in cold weather. Stretching of affected muscles likewise effects spasm, and for this reason the provision of a toe-raising spring to combat foot-drop in a hemiplegic patient tends only to increase the flexion which it attempts to counteract.

Mental factors as well as physical ones influence the degree of spasticity which a patient exhibits at any one time. Conditions of stress and strange surroundings exert an unnaturally potent effect upon the labile emotions of the stroke patient and are likely to increase spasm.

Many of the techniques of physiotherapy introduced in recent years attempt to employ spasticity on the one hand and to inhibit in on the other. It is sometimes necessary to teach the patient to use, for example, an extensor spasm to achieve standing or walking. More frequently, the physiotherapist attempts to reduce spasticity in order to achieve some more functional movement, or to increase the muscle power of those muscles which can oppose the effect of the spastic ones. The use of ice, the use of relaxation techniques, and many of the 'proprioceptive neuromuscular facilitation' techniques are directed towards this end. Biofeedback techniques, especially those using electromyographic recordings, may offer a useful technique of helping the patient reduce spasm.

The use of drugs, such as diazepam, during the day, will often enable the physiotherapist to achieve more active function and will also reduce uncomfortable nocturnal spasm. This drug's value must, however, be balanced against its soporific effect, and its tendency to inhibit intellectual activity and produce intractable lethargy. Its withdrawal frequently produces several days of malaise and depression. Nevertheless sustained stretching of a spastic muscle during 8–9 hours' sleep appears to be of more value than a few minutes' stretching two or three times a day. Thus adequate night doses of diazepam and the use of a lightweight plaster splint with some dorsiflexion of the ankle (vide infra) is more likely to prevent contractures of the calf muscles than intermittent treatment in a physiotherapy department. During the day, ice will often relax spasticity enough to allow the physiotherapist to assist active exercise for the antagonists of the spastic muscles.

Injections of alcohol (40–45 per cent) into the muscle belly near motor points often give some temporary relief. More accurate injection of the motor nerves with small quantities of 2 per cent aqueous phenol will usually have a more prolonged effect. Intrathecal phenol will destroy large motor and sensory nerve fibres with consequent reduction of voluntary power as well as interruption of the stretch reflex arc.

The presence of continuing pain or discomfort, or persistent interference with active function in an otherwise well-rehabilitated patient, should be an indication for considering surgical procedures to produce a more permanent reduction in the spasticity or its effects.

Speaking and writing
Right-sided hemiplegia is frequently accompanied by aphasia or dysphasia. The effects vary from complete inability to understand the spoken or written word, with failure to express thoughts and needs in speech and writing (global aphasia) to a mild difficulty in finding the right word or a slowing in the formulation of sentences, slight spelling difficulties or slowness in reading. Some speech defect is present in about 50 per cent of strokes.

Persistent aphasia (or dysphasia) – particularly global or receptive asphasia – has an adverse effect on rehabilitation. This accompanies about 15 per cent of strokes, and for these patients formal speech thereapy appears to be useless.

In the treatment of aphasia other than the global variety, the precise contribution of the speech therapist in re-establishing a patient's ability to speak has not been clearly established. There are some indications that it may be a supraliminal barrage of afferent visual and auditory stimuli which recalls speech in some cases; in others, the painstaking teaching of speech and reading from first principles may be needed as well.

Aphasia presents considerable problems as it is often accompanied by intellectual impairment shown even in a non-verbal test of intelligence. Repetition of words, with persistent use of wrong words, is common. Occasionally, there may be true anarthria or dysarthria when the muscles of speech are neurologically affected.

In all circumstances of difficulty after a stroke, it is important to establish a sympathetic, encouraging and stimulating environment; this means that all the personnel working with the patient, including nurses, physiotherapists and relatives, should collaborate with the speech therapist in working towards re-establishing normal speech.

For each patient, it is necessary to assess the level of understanding of speech and the written word and to establish a simple method of communication (sign-board writing, pad and picture). Difficulties in comprehension (receptive dysarthria) can be helped by training with visual clues accompanying spoken or written instructions. Executive dysarthria (difficulties in formulating words in the presence of normal understanding) can be helped by formal speech training using oral exercises (e.g. reading, word games and general social activity with friends, relatives, staff and other patients). Defects in reading *(alexia* or *dyslexia)* are difficult to treat but can sometimes be helped by simple practice in reading. The more severely affected patients require special techniques.

Agraphia or *dysgraphia* is in part due to the muscular paralysis of the right arm and in part due to central defects. Some dysphasic patients without paralysis have dysgraphia which may improve with practice. Writing practice is however very boring, and it is necessary to devise ways of maintaining interest, e.g. writing letters and compiling records of activities. There is a general belief that speech and writing ability will either recover, or not recover, whatever treatment is given, and there is little objective evidence of the benefits to be derived from speech therapy. However, most rehabilitation units treating hemiplegics find that speech and writing therapy are an important part of the patient's programme. These activities are often a reflection of the general active and encouraging approach of such a unit. Co-operation and collaboration between physiotherapist, occupational therapist and speech therapist is essential if optimal results are to be obtained. Patterns of activity are so interdependent that each therapist must have an understanding of the skills and contributions of the other.

Mental status

Successful rehabilitation depends upon the patient's ability to comprehend, accept and adjust himself to the level of physical disability and inconvenience inherent in any particular stage of recovery, as well as upon his ability to co-operate with procedures designed to improve function, e.g. exercises and use of aids and appliances. It therefore follows that the final functional efficiency of any particular patient is as much a product of his mental state as his physical condition. The patient who has sustained severe intellectual damage from his stroke, with little residual paralysis, may indeed be the more difficult to restore to his premorbid status. The various types of mental impairment which may accompany stroke differ widely in the effects which they have both on the retraining potential of the patient and on the actual retraining programme which is planned for him. Recognition of the particular type of impairment in any particular patient is therefore essential for the therapists and for the doctors who care for him, so that realistic goals of achievement may be set and presented to patient, relatives and employers alike.

The classification of the psychological effects of brain damage into impairment of perception, impairment of intellectual function, and changes in personality (and mood change), is within most therapists' capability to apply in the evaluation of their patients. With the assistance of clinical and educational psychologists, specialized objective techniques may be used to further evaluate and analyse the important variables of motivation, frustration, co-operation and adaptability. Such an evaluation can provide a useful assessment of a patient's residual mental ability.

Personality impairment: loss of drive and vitality, irritability, easily provoked anxiety, dependence and emotional liability.

Psychiatric symptoms: depression or anxiety symptoms, separately or together, are those most frequently occurring.

Intellectual impairment: loss of memory, inability to appreciate and co-ordinate new and previously learned facts, inability to calculate.

From such an assessment it is possible to classify patients as:

Minimally disabled: those with minor memory impairment or transient anxiety/depressive states.

Mildly disabled: those with intellectual impairment permitting adequate functioning in non-intellectual occupations; those with personality change insufficient to prejudice maintenance of family and other relationships; those with depression or anxiety states responding to treatment.

Moderately disabled: those with intellectual deficiency sufficient to impair work status, and/or produce deterioration in personal relationships and subjective well-being, and/or promote severe or prolonged depressions not responding fully to in-patient treatment.

Severely disabled: those with impairment of personality and intellect severe enough to lead to unemployment or marked fall in employment status, and/or to marked deterioration in family relationships and subjective well-being; and those with severe prolonged depression not responding fully to in-patient treatment.

Such a classification is essentially a practical one, grouping patients according to the effect that their mental status may have upon their rehabilitation potential, but there is a very real need for further research into the mental disturbances following strokes.

One further indication of cerebral damage which has a poor prognosis is the persistence of emotional liability. This may be manifested by rapidly changing emotions, temper outbursts or attacks of inappropriate crying or laughing. Although the premorbid personality will determine the emotional reaction of the patient with a major illness, in strokes, the physical and mental effects of the illness must be carefully assessed. It is the patient's ability to change which is important, and much more clinical and psychological data is needed to establish clear guidelines for the clinician and therapist.

Ability of the patient to respond to rehabilitation

Strokes usually occur in older patients who not only have diseased cardiovascular systems, but degenerative disease in other systems as well. The presence of such disease must influence the effort which a patient can put into practising his exercises and may indeed be the limiting factor which decides the final level of functional competence which he attains. Thus, a patient with chronic bronchitis or coronary insufficiency finds that his exercise tolerance is lowered by the early onset of dyspnoea.

The locomotor assistance which the parts of the body unaffected by the stroke are able to give to the affected parts may likewise be limited by their own dysfunction. Thus, a patient with arthritis in the contralateral leg may find that he cannot stand mainly on that leg as hemiplegics tend to do, because of the pain which weight-bearing induces. Similarly, a patient with arthritis in the hand or arm cannot use bars or walking aids effectively to assist the weight-bearing of the paralysed limb. The compensation which one limb can supply for the deficiencies of the other is therefore diminished and the patient's ability to participate in an active rehabilitation programme is diminished accordingly.

A patient with defective special senses such as blindness or deafness is less able to comprehend and is therefore more likely to experience difficulty during rehabilitation. In particular, a blind patient with hemiplegia has almost insuperable difficulties in recovering functional independence. If he needs a stick to enable him to walk, he holds it in his unaffected hand. This leaves him without a hand to feel before him for obstacles and for steadying himself. He cannot use visual feedback information to supplement defective cortical sensory appreciation and he is unable to instigate muscular contraction so as to assist his balance and bolster his confidence.

LONG-TERM REHABILITATION PROGRAMME

From the very early stages of recovery, it is helpful to impose upon the patient (and the hospital staff) a detailed, regularly performed, programme of activity. The programme should involve:

(1) Daily exercise by the patient on the bed, with and without the slings: lying down, sitting up, leaning back on both hands, sitting on the side of the bed, sitting in the chair, getting on and off the chair, wheeling himself in his wheelchair.
(2) A daily visit to the gym for mat work in the lying, sitting, kneeling and crawling positions; bar work to promote arm and hand movement; and parallel bar walking.
(3) A daily sleep on the bed after lunch, followed by a short session of bed exercises.
(4) Alternating periods of elevation of the affected leg on a stool, and periods of dependence with the sole of the foot resting flat and comfortably on the ground.

Such a programme requires that the patient has outdoor shoes to wear for most of the day and certainly for exercise and walking sessions. A tendency to hypostatic oedema in the affected foot and leg may be checked by wearing tubigrip or an elastic stocking, elevating the leg at frequent intervals and performing regular and frequent exercises for ankle and foot. The establishment of such a programme demands liaison between the occupational therapist and nursing staff to teach the patient independent dressing, toilet, grooming, washing and feeding activities, so that independence training is interdigitated with the daily regime from the earliest possible moment.

It may be necessary during the early days of recovery to issue a hemiplegic patient with various simple aids to encourage his independence. There are, however, some who would deny the value of supplying a patient with a reaching aid, such as a 'helping hand' or 'pick-up stick', or feeding aids such as a non-slip table mat, a detachable vertical lip for a plate, a spork, or a drinking beaker with a wide handle and pliable straw. But issue of such equipment may lead to independence for reaching, feeding and drinking, and this will produce an immense boost to the patient's morale.

It is, however, important to stress to the patient recovering from hemiplegia that he should consider aids and equipment as a young child learning to swim does his water wings. They are a necessary part of learning and should be dispensed with once it is possible to manage without them.

Dressing

Minor alterations in the clothes of a hemiplegic patient will often make independent dressing possible relatively early in recovery. The substitution of velcro fastenings for buttons and the strategic resiting of zips, with the addition of a curtain ring to the zip opening, when necessary, are useful for the clothes of both men and women alike. Men find shirts and coats difficult to manage and need to be shown how to lay them on the bed and how to get into them and out of them again. They also usually need to be shown how to put socks on. The use of elastic shoelaces instead of cotton ones eliminates the difficulty of trying and untying laces one-handed. Women have special difficulties with brassieres, corsets, pants, and stockings or tights. If possible it is far better to accept that these difficulties exist, and to select a form of apparel which will avoid incurring them. The fashionable long trousers in non-iron man-made fibre with tunic tops now available for women are ideal for the hemiplegic patient. Worn with knee-length socks, panti-girdle and front-fastening brassiere, they provide a form of apparel which is easy to manipulate, easy to wash and needs no ironing, besides looking well on the older woman. Lowheeled shoes are essential, and if a caliper is to be worn, the shoe to which it is fixed must be strong and well made.

If a woman will not accept an alteration to her mode of dress, she will usually have to accept some assistance with getting in and out of her clothes, since the average corset of an elderly lady is beyond the ability of a hemiplegic patient to manage, and the use of conventional stockings held up by back and front suspenders necessitates twice-daily feats of agility which try the able, let along the disabled. A stocking aid is helpful to get the stockings on and up, but nothing except sheer manual dexterity will cope with a suspender.

Even when possible to achieve, dressing may be very tiring to the more disabled hemiplegic patient, and it may be expedient to accept some help in order to avoid unnecessary fatigue and exasperation. When independent dressing is a practical proposition, the occupational therapist will show the patient how to lay his clothes down in the reverse order to that in which he will require them next day to dress. He will be shown how to place them by the side of the bed or chair opposite to the hemiplegic side, to prevent him from falling over when he reaches for them.

Washing and grooming present fewer difficulties to the hemiplegic patient and can usually be performed one-handed with little special equipment other than that designed to stabilize the soap.

Visiting and using the lavatory demands far more co-ordination than is generally appreciated. Hemiplegic patients may have difficulty in getting their pants up while standing after defaecation or micturition. The use of braces for men prevents the trousers falling down too far for the patient to be able to retrieve them one-handed. Velcro-fastening or zip-fastening flies help those with urgency of micturition and will give a patient a small but valuable addition to personal dignity by preventing the need for assistance with refastening fly buttons.

Returning home
Once it is apparent that sufficient recovery of physical and mental power is likely to make living at home a realistic possibility, the home circumstances of a hemiplegic patient must be discussed and assessed. This may be done by the occupational therapists and medical social workers liaising direct with the domiciliary occupational therapist, or with the health visitor attached to the practice of the patient's general practitioner. A trained person *must* actually see the patient's home to determine whether any equipment or minor structural alterations are needed. Both patient and relatives are apt to prove biased and uninformed, and the information they proffer needs confirmation by a dispassionate third party.

Often neither equipment nor structural alteration is necessary apart from the removal of slippery rugs and the advice to avoid overpolishing the floors. Heights of bed, chairs and water closet pedestal may however be critical, and the supply of sets of blocks of the requisite height for bed and chair, and a raised toilet seat attachment may be indicated. The *lavatory* itself needs careful checking. A grab rail and an outward opening door may need to be installed. If the lavatory is indoors and easily accessible, only the supply of a night commode beside the patient's bed may be necessary. When access to the lavatory is difficult, as for example when it is upstairs, and the patient is unable to climb stairs, then arrangements will have to be made to convert a downstairs room for the patient's bedroom and for him to use a commode both by day and by night.

Kitchens
Sometimes the question at issue is not merely whether a patient can live at home, but whether she can manage to cope with the running of the home. Active participation in domestic tasks obviously demands a higher degree of functional competence than merely living there as part of the furniture, and the *kitchen* is likely to prove the stumbling block in attaining this competence. Appropriate alteration of heights of sink, stove and working surfaces, so that pots and pans may be slid rather than lifted, does much to facilitate the preparation and cooking of meals, and here a split-level cooker is particularly helpful. For the younger hemiplegic patient, alterations of structure and equipment in the kitchen and other parts of the home are amply justified. But for the older hemiplegic, a drastic refashioning of the kitchen is usually an unrealistic solution to the problem.

Whenever possible the patient should be assessed in a well-equipped occupational therapy department kitchen, or in the assessment flat of a Disabled Living Unit, so that the requisite alterations may be determined and effected before she leaves hospital for home.

When alterations to the kitchen are not contemplated in the case of the elderly hemiplegic man or woman living alone, or that of the elderly hemiplegic spouse, whose marital partner is incapable of increasing assistance, then outside care such as home help, family help and meals-on-wheels may be the only alternative.

Care in the home

When there exists adequate and willing family backing or outside help, a hemiplegic patient may remain happily in the home. When the available assistance is inadequate for the patient's needs, this ceases to be possible.

If the hemiplegic patient is attempting to run the house, removal to a purpose-built downstairs flat or bungalow may make this a feasible proposition. If not, then a warden-assisted flat or Part III accommodation are the only other alternatives. If the patient is not attempting to run the home, but is living as a guest in the home of a relation or with an able-bodied spouse, the ratio of patient's needs to help available is equally critical. With the best will in the world, a busy young mother or the elderly spouse or sibling of the patient can only integrate a certain amount of extra work into the existing daily routine. If the hemiplegic makes too much extra work, he can no longer be cared for at home and must be transferred to Part III accommodation.

If all this information is available for a discussion in case conferences between all the medical and paramedical members of staff looking after the hemiplegic patient, a realistic decision can be made before discharge from hospital is arranged and the possible distress of a failed attempt at independent living may be averted.

When the hemiplegic patient *does* return to live at home, both patient and those giving care will need considerable support from the social and health services. This takes the form of regular visits by the district nurse for bathing and catheter changing; regular visits by the health visitor to detect need for further assistance whether monetary or in kind; regular visits to the nearest day hospital to give relief to those giving care; monthly chiropody, when needed, at the day hospital − this can substitute for the traditional follow-up at the out-patients' department of the unit which was responsible for his in-patient care. Frequent follow-up attendances at a hospital physiotherapy department are essential for the maintenance of the continuing well-being of the stroke patient *only* when adequate care is not provided in community-based services.

Regular visits to a local day centre give relief to those giving care. Such visits will enable the patient to be reviewed by the visiting staff, doctor, physiotherapist, occupational therapist and chiropodist. Under ideal conditions, these would be the general practitioner and paramedical workers. They would be responsible for providing the continuing care that is so essential to the well-being of the stroke patient.

Stroke is not a notifiable disorder and its true incidence has never been determined. Certainly it is very common and its incidence is probably around 2/1000 head of population per annum.

Undoubtedly many strokes are treated at home by the patient's general practitioner. Factors making home treatment difficult even in the presence of adequate nursing facilities are incontinence, dementia and prolonged unconsciousness. All survivors of the actual stroke who exhibit these features will usually be admitted to hospital. Others will also be best treated in hospital because of concurrent illness (e.g. diabetes mellitus) or so as to avoid stressing unduly other members of the family.

The vast majority of these patients are elderly and require predominantly nursing care. This can often be provided in a community hospital near to the patient's home and staffed by people known to him. (Of course, this can only be second best to his own home where, surrounded by familiar objects and familiar faces, he has maximal incentive towards recovery.)

Ideally, each community hospital and each general practice should have the part-time services of remedial therapists seconded from the district general hospital. Their activities should be co-ordinated by the general practitioner and dovetailed into the patient's management. Provided that the therapists work in both community and district hospitals, and provided that there is good liaison between general practitioner and rehabilitation consultant, it should be possible to rehabilitate a large number of strokes in the community. Those patients creating difficult problems could be moved to the district hospital rehabilitation centre under the care of the same remedial therapists.

Following discharge from either the community or the district hospital, the patient would continue his rehabilitation at home under the guidance of the general practitioner and the remedial therapists. Regular domiciliary visits by one of the members of the team, coupled with the patient's regular attendance at the day centre will ensure the essential continued care, repeated assessment, and support for the family as a whole.

TREATMENT OF THE RESIDUAL PARALYSIS OF THE LOWER LIMB

Most hemiplegics will require a walking aid for some weeks or months, and the elderly hemiplegic will often be unable to give up such an aid. Initially, the best aids are 'quadrupeds' or 'tripod' sticks with a wide spread (some 'tripods' tend to be unstable in some circumstances) or walking frames. Later some patients will graduate to the use of a walking stick. It often appears to be a false move to encourage over-rapid progression from walking frame to quadruped, for the use of the frame encourages the use of the hemiplegic hand, and encourages a better balance.

The patient should continue for many months to have periods of prone-lying each day in order to prevent the development of hip flexion contractures. Similarly, the bed foot-board should be retained for some months to prevent foot drop.

Braces, calipers and splints

Occasionally, the leg remains flaccid and a full-length caliper appears to be necessary, but the weight and complexity of the conventional device usually outweighs its usefulness. In early stages, a back-splint to brace the knee is a useful aid for walking training.

Some hemiplegics need some immobolization and support for the ankle because of instability. A boot with a T-strap may suffice, but the more unstable will need a double iron and a drop-foot stop.

As far as below-knee splints are concerned, the problem is usually that of controlling an equinovarus spastic foot. The type of short leg-brace used is determined by the severity of the spasticity. If it is mild, with no clonus, and gives easily, simple piano-wire splints are suitable. But usually the spasticity is too great and any stretching of the spastic muscles tends to increase their spasticity. In these circumstances, ankle dorsiflexion (toe-raising) springs have little value. The spring accentuates the spasticity and only serves to distort the shoe. Thus the lower-leg braces usually need to be 'holding' braces, maintaining the foot and ankle in a functionally optimal position. However, if the foot is not dorsiflexed, there will be a tendency for the knee to hyperextend during the stance phase (if weight-bearing occurs) because of the tight Achilles tendon.

The solution is to get the ankle correctly positioned and 'stop' the caliper. If dorsiflexion can be achieved without increasing spasm then this is an advantage. If, however, Achilles-tendon shortening is present and the patient cannot stand on the hemiplegic leg because of weakness around the knee, a wedged heel-raise will prevent hyper-extension of the knee.

The varus deformity can be corrected by an outside iron which is cranked into valgus at or above the ankle, or by an inside iron with an outside T-strap.

In all instances, it is essential that the shoes fit properly. The heel of a suitable shoe is firm and well shaped so that it holds the heel of the foot firmly and prevents it lifting out of the shoe. An instep strap is sometimes necessary to assist in this, yet the shoes need to open widely to admit the foot easily and thus avoid stimulating a full Babinski response when pulling the shoe on. Furthermore, the shoe needs a firm sole-plate which cannot be deformed by the caliper or toe-raising device. Finally, the brace must be firmly attached to the shoe.

Hemiplegics, it must be remembered, are usually elderly and are one-handed. It is very unusual for a hemiplegic patient to manage to put on a below-knee caliper, and it is virtually impossible for him to manage a full-length caliper. This means that calipers and braces must be very simple or must be accepted as therapeutic training devices to be put on for walking exercise by the physiotherapist.

For all these reasons, it is strongly recommended that, whenever possible, simple lightweight plastic splints are made. New rigid plastics (e.g. polypropylene) have made it possible to produce aesthetically acceptable lightweight drop-foot splints. Their manufacture entails very careful casting, for a plastic moulded splint is only as good as the cast allows it to be. For below-knee walking appliances, it is essential to cast the foot and the lower leg with the distortion created by weight-bearing. Technicians skilled in plaster work can reproduce this by the use of a board placed on the sole of the foot and held in longitudinal compression while casting; others may use an impression-taking machine. Providing the splint is accurately shaped and the foot-piece is correctly positioned, the ankle can be held in a position of slight dorsiflexion to suit the patient's requirements. Plantar flexion is completely stopped, but some increase in dorsiflexion should be possible.

Walking training

Much time is wasted in walking training. The spastic gait is always ugly and awkward looking, but it allows the patient to cover the ground well, and walking is stable. It matters little if the leg is circumducted and there is some degree of foot drop. Even if a patient does achieve a relatively normal gait under supervision, he usually relapses into the typical spastic gait when he returns home. Thus, it is more important to teach the patient to use extensor spasm than to overcome it, e.g. step up stairs off the affected leg and step down on to the affected leg, taking one step at a time.

Evaluation of walking potential is less important than evaluation of potential for total mobility and this must include not only those factors which are obviously directly related to the motor aspects of walking, but also such features as sitting and standing balance, visuospatial perception, weakness or spasticity in the appropriate muscle groups, competence in walking under different conditions (levels, slopes, rough ground, steps), and contractures of hips, knees and ankles.

Furthermore, the evaluation should include a reappraisal of the general clinical status and exercise tolerance, since it may be that correction of some other pathological conditions unrelated to the stroke may be of the utmost value in improving the total capability of the patient.

TREATMENT OF THE RESIDUAL PARALYSIS OF THE ARM

The spastic arm is more difficult to manage than the spastic leg, and its chance of recovery is slim.

Inability to abduct the shoulder is a serious and often painful handicap, interfering considerably with almost all activities of daily living. The spastic adducted shoulder can be mobilized by a combination of passive and active movements, particularly while in the warm treatment pool or after injections of local anaesthetic and hydrocortisone if pain is a predominant feature. Ice packs are often useful in relieving spasm and may be followed by several hours of reduced spasticity, during which time active and passive movements can be achieved. Pulley exercises combining active and passive movements can be carried out as part of the regular daily routine at home.

At all stages, it is important to prevent, and if present to treat, oedema of the hand and fingers. Gravitational drainage, the use of the high sling and passive movements will all have this object in view in the early stages. Unless oedema is prevented, stiffness will inevitably develop.

Hand splints to assist extension of wrist and fingers, e.g. banjo splints, are ungainly devices. They have to be complex and large, both to overcome the powerful flexion spasticity and to pull the fingers in the correct direction. Most lively splints seem only to hyperextend and sublux the metacarpophalangeal joints, and stablizing splints are usually more helpful.

There are few procedures which will improve the upper limb. Relaxation of the entire flexor muscle mass with phenol or alcohol will often improve the appearance of the hand and facilitate the use of splints, since splintage of a flail hand is easier than splintage of a spastic one. Similarly, injection of the biceps and brachialis relieves the flexor spasm of the elbow, and prevents the ugly reflex flexion of the elbow which so often occurs during walking.

Most recovery will occur early, and deformities which are present at 3 months will usually persist. Indeed, many authorities believe that if there is no voluntary control at 3 weeks, there will be no useful recovery of function. Surgery can achieve permanent correction of such deformities, but is usually reserved for the younger hemiplegics whose clinical condition is unlikely to deteriorate.

SURGICAL INTERVENTION

Distinction must be made between spastic deformity and structural contracture. The spastic deformity disappears in sleep, and can be relieved by positioning or a slow passive stretch. Spastic deformity can be controlled by braces and splints, but no braces, whether static or dynamic, will control progressive spasticity. Surgical procedures aimed at rebalancing muscle power are equally doomed to failure. Infiltration of the muscle with local anaesthetics will enable the deformity to be analysed, and temporary reduction of spasticity by infiltration with 40—45 per cent alcohol can allow active rehabilitation to proceed. Non-progressive spasticity of fixed contractures is amenable to corrective surgery. Tendon lengthening, direct injection of the motor points or selective neurectomy are the procedures of choice. Achilles-tendon lengthening for the spastic drop-foot, associated with tenotomies of the flexors, if necessary, is often helpful. Split anterior-tibial transfer can compensate for lateral dorsiflexion. Hamstring release for knee flexion contractures is more successful than Eggars procedure. No surgical procedures will improve weak hip abduction, and no surgical procedures will restore normal gait, for hemiplegia is a disorder in which imperfect motor control is inherent and perfect co-ordination cannot be regained by surgical procedures. Thus reconstructive procedures should aim at reducing deformity and improving standing and walking stability, rather than aiming at an unrealistic normality.

WHEELCHAIR USE

Some hemiplegics are so immobilized by the total effect of the stroke that they cannot walk and need to lead a wheelchair existence. Recovery is invariably greater in the leg than in the arm, and thus concentration on the walking re-education dominates the first phase of active rehabilitation. About one in five of survivors will not achieve independent walking and will require a wheelchair.

The provision of the most suitable wheelchair or wheelchairs for a hemiplegic patient is a matter which presents some difficulties.

Severely disabled: The most severely disabled group of patients, e.g. those with dense hemiplegia or dementia, will be completely unable to propel a wheelchair, and for them a transit chair with 4 small wheels and a perambulator type handle is required. Unless seat height is critical, a 2-inch soft cushion, with or without a half sheepskin or other special cushions, should be supplied with this type of chair, since the patient sits in his chair throughout the day, and may well become sore. The chair is used to transport the patient about his home or residential institution.

Moderately disabled: These patients are able to propel themselves with varying degrees of success. Some patients, in whom spasm is not severe, are able to propel themselves with both hands, provided sensation is adequate to prevent damage to the hands on the wheels. For them, the lightest, smallest standard wheelchairs with rear-wheel propulsion, which are consistent with comfort and stability, are indicated.

Patients in whom severe spasticity, or lack of sensation, prevents propulsion by the hemiplegic arm, have two alternative methods of propelling themselves. In the first, a lightweight standard chair is provided which a patient propels with the unaffected arm and one foot, or else with the unaffected arm and both feet. As the arm propels the large rear wheel on the unaffected side, the feet either 'walk' the chair along, or else the unaffected heel is dug into the ground and the chair approximates towards it. The foot or feet here act both as pivots and propelling agents, and prevent the chair from merely travelling the circular path along which one-armed propulsion directs it.

In the second, a single-armed propelling chair is provided, to be propelled by the unaffected arm. Although such a chair seems the obvious answer for a man with only one functional arm, it may in fact be of little use, particularly for a stiff, elderly person in whom there may be some intellectual deficit, since most available models are big, heavy and need a considerable space for manoeuvring. Front-wheel propelling chairs are particuarly suitable for a hemiplegic who has hemianopia, since the complete steering rims are more easily kept within his field of vision while he is learning to manipulate them. The Ministry Standard Model 3 and Model 1 are both front-wheel propelling chairs which can be modified for one-armed control. The former chair is 4-wheeled and needs a large space to stand and turn; the latter is 3-wheeled and is easily manoeuvrable indoors.

When hemiplegic patients are being taught to use their chairs, it is helpful to put them to practise in a gym or hall with a large full-length mirror at one end of it. They are urged to do some runs under direct visual control, watching their hands and feet as they operate the chair, and some under indirect control, checking the movements of the chair and their limbs in the mirror. This adds to the total sensory impact by which a hemiplegic must reorganize his damaged motor function, and it increases the facility with which he manages the chair.

Some younger hemiplegics can become very skilful with single-handed control chairs, used indoors, but few can achieve outdoor mobility involving any slopes or rough ground with this type of chair.

Most elderly hemiplegics are not going to achieve a high level of activity, and their interest will be best served by providing them with a wheelchair early in their disability. This enables them to attain some limited mobility and independence without much expenditure of effort either on the part of those giving care or of the patients themselves. It also enables friends and relatives to take them out into the community and maintain their morale.

RETURN TO WORK

For those who become hemiplegic before retirement age, return to work is of paramount importance in its economic, social and personal effects on the life of patients and families alike.

It is therefore necessary to ensure that this return is achieved smoothly. Often this can be done by direct arrangement between a patient and his employer, particularly if he has been known to them for a long time. Sometimes an appeal to the DRO is necessary to ask the employers for minor structural alterations of equipment used at work to permit its use by a man with one normal arm and one spastic one. Often the best solution is the transfer of a patient from one department to another in which less manipulatory and/or ambulatory skill is required.

When a patient disabled by hemiplegia attempts to return to work in a place designed for the able-bodied, and at a process designed for bimanual participation, difficulties may occur. These may be difficulties of transport, entrance and egress to place of work, relationship of work surface to patient, relationship of patient with workmates from whom aphasia and the slowness of spastic movement now sets him apart, in addition to the patient's inability to walk the distances between a work area and toilet, or work area and canteen, in the time allotted for this.

Hemianopia, partial sensory loss, memory defect and apraxia may also cause a loss of manipulative skill which bars a patient from the use of machinery.

The consideration of the possible difficulties before a return to work is attempted may avert embarrassments, frustration, loss of face and even loss of employment. A formal work assessment is helpful in indicating potential areas of difficulty, and such an assessment must include an estimation of mental, as well as physical, capabilities.

RESULTS OF REHABILITATION

In general terms, it seems likely that the best results following a stroke are to be achieved by intensive rehabilitation during the first 6 to 12 weeks after the cerebrovascular accident, during the phase of the greatest and fastest recovery. Thereafter, the patient's activities should be, as far as possible, self-determined and self-administered. The rehabilitation period therefore attempts to make regular performance of the more important exercises an unquestioned habit; so that a patient will carry on with shoulder, hand and finger exercises and walking, speech and writing practice, making them a part of his daily life, even when he no longer has the supervision of his therapists to encourage him to do so.

Not only his self-discipline but his own motivation must be stimulated so that formal exercises are supplemented by and incorporated into creative and social activities.

Active exercises to be performed almost indefinitely are frequently prescribed for the treatment of the paretic limbs after cerebrovascular accident, but functional improvement is more likely to be achieved through:

(1) Improvement and co-ordination.
(2) Prevention of contractures.

Many patients are unnecessarily attending physiotherapy departments when they could be better occupied attending social clubs and day centres where general activities would combine exercise with interest and entertainment.

Intensive rehabilitation can achieve improved function in the majority of patients surviving the first few months after the acute cerebrovascular episode. About two thirds of the patients should achieve personal independence and one third are likely to be fit for employment. For one patient, rehabilitation potential may mean a change from the bed-bound state to the ability to transfer to a wheelchair, and for another the ability to return to work in the community.

The end results of rehabilitation are influenced by many factors, some of which are related to the patient himself and some to the environment in which his rehabilitation occurs. Age, of course, has considerable influence on the end results which can be achieved in any particular patient, and the older patient, who has the greater chance of have associated disabilities, has the lower rehabilitation potential. Involvement of the dominant hand and the presence of severe speech defects are two other factors commonly associated with poor rehabilitation achievements.

Immediate surroundings, the therapists giving care and the rehabilitation regimes employed are all important factors in determining the end results. At one rehabilitation unit, less than 10 per cent of patients were able to walk independently on admission, but about 50—60 per cent had achieved some useful level of work or contribution to housework before discharge.

The average length of time patients stay in a rehabilitation unit in the United Kingdom is 6 weeks. These units have the advantage of providing comprehensive physiotherapy and realistic occupational therapy, together with speech therapy, psychiatric advice when necessary, and a close liaison with social workers to plan early return to home surroundings. They attempt to channel the rehabilitation activities of patients into normal activities as quickly as possible, since even the most enlightened occupational therapy and physiotherapy are not substitutes for the activities of daily living.

Attendance at a rehabilitation unit should be kept as short as possible, since the longer a patient is away from his usual routine the more difficult it will be for him to return to it. Therefore it is essential that the functional aims are realistic. Unrealistic optimism about a patient's performance and progress leads to an over-long admission in an effort to achieve an impossible degree of functional improvement which brings only discredit to the process of rehabilitation and its proponents.

SUMMARY

There is no better summary of rehabilitation of strokes than that in Bryan Mathews' book, *Practical Neurology* (1970).

> Treatment must still be based on the long recognised principles of mobilisation, proper hydration and feeding, and the prevention of infection. There is simply no virtue at all in the patient staying immobile in bed. From the onset he must be moved repeatedly in bed and at the very first opportunity he must be got out of bed into a chair for rapidly increasing periods. Formal physiotherapy must be given when available but a willing relative can soon learn to provide the essentials of repeated passive movement and attempted active movement. If there is any difficulty in swallowing a nasal tube should be passed as dehydration is most harmful and inhalation of food even more so. An accurate prognosis is hard to give. Early return of movement is a good sign, while adverse signs are extensive sensory loss, prolonged flaccidity, and previous strokes. After a severe hemiplegia, useful recovery of the hand is unlikely, and the utmost attention should be paid to getting the patient back on his feet. Even if the leg is flaccid, some form of supported walking can be attained by the use of a caliper to hold the knee rigid. Dysphasia may prove a major disibility even if good recovery from the paralysis has occurred, for even a mild degree will prevent employment in many otherwise suitable jobs. Patients certainly improve while having speech therapy, but as the natural tendency is to improvement it is difficult to be certain of any indisputable effect. The patient's attitude of mind will greatly affect the degree of functional recovery, but indifference is usually the result of repeated cerebral infarction and severe disability.

It is always necessary to remember that rehabilitation measures cannot succeed in those patients who are not motivated to improve, and persuasion, explanation and cajolery have little effect in such cases.

The management of stroke during the acute stage is concerned with the maintenance of the life processes, the prevention of deterioration of the locomotor system while its control is no longer properly co-ordinated, and the diagnosis of the causative lesion of the stroke itself.

Concurrently with such management, regular assessment of the clinical picture is necessary, so that the rate and pattern of progress may be perceived. Only through such assessment may the programme of rehabilitation be tailored to the individual abilities and disabilities of each patient. Such tailoring is particularly necessary for stroke patients, when the locomotor symptoms and signs actually manifest may be caused by such a wide variety of cerebral lesions.

Motor recovery and functional capability are the final yardsticks for judging the success of rehabilitation, but there are marked discrepancies between physical ability and functional independence. The major barrier will be any impairment of the patient's mental state.

The peculiarly fascinating yet exasperating quality about stroke rehabilitation is the large element which chance plays in its success. There is still no standardized, universally accepted form of progressive therapy. Encouraging results are obtained with patients treated at one centre which specializes in proprioceptive neuromuscular facilitation techniques; equally encouraging ones at another which follows the Bobath techniques. Some centres provide light and well-balanced splints and calipers which apparently stop flexion contractures and enhance the recovery of less spastic muscles; others forbid splints and calipers as pieces of equipment designed to reduce the proprioceptive sensory input of the joints and muscles which they stabilize. Some centres claim good results from routine use of speech therapy for their aphasic hemiplegics; others believe that speech therapists are useful in the diagnosis of aphasia but not in its treatment. Would a patient from one centre have recovered equally well in another? It is not only the treatment which varies, but the patient, the therapist, the associated features of the hemiplegia, and the atmosphere of the centre as a whole.

One of the few constant findings which can be extracted from the many reports and accounts of stroke therapy is that any treatment designed to increase the sensory input and facilitate motor output of the brain will benefit stroke patients. The degree of benefit will depend upon the expertise of the therapist in applying the treatment, the empathy which she can establish with the patients she treats, and the co-operation and motivation with which they are capable of responding.

There are almost certainly right and wrong methods of treatment for any particular state of recovery of any one patient. Equally certainly, therefore, there must be a correct pattern of treatment for each patient and it cannot be right to treat all patients by the same method. Principles of treatment hold constant, but not the treatment itself. The catalytic affect which enthusiasm and expertise in the application of any chosen technique has upon the recovery of patients makes it difficult to evaluate that technique in absolute terms. Yet it must eventually be possible to select the appropriate technique or combination of techniques which will assist the recovery of functional competence to the highest degree permitted by the absolute brain damage which has occurred in any particular patient. Until this time, we are still shooting in the dark. Until then, we should preface all advice on treatment of stroke with, 'We do not know, but we think that . . .'.

Little has yet been done to study and classify the behaviour patterns of patients during the stages of functional recovery. It is appreciated that the absolute motor paralysis following stroke corresponds to the size and site of the causative cerebral necrosis and the number and location of nerve cells and tracts thereby destroyed. It has long been appreciated also that areas of potential recovery exist in the brain immediately following infarction or haemorrhage, and that the final degree of destruction of brain tissue depends on the ability of the collateral circulation to compensate for the circulatory insufficiency caused by the initial vascular catastrophe. What has not yet been determined is how the actual pattern of recovery is related to the pathophysiology of the causative brain lesion.

It may be that when techniques for diagnosing the site and extent of the causative lesions of stroke are perfected, it will be possible to specify the pattern along which recovery will occur in any one patient, and to adjust the programme of rehabilitation accordingly.

BIBLIOGRAPHY AND REFERENCES

Adams, G.F. and Hurwitz, L.J. (1963). 'Mental barriers to recovery from stroke.' *Lancet* **2**, 533

Adler, E. (1969). *Stroke in Israel, 1957–1961.* Israel; Polypress

Andrews, K. and Stewart, J. (1979). 'Stroke recovery: he can but does he?' *Rheum. and Rehab.* **18**, 43

Brocklehurst, J.C., Andrews, K., Richards, B. and Laycock, P.J. (1978). 'How much physical therapy for patients with stroke?' *Brit. Med. J.* **1**, 1307

Carter, A.B. (1963). 'Strokes.' *Proc. R. Soc. Med.* **86**, 483

Harris, R., Bruk, M.I. and Copp, E.P. (1964). 'Rehabilitation and resettlement in hemiplegia.' *Ann. phys. Med.* **7**, 209

Hurwitz, L.J. (1969). 'Management of strokes.' *Br. med. J.* **3**, 699

Lenman, J.R. (1959). 'A clinical and experimental study of the effects of exercises in motor weakness in neurological disease.' *J. Neurol. Neurosurg. Psychiat.* **22**, 182

Matthews, W.B. (1970). *Practical Neurology.* London; Blackwell

Millard, J.B. (1966). 'Rehabilitation and the hemiplegic patient.' *Ann. phys. Med.* **8**, 244

Rusthworth, G. (1964). 'Pathophysiology of spasticity.' *Proc. R. Soc. Med.* **57**, 29

Storey, P.B. (1968). 'Some psychological aspects of disability and resettlement.' *Physiotherapy* **54**, 54–57

Working Group on Strokes of Geriatric Committee, Royal College of Physicians (1974). 'Stroke disability in Great Britain.' London; Royal College of Physicians

Yates, G. (1968). 'A method for the provision of lightweight aesthetic orthopaedic appliances.' *Orthopaedics: Oxford* **1**, 153

Zankle, H.T. (1971). *Stroke Rehabilitation.* Illinois; Thomas

11 Rehabilitation After Head Injury

MARTYN ROSE

INTRODUCTION

Rehabilitation begins as soon as the trauma has occurred. Early care is aimed at limiting the development of complications especially of the chest where problems may lead to secondary brain damage, and of the limbs (spasticity and posture).

Later, when the acute problems have passed, careful assessment must be made by a team in which the psychologist should play a prominent part. Appropriate treatment regimes may then be started or continued and maximal use made of spontaneous recovery. At as early a stage as possible the relatives of the head injured patient must be brought into discussions, as they will have an important role to play.

Head injury is common. The associated brain damage varies from the apparently trivial, with few sequelae either physical or psychological, to the most severe with early death. Rehabilitation, when available, tends to be concentrated on those patients with severe (major) injury. The management of moderate and mild (minor) injuries has yet to be seriously considered as a rehabilitation commitment by the majority of doctors.

Rehabilitation of brain-damaged people presents special problems, but there are also certain advantageous aspects. Severe head injury is commonly associated with other serious injury which may complicate recovery, but occurs most often in fit young men. They possess previously normally functioning nervous systems, and their bodies do not show the deterioration associated with ageing processes.

Much of the management of these brain damaged people parallels that of the stroke patient, but the disorders of 'higher cerebral function' associated with head injury present added, different and long-lasting problems.

Incidence

There are more than 140 000 people admitted to hospital in England and Wales with head injury each year, nearly 12 000 of whom will have more serious types of head injury. It has been suggested that in the same period between 550 000 and 700 000 will be treated in Accident and Emergency Departments and estimated that 70 000 people will consult general practitioners (a very small proportion of whom will be admitted to hospital).

Admissions to hospital for head injury have increased steadily. In 1972 there were more than twice the number in 1957, but the incidence of more severe head injury has declined from a peak reached in 1965 and it seems likely that the increase in admission is due to changes in admission policy rather than an increase in numbers of head injured.

A majority of people with head injury are young — just under half of those admitted to hospital are people under 20 years of age — and the majority are male.

Males with head injury outnumber females by 2:1, but between the ages of 15 and 34 years the ratio of male to female is more than 3:1. An important factor influencing rehabilitation is the fact that males of social class V (unskilled) at any age are at an appreciably greater risk of head injury than all other social classes. Resettlement in work is much more difficult for the unskilled manual person.

Cause

In adults under 65 years road traffic accidents are a major cause of head injury producing about 50 per cent of hospital admissions. Such accidents are commonly associated with other severe injuries which complicate rehabilitation. In the elderly (over 65 years) falls are a more important cause of injury and in these patients the other features of ageing complicate rehabilitation.

People with head injury do not form a representative sample of the general population. It is suggested that a large percentage of the head-injured group will have been previously mal-adjusted, and the incidence of chronic alcoholism and previous psychiatric disturbance may be higher.

Classification

Brain injury is commonly classified as severe (major), moderate or mild (minor). This must not be confused with severity of outcome because there is surprisingly little useful correlation between the two.

The severity of injury is usually measured in terms of Post Traumatic Amnesia (PTA). This is the length of time following injury during which events are not recorded in the memory. There are difficulties in using PTA:

(1) It is retrospective.
(2) Its endpoint is rarely clearly defined (or recorded).
(3) It takes no account of penetrating injury, where consciousness may not be lost.
(4) It takes no account of focal brain and cranial nerve damage.

These factors have led some clinicians to use the length of unconsciousness, and others length of hospital stay as measures of severity. At present a severe head injury is defined as one with

(1) A PTA of more than 24 hours.
(2) A period of unconsciousness of more than 4 hours.
(3) A hospital stay of more than 7 days.

Minor head injury (a term used to cover both moderate and mild groups) involves PTA of less than 24 hours, unconsciousness of less than 4 hours and a hospital stay of less than 7 days.

Head injuries may also be classified as 'closed' (with or without fracture), or 'open' where there is either a laceration communicating with a fracture or a fracture crossing one of the air sinuses. The nature of the injury may be 'blunt' or 'penetrating', and any fracture may be linear or depressed. Penetrating injury may not cause loss of consciousness, despite considerable focal damage, but in common with fractures involving air sinuses may result in intracranial infection including abscess formation.

PATHOPHYSIOLOGY OF HEAD INJURY

The trauma which produces the head injury causes primary brain damage. Complications may then develop leading to the development of secondary brain damage. Acceleration/deceleration injuries – the commonest type – if severe enough produce loss of consciousness. There is movement of the brain within the skull, and as a result of differing tissue densities shearing forces are set up at all levels, but especially at the level of the tentorium cerebelli where there is relative fixity of brain stem and also differing tissue density. As a result there is damage which may be evident macroscopically or visible at cell level only. All blunt injuries produce some diffuse brain damage, but there may be more local damage directly under the site of impact and at the opposite side (contrecoup injury). Injury causing acceleration/deceleration in the saggital plane may cause more damage owing to the configuration of the skull (especially the petrous temporal and sphenoidal ridges).

The main early complication following head injury is the development of raised intracranial pressure. This may be due to

(1) Cerebral oedema.
(2) Intracranial haemorrhage.

Epilepsy, which may follow head injury early (in the first seven days) or later can produce difficulties in resettlement and employment at a later stage. Hydrocephalus may also occur and produce abnormalities which are only recognized at a later date. Infection is a problem of 'open injury' and may complicate recovery.

Trauma is associated with oedema and haemorrhage on a large or small scale. There is some irreversible neuronal (nerve cell) loss, axon degeneration and disruption. There is also an element of dysfunction which is reversible perhaps owing to the effects of oedema, haemorrhage, electrolyte imbalance or demyelination. In severe head injury, where there is always major irreversible damage, the brain lesion results in a cutting off of higher cerebral centres from lower ones. As the human develops from neonate to adult there is a gradual replacement of mass uncontrolled activity by more and more sophisticated responses. It is generally assumed that the major effect of the higher centres is to inhibit normal reflex reactions of lower centres, so that the effect of brain damage is to free the lower centres from inhibition and thus release normal reflexes which are observed as abnormalities of posture and response in the recovering patient.

The basis of recovery
Virtually all people with head injury who survive show some degree of improvement and indeed the great majority make a good recovery. The questions that need to be answered are:

(1) What happens in the central nervous system as recovery occurs?
(2) What can be done to assist this?

The old idea was that recovery from a clear destructive lesion had to be explained in terms of an existing structure which reorganized itself physiologically. It is now accepted that morphological changes occur which can bring in previously non-existent or ineffective connections. The central nervous system exhibits plasticity.

There are a variety of mechanisms by which recovery could occur and some of these are outlined below:

(1) Dispersal of oedema.
(2) Correction of electrolyte imbalance.
(3) Remyelination.
(4) Regeneration of cut axons.
(5) Collateral sprouting and switching of inputs.
(6) Improved synaptic action.
(7) Spare capacity in the brain with re-routing.
(8) Division of nerve cells.

There is experimental evidence for the existence of most of these mechanisms, but little evidence concerning the role of any of them in recovery. There is good evidence from animals that switching of inputs occurs. For example it has been shown that if the nerve cells sending impulses to a region of the thalamus are removed then that area of thalamus is rendered silent initially, but later begins to show response to input from other areas. The input to the cells has been switched from one area to another.

In children there is observational evidence that switching of function can occur. Under the age of 8 years it is certainly possible for speech to return after destruction of the dominant hemisphere speech areas. It is suggested, however, that the gain in this activity (speech) may result in the loss of some other function.

It is possible, of course, that not all changes in the central nervous system after damage are beneficial to the patient and that at some future time we shall be able to advance helpful change and retard others.

PROGNOSTIC FACTORS

While we are unsure of the mechanisms by which recovery occurs, we can recognize some of the factors which are of importance in determining outcome.

Age has a major influence on survival, morbidity and rehabilitation. The outcome is better in those under 20 years compared with the over 20's.

The *place* of the lesion, its site and size is of obvious importance. There are surprisingly large areas of the brain which can cease to function with little in the way of external evidence. A further factor here is the method of production of the completed lesion. Several small lesions have a better outcome than an equivalent injury caused by one insult.

Premorbid intelligence and personality (rarely well documented before injury) have undoubted prognostic significance ('it is not only the kind of injury that matters, but also the kind of head'). While many authorities refer to personality change after head injury others believe the difference to be simply less inhibition of the old personality.

Pre-injury occupation, which correlates fairly highly with intelligence, is also important. Unskilled workers do badly, especially with regard to return to former employment. However, one wonders if the high percentage of return to former employment shown by skilled and professional workers does not in part reflect the relative ease with which disabled people can be 'carried' in these jobs.

Social factors too play a part in determining outcome. The family, its response to stress and ability to support the patient appear to have a crucial effect on the degree of recovery regardless of the disability.

The rehabilitation team aims for improvement in four main ways:

(1) By limiting deformity and spasticity.
(2) Retraining and hopefully encouraging the mechanisms of recovery by, e.g. building up patterns of movement.
(3) Teaching ways of utilizing the recovery that occurs to the full.
(4) Teaching ways of compensating for losses.

After head injury the contribution of physiotherapist, occupational therapist and speech therapist must be complemented by the assessment of a clinical psychologist (preferably with experience of neurological problems). Brain damage is diffuse; neurological deficits, especially aspects of memory and data processing, may be small but make a major difference to planning of and response to the therapist's rehabilitation programme.

It has been found difficult to set up adequately controlled trials in a clinical situation aimed at assessing the specific effects of rehabilitation in brain damaged people. We do not know which of our present techniques are of value. Indeed the answers to such questions as 'who to rehabilitate, where, when and for how long' are also unknown.

Many workers are trying to evaluate the contribution of the various parts of rehabilitation techniques using animal experiments, as both management and lesion can be controlled. These experiments suggest that early training produces better results than delayed treatment and that including the contralateral limbs (normal side) in the training routines does not enhance the response of the affected side. Other work comparing the outcome of different managements suggests that the functional results are better in brain-damaged animals treated with apparatus (such as treadmills and levers to pull) and in groups, than those treated singly or not treated at all. It is suggested that the animals in the first group mentioned are given the equivalent of good rehabilitation.

It would be rash to extrapolate directly from animals to humans for many fairly obvious reasons, but this work may provide some impetus for studies in human rehabilitation.

OVERALL MANAGEMENT

Once the primary brain damage has been sustained it is important to be able to recognize the development of rising intracranial pressure (see later). It is also important to recognize the people most at risk of developing the complication. Ideally those at risk will be admitted to hospital, although there is constant pressure to limit admissions to hospital especially as complication rates even in the selected 'at risk' group are very low. However, Jennet has suggested that too many patients with apparently 'minor' head injury who talk coherently after injury die, often with surgically treatable lesions (e.g. intracranial haematoma). This problem of recognizing the deteriorating patient occurs at all levels of care from general practice to specialist hospital units.

Problems which may particularly (though rarely) trouble those attending the less severely head-injured are:

(1) Extradural haemorrhage with the classical story of a minor injury and lucid interval followed (usually within 24 hours of the injury) by unrelenting decline and death unless treated.
(2) Leakage of cerebro-spinal fluid (CSF) — sometimes presenting as the permanent 'cold' after head injury.
(3) Epilepsy — This can cause sudden changes in response level which, if the fit is not observed leads to unnecessary concern over the possibilities of raised intracranial pressure.

MINOR HEAD INJURY

Initial care

Diagnosis is all important in the apparently minor head injury and the attending doctor must discover what happened, including the nature of the trauma.

The first question to answer is whether or not admission to hospital is required. The guide lines for this at present are to admit:

(1) Those who have been unconscious.
(2) Those with post traumatic amnesia — however short.
(3) Those with evidence of skull fracture (especially a boggy superficial haematoma).
(4) Children brought to hospital.

Progress

Patients with minor head injury will have diffuse brain damage. The majority can confidently be expected to make uneventful recoveries, but a proportion do complain of a variety of symptoms, including headache, dizzyness and lack of concentration. In the past this has been described as 'the post-concussional syndrome' and some authorities have commented on its relationship to compensation neurosis. The present opinion is that there is an organic basis for the symptoms. There are no distinguishing features in the first few days, but by one week some signs have appeared. The problem appears to be related to handling or processing anything more than the simplest data. *Special* psychological tests can reveal the defect. It is suggested that the appropriate management (rehabilitation) can improve the prognosis for this group.

On similar lines Relander and his colleagues have tried to show that organized care of minor head injured people (same doctor, same physiotherapist and an explanation of the problems) produces better results in terms of return to work than standard care which regrettably often appears to fall below even the minimal level of organization in Relander's treatment group. (This is the only *controlled* trial of any rehabilitation regime in head injury, in that two treatments were compared). The results of this trial, although not entirely satisfactory, are particularly relevant for general practitioners and doctors in Accident and Emergency Departments where the majority of minor head injuries are managed.

The optimal management of minor head injury has yet to be decided but the basic principles of early and progressive mobilization are well known and appear to give good results. It is likely that with a small amount of organization the great majority of people with minor head injury can be rehabilitated adequately.

Return to work
Ideally all people with minor head injuries would be followed up regularly, receiving clinical supervision and psychometric testing. Return to work could be staged to coincide with the return to normal of the psychometric test results. A cheaper, perhaps more expedient method would be to wait for the development of symptoms and then speedily offer treatment. Unless one of these approaches becomes accepted policy a useful rule of thumb to apply is that described by Cairns in 1941.

Length of PTA	Time off work	
5 – 60 minutes	4 – 6 weeks	Minor injury
1 – 24 hours	6 – 8 weeks	
1 – 7 days	2 – 4 months	Severe injury
Over 7 days	4 – 8 months	

SEVERELY HEAD-INJURED PATIENT

Initial management
Any patient with a lowered response level needs urgent protection of the airway. Neck injury may accompany head injury, and this must be remembered particularly if endotracheal intubation is required. A check list for cases of severe head injury is outlined below:

(1) Airway.
(2) Neck.
(3) Chest.
(4) Circulation.
(5) Abdomen/pelvis (signs of haemorrhage especially).
(6) Limbs for fractures.
(7) Head (including face and eyes).
(8) Central nervous system.
(9) Other.

The airway is especially important in brain damage as hypoxia and hypercapnoea lead to cerebral oedema, producing raised intracranial pressure and secondary brain damage.

Limb injury is important for three reasons:

(1) As a source of significant haemorrhage.
(2) As a cause of limited movement (which can confuse later examination of the central nervous system.
(3) It needs treatment in its own right.

The circulation is important too. Undiagnosed haemorrhage in the unconscious patient may lead to hypoxia (and secondary brain damage) or death, even when the primary brain damage is relatively trivial.

Inspection of the head may give clues about the type of injury and the direction in which the trauma occurred. Lacerations may communicate with (depressed) fractures and boggy haematomas may alert one to the presence of intracranial bleeding. In some cases brain presents itself at the surface — this does not necessarily indicate a poor prognosis especially if the cause is a localized penetrating injury.

Initial CNS assessment
Head injury produces primary brain damage. Complications which may follow can lead to the development of secondary brain damage. Initial assessment provides the base line from which further management decisions are made.

The end result of complications is to produce raised intracranial pressure (RICP) which is most readily recognized by a progressive lowering in response level (often unhelpfully called conscious level). Changes do occur in pupil size and response, pulse, blood pressure and respiration, but all are *late* signs of rising intracranial pressure.

Early management
The primary concern for the physiotherapist is the patient's chest. Adequate gaseous exchange is essential and physiotherapy aids this by concentrating on the treatment of any initial condition and preventing the development of problems. A blocked bronchus for instance, can produce sufficient change in the concentration of blood gases to cause rapid deterioration in the patient's response level. Chest physiotherapy may be able to correct this and minimize brain damage. The occurrence of chest problems despite adequate physiotherapy should lead to the consideration of tracheostomy.

Care must also be given to the limbs. In later stages of management the problem is likely to be one of spasticity coupled with deformity. Early management aims to minimize both.

It is generally accepted that limbs should be placed in positions where spasticity is least likely to develop. When the patient is lying in bed the leg is placed in flexion, the arm partially flexed at the shoulder in external rotation, with elbow and wrist extended. External rotation of the humerus is thought to be particularly important. Passive movements through as full a range as possible are performed several times each day and again this is felt to be of value. The mechanism of action is unclear but there are many observations of the improvement in function after initial passive movement of a limb.

It is possible that more attention should be placed on limb position at all times if the best patterns of movement are to be encouraged. Nursing staff may need more information about limb posture and spasticity and this is an area for close collaboration between nurses and physiotherapists.

Later management

Each patient needs individual assessment by each specialist (the therapists, psychologist and social worker), but a planned programme of treatment with each member of the team complementing the efforts of the other. Physical assessment is relatively straightforward (although there is no universally accepted standard form of assessment and this makes communication between therapists difficult).

The basic questions to answer are:

(1) Does the patient present the problem of hemiplegia or quadriplegia?
(2) How much motor loss is there?
(3) How much sensory loss is there? What is its pattern? Does it include inattention (of hearing, vision or ordinary sensations).
(4) Is spasticity a problem? (a 'pure' cortical lesion for instance produces flaccidity).
(5) Is ataxia a problem?

Of greater importance is the assessment of higher cerebral function — especially memory, perception, speech and behaviour. Is there flatness of affect, emotional lability or euphoria?

Active physiotherapy *can* start before there is any major improvement in response level. Re-education of normal postural reflex mechanisms can begin early. The patient is taken, in sequence, through a pattern of positioning and movement designed to follow the stages of development shown by the normal human infant — neck control, righting reflexes, overcoming of gravitational forces up to and including walking. A high degree of re-education of postural reflex mechanisms can be achieved whilst the higher cerebral functions, which commonly take longer to recover, are more slowly improving.

The detailed timing of the introduction of more active physiotherapy depends on the individual patient and therapist. There are no hard and fast rules once the basic chest problems, in particular, are stable, but in general early mobilization is favoured.

Mobilization and re-education is continued at a rate appropriate for the individual. Generally this means without the production of complaint of dizziness, undue fatigue or headache.

Occupational therapy is particularly concerned with the re-education of activities of daily living (ADL) and the assessment of work potential. However, perceptual training is undertaken in some units (a particular non-dominant hemisphere function) although its value is uncertain. After careful assessment to discover the major perceptual problem, patients with disorders of, for example body image or sensory inattention are 'trained' using a graded series of tasks in which the level of perception necessary to complete the task is gradually increased. There is some evidence that early introduction of occupational therapy helps to mould recovery of mental function leading to a reduction of neurotic disability later. The physical problems associated with head injury are usually less disabling than the psychological/psychiatric factors.

Behaviour problems occur commonly, particularly in the early stages or on admission to a rehabilitation unit. The latter situation is brought about by disorientation caused by change in surroundings and personnel. It is best managed by patience, passage of time and efforts to obtain clear channels of *communication* between some staff members and the patient. Occasionally sedative drugs must be used, but with caution. We do not know the effects of these drugs on recovery and once prescribed it is difficult to decide when to withdraw them. The drugs themselves can produce disorientation and behaviour problems. Transfer from hospital to home is often accompanied by an improvement in behaviour.

Dysfunction of the higher cerebral functions needs particular assessment. Patients who have problems with perception or the processing and storing of information (memory) produce difficulties in rehabilitation. Psychological tests often provide vital information for the correct management of these difficulties. The psychologist may also be able to help with treatment, especially using behaviour modification techniques. Patients are commonly said to be well or poorly motivated (i.e. do or do not do as they are told). A more helpful way of looking at this is to regard them as showing a particular behaviour pattern. Behaviour is largely a response to environment and it is often possible to show why a patient behaves in a particular way. It may then be possible to achieve behaviour modification. For instance a patient who needs assistance in walking, may refuse a wheelchair as this would cut down on the attention received while 'learning to walk'. Once the problem is understood a solution can be worked out. However, there is some work which does suggest that brain damaged patients who work well in the presence of therapists, but not in their absence differ in this respect from other disabled patients.

Recently newer methods for managing particular problems have been considered. Patients may be able to learn to compensate for certain disabilities by using alternative strategies. For instance people with loss of ability to calculate (left parietal lobe) may regain their ability to deal with numbers again by using an abacus (right hemisphere function). This approach needs more investigation. The specific activities undertaken by the various therapists and their limitations have already been discussed more fully in Chapter 10 on Strokes and this should be consulted.

OUTCOME

There is no generally agreed classification of outcome other than death, although there has been a lot of discussion about the topic. One recently suggested scale has certain merits and it is outlined below.

(1) Death.
(2) Persistent vegetable state — describing the patient who remains *unresponsive* and *speechless* for weeks or months until death. Other states including akinetic mutism and the 'locked-in' syndrome where communication using the eyes is possible, must be excluded.
(3) Severe disability (conscious but disabled). Patients in this group are dependent for daily support by reason of physical, mental or combined impairment.
(4) Moderate disability (disabled but independent).
(5) Good recovery. This implies return to normal life with or without some impairment.

The great majority of head injured people who survive recover to grades 4 or 5. On the basis of an estimated 107 000 people admitted to hospital with head injury in 1963, there were 7 500 with severe head injury. Of these 6 000 (80 per cent) could be expected to return to their former employment, although recovery may have been delayed for some months. The remaining 1 500 included 900 who would return to some (simpler) employment, but 600 would never work again — mostly males and mostly under 20 years of age. This group of 600 would include most of the severest head injuries with unconsciousness for one month or more.

The life expectancy of these survivors of severe head injury is less than that for uninjured people. Patients in the persistent vegetative state rarely live one year (but some do — surviving repeated episodes of broncho-pneumonia on the way). The more seriously disabled people who nevertheless return home still show a shortened life expectancy, although the reasons for this have not been clarified.

Information on people with minor head injury is not available although it has been estimated that 10–15 per cent of people with PTA of less than one hour and without immediate complications will develop the 'post concussional syndrome' or epilepsy.

Return to work is probably made easier and more successful if there is:

(1) Early contact and assessment of patients.
(2) Early contact with the employer and an early job assessment.
(3) Continuing contact until the problems are settled.

This work is done principally by Resettlement Officers and involves not only assessment but where necessary re-training for former job or new employment and placement. Early contact should inspire the patients and encourage employers to expect them to return to work.

Generally speaking the recovery from paresis, sensory disturbance and cranial nerve lesion is good, but anosmia, the commonest cranial nerve lesion despite the rarity of complaint about it, remains. (In fact, of course 'cranial nerves' one and two — olfactory and optic — are extensions of the brain and not nerves).

Ataxia and visual defects have a poorer prognosis while epilepsy tends to lessen with time in terms of frequency and severity of fits.

Cognitive Sequelae

Brain damage is almost always accompanied by some abnormality of higher cerebral function which expresses itself in impairment of:

(1) Intelligence.
(2) Memory.
(3) Perception.
(4) Visuo-spatial organization.
(5) Language and communication.

Little work has been done on any of these aspects, but it is generally considered that improvement is the rule, but mostly within the first six months after injury.

Psychiatric sequelae

Again there is insufficient work in this field, but it is thought that brain damage accounts for only a small part of psychiatric morbidity after head injury. The disability increases with the degree of brain injury and depends to some extent on the site of the lesion.

Behavioural disorders are particularly associated with frontal lobe lesions, while intellectual impairment is associated with temporal and parietal lesions.

In children there has been found to be a significant lowering of intelligence quotient (IQ) in those unconscious for more than three days compared to those with shorter periods of unconscious. Behaviour problems are the commoner psychiatric sequelae in this age group. The role of drugs (e.g. phenobarbitone, although much less commonly prescribed nowadays) must not be forgotten.

The patient and his family

Behaviour problems create more difficulties than physical impairment, although epilepsy is particularly disrupting.

There are two aspects of the patient's behaviour which create particular problems. Rage reactions — 'uncontrolled and inappropriate response' — fortunately tend to improve with time but other aspects of emotional lability, especially pathological laughter, may remain.

The patient often remains unaware of his problems, but may complain of loneliness. Isolation of the individual is indeed often the way families react to emotional lability. The families of people with brain damage show varying degrees of stress, but denial of any disability by relatives may produce a management problem. Stress appears to be mediated by the relatives, perception of personality change in the patient, and thus the degree of stress shown varies enormously. The worst period of stress for a majority of relatives is the first month after injury with a levelling off by the 6th month. Wives and mothers of patients often require some sort of treatment themselves, especially tranquillisers or counselling. There is a reported high divorce and separation rate, although comparison with other groups has not been made.

Doctors, nurses, therapists and other members of the health care team should note that relatives often complain of lack of information. While this may not reflect a failure to *talk* to relatives it does show an inability to *communicate* and is one area where improvements could be cheaply and easily made.

People suffering the after effects of head injury, and their relatives, need counselling — that is, the opportunity to talk to the people involved in the rehabilitation process. They need the best available advice with regard to the prognosis especially for independence and work, and the likely rate of progress. While realistic advice is essential it should be tempered with kindness and as much useful support as is possible. Advice should be given, whether or not it is sought for and should be repeated often, remembering that the majority of people forget the majority of information they are given by doctors.

Follow-up care, preferably in the form of domiciliary visits, is essential. The old idea that patients almost inevitably function at a higher level at home compared to hospital may not be true and this must be taken into account when discharge from any unit is being planned. It probably does not matter whether the care is by domiciliary physiotherapist, occupational therapist, health visitor or social worker, as long as it is undertaken.

THE FUTURE

Our knowledge concerning the processes of recovery after head injury and the ways in which is can be helped is embarrassingly scanty.

Research to increase the pool of knowledge needs to be on several levels. While work into the patholo-physiology of damage, dysfunction and recovery is vital, there is also the opportunity for clinicians to organize trials to answer simple questions. To which patients should we offer our scarce rehabilitation resources? Is this necessarily the group that will do best? Where should rehabilitation be conducted and should specialized units be encouraged? If special units are to be used, at what stage in the disease should the patient be transferred to them? What are the best treatment methods and for how long should they be continued and how should they be given — in short bursts or over a prolonged period until the patient's improvement rate plateaus out? Does rehabilitation do more than teach patients (and relatives) to use the recovery that has occurred spontaneously?

In order to help the greatest number of people these and other questions need answers.

REFERENCES

Belmont, I., Benjamin, H., Ambrose, J. and Restuccia, R.D. (1969). 'Effect of cerebral damage on motivation in rehabilitation.' *Arch. Phys. Med. Rehab.* **50**, 507–511

Bond, M.R. and Brookes, D.N. (1976). 'Understanding the process of recovery as a basis for the investigation of rehabilitation for the brain injured.' *Scand. J. Rehab. Med.* **8**, 127–133

Cairns, H. (1941). 'Rehabilitation after injury to the central nervous system.' *Proc. R. Soc. Med.* **35**, 299–302

Daniel, J. (July 1978). Paper given in Basle. IRMA III

Gronwall, D. and Wrightson, P. (1974). 'Delayed recovery of intellectual function after minor head injury.' *Lancet ii* 605–609

Hook, O. (1969). 'Comments in rehabilitation of brain injury.' In *Late effects of head injury* Eds. Walker, A.E. Thomas, Springfield Ill., 398–407

Jennet, B. and Bond, M.R. (1975). 'Assessment of outcome after severe brain damage.' *Lancet i* 426–484

Kaales, M. (1971). 'The role of the occupational therapist in the early stages of rehabilitation after head injury.' *Occupational therapy*, Feb., 30–35

Lewin, W. (1970). 'Rehabilitation needs of the brain injured patient.' *Proc. R. Soc. Med.* **63**, 8–12

Oddy, M., Humphrey, M. and Uttley, D. (1978). 'Stresses upon the relatives of head injured patients.' *Brit. J. Psychiat.* **133**, 507–13

Panting, A. and Merry, P.H. (1970). 'Long-term rehabilitation of severe head injuries — social and medical support for the patient's family.' *Injury* **2**, No. 1, 33–37

Potter, J.M. (1973). 'Hospital admission after head injury.' *Lancet ii* 1381 (Letter)

Reilly, P.L., Graham, D.I., Adams, J.H. and Jennet, B. (1975). 'Patients with head injury who talk and die.' *Lancet ii* 375–377

Relander, M., Troupp, H. and Bjorkesten, G. (1972). 'Controlled trial of treatment for cerebral concussion.' *B.M.J.* **9**, 777–779

Ritchie Russell, W. and Smith, A. (1961). 'Post traumatic amnesia in closed head injury.' *Arch. Neurol.* **5**, 16–29

Series, C. and Lincoln, N.B. (1978). 'Behaviour modification in physical rehabilitation.' *Occupational therapy* **41**, No. 7, 222–224

Wall, P.D. (1976). 'Plasticity in the adult mammalian central nervous system.' in *Perspectives in Brain Research* Eds. Corner, M.A. and Swaab, D.F. Elsevier. Vol. 45, 359–383

BIBLIOGRAPHY

CIBA Foundation Symposium 34: (1975). *Outcome of severe damage to the central nervous system.* Amsterdam; Elsevier. Excerpta Medica. N. Holland

Field, J.H. (1975). *Epidemiology of head injuries in England and Wales.* London; HMSO

Jennet, B. (1972). *Epilepsy after non-missile head injuries.* 2nd edn., London; Heinneman

Johnstone, Margaret (1976). *The stroke patient: principles of rehabilitation.* Edinburgh and London; Churchill Livingstone

12 Rehabilitation Following Amputation

ANN HAMILTON

INTRODUCTION

Any person who because of amputation or congenital deformity has a short limb will face physical, psychological and social difficulties through his or her life.

These difficulties are somewhat lessened by the provision of artificial or prosthetic limbs — lessened but not solved. Even with efficient prostheses, loss of an upper limb always results in reduced dexterity, loss of a lower limb in reduced mobility. Quite apart from this, the absence or loss of any limb has an adverse effect on self image.

Functional recovery following amputation may be complicated in a number of ways. For example, patients who lose a limb following trauma may have other associated injuries — such as fractures of other limbs, or brain damage following head injury: patients who have a limb amputated for neoplasm may require cytotoxic therapy or radiotherapy and are likely to experience periodic debilitating malaise.

Whatever the cause of amputation or the nature of the complications which accompany it, rehabilitation of the amputee entails the closely integrated efforts of the patient and his family, the hospital staff, the community services, the limb fitting service and Social Services if it is to be of optimal effect.

It is convenient to consider first the rehabilitative care of young amputees. The rehabilitation of the older and ischaemic amputees is dealt with in a subsequent chapter, since the greater age and generalized peripheral vascular disease of this latter group of patients produce problem complexes very different to those associated with the amputation of the limbs of younger patients, and necessitate a modified rehabilitative procedure.

Various problems of rehabilitation are of course common to the younger and the older amputee, and occur following upper and lower limb amputation. To save reduplication, these problems will be considered in the chapter in which their inclusion seems most appropriate.

REHABILITATION FOLLOWING UPPER LIMB AMPUTATION

Congenital amputation

Patients with short or phocomelic limbs from intra-uterine maldevelopment are also referred to as amputees although their amputation is developmental and not acquired. Amputation of the upper limb in infancy and childhood is almost always congenital in origin, and the usual amputation level is below the elbow.

There are a number of factors which determine the acceptance of a prosthesis by the congenital amputee, the degree to which it will be incorporated into his lifestyle, and the extent to which he will overcome his handicap and realise his full potential in later life.

(1) Parental attitude and co-operation.
(2) Ready availability of appropriate prostheses.
(3) Early integration of prosthesis with patient's self image.
(4) Length and strength of stump. Overall health of patient.
(5) Motivation of patient.
(6) Early start on a realistic and forward-looking programme of rehabilitative care.

Parental Attitude and Co-operation
The initial reaction of most parents to the birth of a baby deformed by the presence of a short or absent limb is one of disbelief, horror and repugnance. Resentment follows, regret and sometimes psychological or actual physical rejection. Then grief and guilt supervene, and it is in the alleviation of these destructive emotions that the early referral of a phocomelic babe to a Limb-fitting Centre can be helpful. Family doctor, gynaecologist, pediatrician and nursing staff will all have attempted to give counsel, but the practical advice of a limb-fitting doctor and his introduction of the newly referred parents to the parents of an older and well adjusted child with a similar amputation will alone give them the reassurance they need.

Once they can be helped to accept the phocolemic arm as a part of their child, and not to consider it as an unacceptable appendage with which he is encumbered, they are then able to transmit this attitude to the child himself. Instead of considering the short arm as an excuse for non-participation, he is encouraged to think of it as a spur to high achievement, and the provision of an effective prosthesis as the means to help him attain his objective.

A child does not automatically dislike and reject an artificial arm. So long as the functional benefit which it provides exceeds its disadvantages it will be accepted. But the enthusiasm and encouragement of his parents, and their appreciation of his efforts to use it will encourage him to persevere until he has attained maximal expertise.

Parents themselves need continual encouragement initially to develop an optimistic and outward looking attitude, so that they allow their child to attempt anything that other children do, unless his prosthesis makes it frankly dangerous.

Equally, they need to be advised that forcing a prosthesis on an unwilling child can only make him hate it, and will effectively prevent him integrating it into his self-image. He needs always to have some time each day without his prosthesis, so that the afferent stimuli which the skin of his phocomelic limb transmits to his brain can enlarge his sensory picture of the outside world. There will be some things which he prefers to do with his prosthesis, and some with his phocomelic arm, and effective rehabilitative care helps him to establish the optimal usage of both.

Readily Availability of Efficient Prostheses
Early Integration of Prosthesis with Amputee's Self-image
Many authorities hold the view that it is important to supply a prosthetic arm to a phocomelic child at a very early age, even as young as three to six months, and many limb centres in the UK fit a simple one-piece plastic arm at this stage so that the child has two limbs of equal length when bimanual movements become important to his development. Early fitting of a prosthetic arm is thought to increase the likelihood that the child will come to accept a more useful prosthesis at a later date, because he has integrated the presence of an arm-substitute with his self-image.

Most infants soon realise the advantages of the simple plastic arm as an arm lengthener, a holding mechanism and an aid to balance, and provided the parents accept it and encourage its use by putting it on regularly and removing it whenever it becomes a source of annoyance, its presence becomes a part of the daily routine.

As the phocomelic child grows, he is ideally brought up to his Limbfitting Centre every three months to have his prostheses repaired or new ones fitted. Once his understanding and co-ordination are sufficient, a split hook is fitted onto a light working arm, and he is taught to use the hook for feeding and playing. Alternatively a cosmetic hand may be fitted onto the working arm for social occasions, or if the child prefers it.

Parental enthusiasm is especially needed to promote the child's use of the split-grip or hook, rather than the cosmetic hand, as a terminal device on his prosthetic arm. Despite the decrease in functional efficiency which the passive hand entails, parental distaste and dislike of the appearance and associations of the split-grip can effectively prevent its acceptance and utilization, and so degrade the prosthetic arm into an appendage rather than a multi-purpose tool.

Length and Strength of Stump. Overall Condition of Patient
If other factors are equal, the usefulness of a phocomelic arm, with or without a prosthesis, is directly proportional to its length, and to the efficiency of its joints and muscles. Thus the child born with complete absence of an upper limb will have minimal functional benefit from the provision of a prosthesis, since he only has the shoulder girdle to effect its active movement. The usefulness of this prosthesis is therefore limited — partly cosmetic, to produce apparent body symmetry, and partly as a stabilizer to fix objects for manipulation by the remaining hand.

An above-elbow amputee with an intact gleno-humeral joint fares better, and the amputee with a below-elbow stump — the commonest type of congenital upper limb abnormality — better still.

Motivation of Patient.
Early Start on a Realistic and Forward Looking Programme of Rehabilitative Care.
However co-operative the parents or willing the child, short intervals of training in prosthetic usage by a skilled occupational therapist can be of inestimable value in teaching a child how to make the best use of his prosthesis and himself. Admission to a Rehabilitation Centre or Disabled Living Unit for a few days at a time — initially with and later, when he is willing, without a parent — is arranged. Such admission may be timed to coincide with the issue of a more sophisticated type of prosthesis, or else to solve a particular problem of daily living.

Toiletting, dressing and feeding are particularly important regimes in which independence needs to be established early and effectively, so that attention is not constantly being drawn to the prosthesis and phocomelic arm by slow or conspicuous behaviour.

The wise therapist adds her expertise and appreciation of the child's efforts to the task of building up his self-image, and the equally important task of facilitating symmetrical physical growth by encouraging maximal use of the prosthetic arm. She, too, constantly advocates use of split-grip rather than cosmetic hand, because of the greater functional efficiency of the former as a hand-substitute. A child who uses his split-grip well will use his prosthesis as an arm/hand complex: the child who uses only his cosmetic hand is limited to *arm* use only, since he gets little or no functional benefit from the passive cosmetic hand. The good split-grip user thus becomes bi-manual in his activities, and the range and power of the consequent movements of his phocomelic arm act as a constant stimulation to the growth of the phocomelic arm itself, the shoulder girdle, the thorax and the spine.

Throughout childhood the young child continues to be seen at his local limb-fitting centre at three to six month intervals for supervision of his growth, activity and prosthetic fitting. Many centres have an occupational therapist attached to them, who advises outpatients attending limbfitting clinics, and arranges admission when needed to her unit. By medical officers, prosthetists and parents, therapists and teachers, the phocomelic child is constantly urged to acquire new skills.

Swimming and other sports are advocated to help symmetrical use of the limbs and good trunk development, dancing to help poise and balance. Early instruction in unarmed combat is suggested if the child lives in an area where he may have to defend himself against attack by other children. Phocomelic children are encouraged to learn a musical instrument at the earliest possible age – the French horn and trumpet only need one hand to play them: the guitar, cello, viola and banjo can be played with one hand to finger the strings while the split-grip is used to hold a bow or plectrum. Disability isolates. Without such a skill or some comparable prestigious ability the phocomelic child may become shy and withdrawn.

Before a child with an artificial arm starts school or when he changes schools, the parents should if possible visit the headmaster to explain the limitations of the prosthesis. Some headmasters prevent the bullying and ragging which normal children frequently offer to a split-grip using phocomelic child by demonstrating how the prosthesis works to the whole school. For other children a quiet word with the form teacher is better.

Sometimes a child will use a prosthetic arm with its split grip quite happily until he reaches his teens, when he may insist on wearing only a cosmetic hand or arm. This phase corresponds to a period of high sensitivity about self image and is usually only temporary. In due course he will perceive the split-grip's advantages and will again accept the issue of a 'working arm'.

Acquired upper limb amputation
Upper Limb Amputation in the Child
When upper limb amputation in the child follows trauma, infection or malignancy, the rehabilitation programme is similar in most aspects to that advocated for the congenital amputee.

The supply of a prosthesis and institution of effective instruction in its use are matters of urgency, to enable the child to re-establish a pattern of activity as similar to his premorbid pattern as possible.

AcquiredAmputation to the Upper Limb in the Adult

HOSPITAL CARE

Following amputation for neoplasm or injury, the upper limb amputee feels horror and despair. It is an irretrievable loss and he will need help to accept it. The attitude of the nurses who dress the amputation stump and the physiotherapists who mobilise it are important in helping him to overcome his grief, and their willingness to examine and touch the stump will be vitally important in the initial rebuilding of his self-image. As soon as possible he should examine and touch the stump too, and should do some of his daily exercises in front of a mirror.

During the early post-operative days he should have sufficient analgesia to keep him comfortable, and nurses giving care need to ensure that he is never left in pain just because 'he is not written up for anything'. A patient who experiences severe unrelieved pre-operative and post-operative pain is more likely to have intractable and prolonged phantom pain after the stump has healed. Careful supervision of the stump detects early onset of infection and permits prompt prescription of antibiotics: meticulous bandaging avoids stump constriction with terminal engorgement and swelling.

The occupational therapist advises the amputee on daily living activities, and in the absence of other injury, he can become completely independent within two weeks of amputation. Minor clothing adaptations such as Velcro fastenings, elastic-stalked buttons, stretch nylon sweaters, made-up ties and elastic shoelaces assist him in this.

The hospital medical social worker will ask about family circumstances and relationships. She will also see the amputee's girlfriend or wife and explain how important it is that she accepts the amputation and is willing to touch and be touched by the stump.

Phantom pain, the impression of pain in the amputated hand and arm, is almost always present immediately after the operation but gradually becomes less severe and is less often experienced during the first few post-operative weeks. If the severed nerves of the stump adhere to the amputation scar, the pain persists, and sometimes refashioning of the stump is necessary to relieve it. Sometimes nerve fibres at the site of a severed nerve proliferate to form a tumour-like mass (neuroma), which can also give rise to stump and phantom pain; injection of local anaesthetic, ultrasonics, percussion or surgery may be effective in providing relief. Hypnosis can often lessen or abolish this pain and so can behavioural therapy. Electrical stimulation is also sometimes helpful.

Stump tenderness is a different entity although it may coexist with phantom pain. It is caused by infection or ischaemia in bone or soft tissue, or by the presence of one or more neuromata. Unless properly treated, stump tenderness can prevent the wearing of a prosthesis.

PROSTHETIC CONSIDERATIONS
Immediate Post-operative Fitting. Some centres advocate immediate post-operative fitting for suitable cases. With mid-forearm or wrist-level amputations,

a light plaster of paris cast is often applied over the dressed stump at operation. A steel hook is embedded in the plaster and is usable as soon as the plaster is set.

In other centres a cast is taken of the stump as soon as the stitches are out and tenderness and swelling have subsided sufficiently. A light-weight working arm is ordered and arm training arranged.

Prophylactic Effect of Prosthesis.   Although a one-armed man can become independent, the long-term over-usage of the normal limb does appear to lead to the development of arthritis in shoulder, elbow, wrist and hand, and some older amputees who have never worn a limb or only accepted a cosmetic one will in later life request a working arm to relieve the strain on the normal limb. Every effort should be made to persuade the new amputee to wear a prosthesis to prevent this over-usage, unless the amputation stump is long enough and strong enough to make the use of a prosthesis unnecessary.

Dominance.   When the arm on the dominant side is amputated, the functional gain which a prosthetic arm can supply is far less than when the amputated arm is on the non-dominant side. The patient has then not only to master the intricacies of using a prosthesis, but also to acquire maximal skill with the remaining limb.

Usefulness of Prosthetic Arm.   The usefulness of an artificial or prosthetic arm to an adult with acquired amputation of an upper limb will vary with

(1) level of amputation
(2) condition of stump
(3) occupation and motivation
(4) economic and family circumstances
(5) type, fit and efficiency of prostheses.

(1) LEVEL OF AMPUTATION
Unlike amputation of the lower limb, amputation of the upper limb is seldom performed for peripheral vascular disease, but usually follows trauma or neoplasm, the site of which largely determined the level of amputation. Not all amputees need or want to wear a prosthesis. The higher the level of amputation, the greater the need for a prosthetic substitute. With a below-elbow stump an amputee may achieve bimanual dexterity without a prosthesis, particularly when wrist and palm are present. An above-elbow or short below-elbow amputee needs a prosthesis to correct his body outline and provide a limb lengthener and a tool bearer.

At operation it is not necessarily the wisest policy to preserve the longest possible fragment of limb if the patient is planning to use a prosthesis. Amputation in the middle third of the forearm provides a sufficiently long lever to work the prosthetic arm adequately yet leaves room for the wrist mechanism. Above-elbow amputation is likewise sited within the middle third of the upper arm to ensure adequate leverage and room for the elbow mechanism. It is only when through-hand amputation is performed that conservation of length is vitally important — a stump of finger which can achieve a pinch grip with a thumb is worth saving. But to preserve tissue which is ischaemic, anaesthetic and paralysed or painful just for the sake of conserving the maximal length of stump is to have a legacy of continued trouble.

When amputation is above-elbow and is accompanied by permanent damage to the brachial plexus, giving a flail stump, many surgeons permanently fuse the glenohumeral joint in 5 degrees of abduction and 5 degrees of flexion. This provides a stable base for the prosthesis and prevents the discomfort and inconvenience of shoulder distraction or recurrent subluxation.

(2) CONDITION OF STUMP

One of the reasons why the recommended level of amputation is within the middle third of upper arm or forearm is that there is enough muscle bulk at these sites to ensure adequate coverage for the stump end. Enough skin and muscle, a good blood supply and nerve supply, and a well-rounded bone end are the basic characteristics of a good stump. If there is inadequate coverage and when amputation occurs before growth has stopped, the lengthening bone tends to push its way out of the stump periodically, and further operation becomes necessary to remove the protruding bone end. When amputation occurs after growth has stopped, inadequate coverage of the bone end still leads to a tender stump with a sharp end where soft tissues have retracted leaving the bone covered with skin and scar tissue alone. Ulceration plagues the patient, and stump tenderness makes for discomfort when the prosthesis is not worn, while at the same time precluding its use. The ugly and unsightly structure offends both the patient and those around him.

Ulcerated skin, allergic reactions, painful neuromata will all discourage the amputee from wearing his prosthesis, and constant care to ensure a well fitting socket and to locate and eradicate the cause of any allergies — such as protruding, improperly sunk nickel screws in the socket — is important. Neuromata may need treatment by injection or surgery.

Even with faultless surgery, an amputation stump is almost invariably cold, and tends to develop chilblains in the winter. Covering the stump with a woollen stump sock, whether or not the prosthesis is used, is only of moderate help.

(3) OCCUPATION AND MOTIVATION

Occupation. What a patient does for his living and in his leisure hours will greatly influence whether he accepts a prosthetic arm and how efficient he will become using it. A manual worker employing moderate skills tends to fare well, since the split-grip and universal tool holder fitment provide a good range of performance. Those employing fine manipulative skills, such as surgery, drawing and painting, fare badly if the dominant arm is amputated. The appropriate tool on a prosthesis subtended by a strong mobile stump can form an effective functional unit, but it can never replace a normal hand and arm.

People with academic or administrative occupations perhaps fare best of all.

Motivation. Following traumatic amputation and while a claim for compensation remains unsettled, the necessary motivation to learn to use the prosthetic arm and restart work is too often diluted by advice to make the most of the injury and the disability it has caused.

Reform of the present system of compensation is urgently needed, so that an appropriate pension or lump sum is paid as soon as possible after the anatomical and physiological extent of the injury is known. The gain in terms of restored self respect and recovered efficiency would be considerable and should assist a speedy return to employment.

The question of return to work should be raised as soon as the amputee is able to discuss it with the surgeon post-operatively. Help from the medical social worker may be needed to contact the manager or personnel manager at his place of work to request them to hold his job open. If return to his old job is not possible, referral to the DRO may be advisable. For many men however this is unnecessary, since those with extrovert personalities, self respect and determined characters will find their own jobs and make a success of them, integrating the use of their prostheses into their chosen lifestyle with minimal ostentation.

(4) ECONOMIC AND FAMILY CIRCUMSTANCES

Men and women with young families usually are highly motivated to attain rapid expertise and optimal usage from prostheses. Nevertheless, men of low intelligence with amputation at a high level are often hard put to it to find employment. Available jobs for such men are often poorly paid and carry little job satisfaction, and they may actually lose money by accepting employment. Rounds of assessment and retraining centres are abortive for them, if high amputation and possibly a flail stump have necessitated the supply of a prosthesis which is of mainly cosmetic value, and cannot contribute to the two-handed labouring demanded of uneducated men.

Most below-elbow amputees who want work will find jobs and keep them — driving cars and tractors without difficulty and manipulating machinery satisfactorily — because with the provision and efficient usage of a working arm and split grip they virtually become two handed.

The majority of traumatic upper limb amputees are men, who frequently return to operate the heavy machinery which caused their amputation. Women amputees who are married are doubly motivated to become efficient users of their prostheses. The need to care for home and family as well as the need to provide an extra income will decide how well and how often they use their prostheses. Unmarried girls are motivated by the desire to look normal, to re-establish body image, to increase employment value and to find a husband.

(5) SUPPLY, TYPE, FIT AND EFFICIENCY OF PROSTHESES

Supply.   At present a wide variety of upper limb prostheses is available. Some are prescribed for cosmetic purposes, some for work and they may be powered or non-powered. In the UK a selection of prostheses is prescribed by the DHSS and a further selection may be purchased privately. The financial commitment of the DHSS to prescribe prosthetic limbs free from birth till death to a phocomelic child is an immense one.

Type of Prostheses.   A prosthetic or artificial arm consists of a few basic parts which can be varied in construction and control to suit the needs of the individual. There is a socket to enclose the stump or phocomelic arm, an outer casing to complete the outline of the arm and to bear a prosthetic hand or tool, and some form of attachment to the upper arm or trunk. Depending on the length of the stump, the prosthesis may have a hinged elbow joint, a wrist rotation joint, or neither.

The socket fits the stump exactly. It is constructed from a cast taken from the stump, and is made of plastic or leather. Some amputees wear a cotton nylon or woollen sock over the amputation stump to protect it from rubbing the socket: others wear no protection.

Amputees are usually issued with two artificial arms, so that if one breaks, they have the other in reserve while the broken prosthesis is repaired or replaced. Frequently one prosthesis is a working arm with split grip and various other attachments, and the other prosthesis is a cosmetic arm.

Cosmetic Arms are lightweight models of the human arm and hand, made of plastic and foam, with the hand covered by a plastic glove tinted to resemble human skin.

They have no useful purpose other than to preserve the normal appearance of the patient. They are attached by a strap, light corset or elasticated cuff, except if amputation is in the upper arm, when a trunk harness is essential.

Working Arms   are strong prostheses made of leather, steel or specially strong plastic, and carry a steel wrist-unit into which may be screwed a variety of terminal devices. For above-elbow amputees, an elbow joint is also incorporated. A strong harness attaches the arm to the trunk, passing under the opposite axilla and acting as a counterpull. The amputee uses a split-grip for most purposes, but the appropriate devices are available for various specific tasks, so that most types of work and sport are open to him. he may also attach a cosmetic hand to the wrist unit for social occasions.

Myo hand or Bionic Arm.   Powered prostheses were prescribed extensively during the early years of many children made phocomelic by Thalidomide. Some were gas-powered and some battery-driven. By and large they were all discarded except by those children whose lower limbs were unable to substitute as arms because they were too deformed.

The myo-electric hand or bionic arm, pioneered in Sweden, has an electrically powered hand which works by the amplification of the myo-electrical impulses generated by contracting forearm muscles to activate a powered unit concealed in the prosthetic hand.

The limb currently being evaluated in the UK and Sweden makes only a single movement consisting of a three-point grip between the index and middle fingers and the thumb. But more advanced prostheses have already been designed allowing both pronation and supination of the hand and wrist flexion.

A small number of children have been selected to receive this type of prosthesis in the UK, financed by the DHSS, and their subsequent progress is being assessed. Other children and young adults have purchased myo-electric prostheses privately, at the cost of £1–2000 per limb.

Disadvantages. The disadvantages of the models currently available are that they break down frequently: their construction entails long waits for child and parents during fitting sessions, followed by numerous hospital attendances for training purposes. the fit of the prosthetic socket to the stump has to be exact, and is so tight that normal growth soon makes any particular limb unwearable: the tight fit needed tends to cause skin soreness and excoriation, particularly in those who sweat a lot: use of the myoelectric arm demands the continued co-operation and training assistance of the parents, and considerable patience from the child: in addition, a battery has to be warn on a harness worn round the waist, with leads passing to the prosthesis. The currently assessed DHSS limbs are only suitable for children with below-elbow stumps, and with ages between 2 and 4 years.

The *advantages* of the myoelectric hand are that it looks like a hand: it needs no harness round the chest (although it *does* have a waist harness): it gives the user the satisfaction of operating the hand as part of a natural movement pattern: self image and social acceptance are said to be improved for the child who wears it.

So long as children retain their natural love for sand, mud and water and their disrespect for valuable equipment, the supply of myoelectric limbs is an unrealistic and expensive exercise.

Time will show whether the simpler split-grip, disguised by a hand-like covering, will not provide a hand substitute which is both more functionally adequate and economically feasible.

REHABILITATION FOLLOWING AMPUTATION OF LOWER LIMBS

Congenital amputation
Infancy

A small number of children are born each year with shortening and malformation of one or both lower limbs.

Such children benefit from referral to a Limb Centre when only a few weeks old, so that the parents can be counselled and informed of prosthetic possibilities.

At the age when the infant would normally walk, he is referred back to the centre, so that a first prosthesis may be made. If he has a suitable hip and good foot on the phocomelic side, a platform prosthesis is made in the first instance to level the pelvis. The platform prosthesis is a strong leather gaiter terminating in a shin-piece and foot: the child weightbears on a platform incorporated in the proximal part of the shin-piece, and learns to walk with his parents' help without any special physiotherapeutic training. If the hip is unstable, the same type of prosthesis is offered, but walking is never as good.

These platform prostheses are replaced as the child grows until he is a few years old, and the rate of growth of the phocomelic limb has become apparent, when the parents are often urged to allow the child to have an appropriate selective amputation with preservation of an end-bearing pad. Following this procedure he has a stable stump and is fitted with a prosthesis, so that he can walk on two symmetrical legs and wear normal shoes and socks. Whenever possible, the amputation is carried out before the child starts Primary School.

Children who have had this rehabilitative treatment do well. They have an almost limp free gait, play any sport, and grow unimpeded by pelvic tilt or scoliotic curve. Their self image appears to be less affected by the possession of an amputation stump than by the presence of a short, misshapen leg. Other children do not mock a stump as they do a deformed leg.

This scheme of treatment is not suitable for all children, and the optimal surgical procedure for any one child is dictated by the length, shape and deformity of the phocomelic limb, and is the decision of the orthopaedic surgeon giving care.

The same regime is followed by bilateral lower limb phocomelia as for unilateral, and the parents of such children are offered platform prostheses or appropriate amputation and the provision of paired prostheses.

Youth

Some children with single or bilateral lower limb amputation are refused by their parents the operative treatment which is offered, and may elect to have their abnormal feet amputated when they become old enough to make the decision for themselves. Some elect to wear platform prostheses for life.

Acquired amputation
Infancy

Occasionally infants have lower limb amputation following trauma or malignancy. Their rehabilitative care involves rapid referral from parent hospital to Limb

Fitting Centre for the provision of prosthetic fitting as soon as post-operative condition permits. Walking training is unnecessary, but frequent visits to the Limb Fitting Centre are essential — as often as three monthly — since no prosthesis has yet been produced which can stand up unscathed to the normal treatment meted out to it by an active growing child, and repair and replacement are almost continuous to keep up with destruction and growth.

Youth

The incidence of amputation following trauma and malignancy rises in older children, particularly in young boys, and early prosthetic fitting and frequent repair and replacement are again the pattern of rehabilitative care. As is the case with upper limb amputees, these children need constant encouragement to attempt new activities, repeatedly expressed appreciation of their achievements, and guidance in education and choice of career.

No special walking training is necessary, but compassion and priority of appointment and limb production are needed and given to young lads on cytotoxic or radiotherapy, and to those with secondary deposits. Malaise and depression frequently complicate rehabilitation, and prosthetic usage may have to be discontinued temporarily or permanently.

Young Adulthood

Trauma, malignancy and ischaemia in that order of frequency are the causes of amputation in young adults.

The nature and order of rehabilitative procedures during hospitalization are similar for young and old amputees, and are considered in detail in the chapter on the latter group of patients. Here, the various characteristics of the amputee and his rehabilitation programme which effect his final functional state are briefly considered.

These are:

(1) Nature of stump;
(2) Physical and mental condition;
(3) Type of rehabilitative care offered;
(4) Type of limb offered;
(5) Persistence of phantom pain.

(1) NATURE OF STUMP

Amputation attempts to produce a viable stump which is strong and mobile, designed to provide optimal mobility, capable of powering a prosthesis, and ready for measurement for this prosthesis in the shortest possible time: a stump free from pain and phantom pain which matures well and stands up well to the continual multiple minitraumata of prosthetic walking.

Stump length, stump site, stump construction and the shape and final steady state of a stump are all important in the achievement of this object.

Stump Length.   It is not always the best policy to conserve as much of a limb as possible. Ideally an amputation stump is deliberately constructed to enable its owner to wear a particular type of prosthesis, and not merely to get rid of the non-viable or malignant distal part of a limb. Over conservation can lead to the prolonged hospitalization of a patient, when healing is awaited in a long stump made ischaemic by vascular trauma or disease. Such a stump may give long term trouble, as well as causing depression, debility and domestic upset in the hospital-bound patient.

The elective sites for amputation of the lower limb are in the middle third of the tibia for below-knee stumps, and in the middle third of the femur for above-knee stumps. The exact levels are dictated by the viability of the tissues and the height of the patient. Tall people need longer stumps than shorter people, to obtain the best mechanical advantage from the ratio $\dfrac{\text{length of stump}}{\text{length of prosthesis}}$.

To take an absolute value for an elective amputation site — such as 5½" below the joint line for a below-knee stump, and 9" from the crutch for an above-knee stump — is unrealistic. Appropriate siting of an amputation either within the middle third of the tibia of the middle third of the femur will provide a stump which clears the mechanism of the prosthetic joint distal to it, is long enough to remain in the socket without constantly slipping out, and long enough to power the prosthesis adequately.

Stump Site.   The rehabilitation and subsequent prosthetic management of patients with *through-foot* amputations is fraught with many problems, and even in young patients, such amputations are seldom indicated. Due to the intricacy of muscle balance in the foot it is difficult to produce a satisfactory stump free from contractures and torsion, and the production of a durable and comfortable prosthetic forefoot is no less difficult to achieve.

Through-ankle   amputation by Symes procedure produces an excellent weight-bearing stump, but is best avoided in older patients with peripheral vascular disease. Prosthetic walking and return to normal work and leisure activities are rapid in the young and healthy.

Below knee amputation   in young and old should always be attempted if there is a reasonable chance of stump viability, since the advantage of retaining the knee is inestimable. Not only is walking easier with a living knee than with a prosthetic one, but also the prostheses for below-knee stumps are more comfortable to wear than those for above-knee stumps. Conservation of the knee is especially important in the older patient with peripheral vascular disease, whose chances of losing his second leg are high. With a double below-knee amputation he stands a reasonable chance of walking on prostheses, but with a double above-knee amputation his chances of achieving prosthetic walking are virtually nil.

Supra Condylar or Gritti Stokes Amputation: The stumps produced by disarticulation through the knee, or supracondylar amputation above the knee by the Gritti Stokes method, are advantageously constructed by swift and relatively bloodless surgical procedures. Nevertheless, the necessity for an abnormally low prosthetic knee which they entail makes them disliked by patients and prosthetists. When the patella is retained it frequently 'wanders' and complicates limb fitting. When endbearing is attempted after disarticulation, skin ulceration tends to occur when weight bearing is attempted on skin which was not constructed to take weight. Spur formation is frequent, marked and troublesome in stumps constructed by the Gritti Stokes technique.

Above Knee Amputation.   Amputation in the middle third of the thigh produces a stump which usually heals well with few complications, and is favoured by prosthetists for fitting with a goodlooking and comfortable prosthesis.

Stump Construction.   Although several alternative surgical procedures may be followed in the construction of any particular stump — such as the use of simple flaps, 'guillotining', a myoplastic or an osteomyoplastic technique —

certain surgical 'constants' are common to all. Sufficiently long skin and soft tissue flaps should be left to provide good coverage of the amputation stump: the scar should be sited to avoid pressure areas and shaped to contribute to the rounded cone-shape of the final stump: the nerves should be carefully cut and their ends buried in muscle well away from the scar and the cut end of the bone (to avoid tethering of the nerves to the scar or the formation of neuromata); a sufficient length of muscle tissue should be left to enable the ends of agonists and antagonists to be sutured together and to provide a good coverage for the bone end: the severed bone should be well-bevelled — sharp ends of guillotined bone are tender to pressure, are effective sources of ulceration, and may jeopardize prosthetic walking: the arterial supply should be adequate to ensure good healing and a stump which is free from tenderness and rest pain.

The ideal stump is one which remains fleshy and rounded, and in which the soft tissues do not retract or fall away from the cut end of the bone. Some surgeons manage to attain this type of stump without also producing such tethering of nerves and skin that persistence of phantom pain is ensured.

Scarring from arterial surgery, burning, skin grafting or trauma may make a stump tender and prone to excoriation during early prosthetic life.

(2) PHYSICAL AND MENTAL CONDITION OF PATIENT

The general physical condition of a lower limb amputee should be improved by regular graded exercise before limb fitting is commenced. The presence of a fracture in the opposite leg may make walking extremely difficult, with one leg stiffened by a plaster cast, and the stump of the other encased in a rigid pylon.

Upper limb fractures may reduce the power to grip rails, frame or crutches. Head injury may cause weakness and spasticity of one or more limbs.

Also following head injury the *mental* condition of a brain-damaged patient may complicate recovery. Loss of communication, reduced span of short-term memory, reduced reasoning power and understanding, perceptual dysfunction and disordered balance may all make it difficult for the young traumatic amputee to master prosthetic walking.

(3) TYPE OF REHABILITATIVE PROCEDURE

IPOF.   Immediate Post Operative Fitting of a lower limb prosthesis is no longer a procedure of choice following amputation of a lower limb, and is seldom, if ever, used in this country. Designed to facilitate speedy post-operative walking, the procedure requires that the amputation stump is encased in a plaster-of-paris cast immediately following operation, with a prosthetic socket embedded in the lower end of the cast. A prosthetic end piece is screwed into this socket when the plaster has set, and assisted walking is permitted as soon as the surgeon requests. The dangers of undetected haemorrhage and infection, coupled with the need to maintain a large and specially trained surgical and paramedical team on constant call have caused this type of rehabilitative care to lose favour.

EPOW.   Early Post Operative Walking has succeeded IPOF as the type of rehabilitative procedure adopted for the majority of lower limb amputees.

With the use of the PAM aid (Pneumatic Post Operative Aid to Mobility), or pneumatic pylon, assisted walking is available for patients with long AK (above knee), TK (through-knee) and BK (below knee) stumps, as soon post operatively as the surgeon requests. (See Chapter 13).

Preliminary Rocker Pylon.   Following elective amputation, pre-operative measurement can ensure that a rocker pylon is ready for use within a few days of operation. Even following routine operation for peripheral vascular failure, patients are usually ready to be referred to the Limb Fitting Centre 10 − 14 days post operatively, and can probably be walking on their preliminary rocker pylons by the end of the fourth post operative week.

A short programme of walking training with the pylon, and then later with the prosthetic leg, is advisable for all patients, (children only excepted). Even young and active men benefit from early inculcation of the correct method of prosthetic useage, to avoid the development of bad walking habits. (See Chapter 13).

When possible the amputee should have this prosthetic training as an inpatient.

(4) TYPE OF PROSTHETIC LIMB AVAILABLE

There is a wide variety of prosthetic design and material currently available to the amputee, and a detailed account of the individual prosthetic limbs is beyond the scope of this book.

The two main types of prostheses are, however, the *conventional prosthesis* which has a handmade socket and is purpose-built to the measurements and specifications of the prosthetist for a particular patient, and the *MAP or Modular Assembly Prosthesis* which is assembled from a kit containing a selection of the various standardized component parts of the prosthesis, integrated with a socket made from the cast or measurement of the stump. This latter type of limb should eventually speed up the production of the prostheses and enable them to be produced at the Regional Limb Centres and not only at a few centralized limb factories.

Patients may sit or kneel on weightbearing areas of their prosthetic sockets, or may have endbearing stumps which take varying amounts of weight. Prostheses are attached to the body by corsets, waistbands, shoulder-harnesses and various suspensory straps, cords and suspenders. When patients are young and their stumps well shaped, they may be able to wear prostheses with suction sockets and no suspension.

An exact fit between stump and socket is essential in the more demanding suction sockets of some AK prosthesis, and the patella-tendon-bearing sockets of some BK prostheses. When stump fluctuation is likely to be considerable, prescription of these prostheses is not indicated.

(5) PERSISTENCE OF PHANTOM PAIN

Severe phantom pain can have such an adverse effect on the rehabilitation of any lower limb amputee that (as in amputation of the upper limb) pre-operative and post-operative care should be deliberately directed towards minimizing its causes. The importance of avoiding *precipitating* causes such as unrelieved pain and undue manipulation of the nerves during operation has already been mentioned. Infection and ischaemia of a stump and tethering of nerves to bone and skin by scar tissue are sometimes inevitable, and then may provide the *perpetuating* causes which can transform phantom pain from a transient and tolerable sensation into recurrent and unbearable agony.

Once established, phantom pain of this severity cannot be eradicated merely by increasing the dose of analgesics. Sometimes behavioural therapy is effective in controlling the pain: sometimes hypnotherapy is the method of choice in suitable subjects. Initially a hypnotherapist but eventually the patient himself induces the hypnotic conviction that pain has been removed. Revision of stump, removal of neuromata, electrical stimulation and even cordotomy have been necessary to alleviate phantom pain in some patients.

Epilogue

If a generalization *can* be made about the rehabilitation of amputees, it is that standardization of prosthetic prescription and patient management can never be successful. People are different, stumps are different. Wise rehabilitation will adapt procedure and hardware to the needs of the individual.

BIBLIOGRAPHY AND REFERENCES

Barber, L. M. and Nickel, V. L. (1969). 'Carbon dioxide powered arm and hand devices.' *Am. J. Occup. Ther.* **23**, 215

British Medical Association Planning Unit Report No. 2 (1969). *Aids for the Disabled.* London; BMA

British Orthopaedic Association (1973). *Report of Committee on Prosthetic and Orthotic Services.*

Brewerton, D. A. and Daniel, J. W. (1969). 'Return to work after injury.' *The Hand* **1**, 125

Brooks, M. and Shaperman, J. (1965). 'Infant prosthetic fitting.' *Am. J. Occup. Ther.* **19**, 329

Carter, I., Torrance, W. N. and Merry, P. H. (1969). 'Functional results following amputation of the upper limb.' *Ann phys. Med*, **10**, 137

Fulford, G. E. and Hale, M. J. (1968). *Amputation and prostheses.* Bristol; Wright

Hamilton, A. (1979). 'Rehabilitation of the Upper Limb Amputee.' *Nursing*

Loughlin, E. (1968). 'Immediate post-surgical prosthetics fitting of bilateral below-elbow amputee: a report.' *Artif. Limbs* **12**, 17

Nickel, V. L. and Waring, W. (1965). 'Future developments in externally powered orthotic and prosthetic devices.' *J. Bone Jt. Surg.* **47B**, 469

Parry, G. R. (Personal communication) Artificial Limb and Appliance Centre and Nuffield Orthopaedic Centre, Oxford

Proceedings of a symposium on basic problems of prehension, movement and control of artificial limbs (1969). London; The Institution of Mechanical Engineers

Robinson, E. (1979). 'Rehabilitation of Arm Amputees and Limb deficient children.' Bailliere Tindall, London

Sarmiento, A. (1968). 'Immediate post-surgical prosthetics fitting in the management of upper extremity amputees.' *Artif. Limbs* **12**, 14

Simpson, D. C. (1969). 'An externally powered prosthesis for the complete arm.' *Biomed. Eng.* **2**, 106

13 Rehabilitation of the Older Amputee

ANN HAMILTON

INTRODUCTION

The successful rehabilitation of the older amputee demands the urgent and closely integrated action of several disciplines.

The problems involved are many and complex. Approximately 4500 people become lower limb amputees every year in the United Kingdom and 65% of these are over 60 years of age and come to amputation because of peripheral vascular disease.

Several recent surveys reveal that 50% of these patients will be dead within 2 years of amputation. It is therefore crucial that their rehabilitation programme should be started early and pressed forward urgently, and that inter-departmental delays of referral and acceptance should be eliminated as far as possible.

Rehabilitation for such patients is not just a matter of fitting the healed stump with a prosthesis and teaching the amputee how to walk on it. The peripheral vascular disease which brought a lower limb to amputation may affect cerebral and cardiac circulation and that of the remaining lower limb, and at any time ischaemia of brain, heart and contralateral leg may complicate convalescence, and make prosthetic walking more difficult to achieve. Degenerative disease or dysfunction of any system of the ageing body may further complicate the attainment of functional competence.

If a large part of the short life span remaining for many amputees is not to be spent in unnecessary and costly hospitalization, all members of the hospital rehabilitation team need to establish close understanding and good communication with each other, with the medical officers and prosthetists of the Limb Fitting Service and with their opposite numbers in the community. Elderly people tend to have elderly partners and live in elderly houses. The support obtainable from the former and the amenities of the latter are likely to be limited. Without careful synchronization and early modification of intended action, the necessary modifications to the home and mobilization of back-up community services cannot be carried out soon enough to enable the patient to be discharged home to the coninuing care his condition demands.

REHABILITATION PROCEDURES

Pre-operative treatment
Medical and Surgical Aspects
Preparation for the rehabilitation of patients with lower limb ischaemia is started pre-operatively, when patients are seen regularly and their circulatory

efficiency is reviewed. They are advised to stop smoking, to lose weight, to limit exercise and to attend scrupulously to the cleanliness, warmth and chiropody of their feet. Pain is controlled as effectively as possible with analgesics.

A lumbar sympathectomy on the affected side may be indicated to increase cutaneous blood supply.

Arterial surgery may improve the circulation of a threatened limb sufficiently to prevent or postpone the need for amputation, but when surgery fails or is inappropriate, amputation becomes inevitable.

It is essential to avoid a prolonged interval before the decision to amputate is made, so that patients may be spared the distress of long weeks of observation at home or in hospital, suffering from acute pain, and apathetic from lack of sleep and heavy sedation.

Patients for whom amputation is delayed overlong in favour of conservative treatment frequently develop hip joint contractures from sitting in bed in the 'knee-up' position, hugging the knee of the painful ischaemic limb in an attempt to gain relief from pain. Stiff joints, weak muscles, reduced respiratory function and mobility, and deterioration of hope and morale contribute to increase the operative risk to such patients, and to reduce their chances of successful prosthetic rehabilitation.

Arteriographic demonstration of the vascular pattern of the limb assists the decisions of when to attempt arterial surgery and when to amputate, and also in the choice of separative procedure or level of amputation.

General medical care pre-operatively attempts: to detect and treat infection – particularly in limb, chest or urinary system: to relieve pain with effective analgesia: to detect and control hitherto undemonstrated diabetes: to support cardiac function: and to explain the need for the proposed course of action to patient and relatives.

Nursing Aspects
Nursing care pre-operatively aims at promoting comfort and preventing or reducing the occurrence of complications for the patient awaiting amputation.

The provision of adequate equipment assists these aims:

(1) A bed of adjustable height with good brakes – such as the King's Fund bed or equivalent – helps physiotherapeutic and nursing care and patient transfers.
(2) A firm mattress facilitates balance exercises and pronelying.
(3) A sheepskin to lie on reduces the risk of pressure sores on buttocks, hips and sacrum, and sheepskin bootees prevent ulceration of heels and malleoli.
(4) A Monkey-pole and bed-end pull help the patient change his posture unaided.
(5) A cradle protects legs and feet from the pressure of the bedclothes.

Physiotherapeutic Aspects
The amputee elect is frequently toxic, exhausted and in pain, and may be too ill or too confused to accept more than a minimal amount of physiotherapy. Pre-operative physiotherapeutic regime therefore concentrates on a few basic essentials:

(1) The prevention of flexion deformities by active exercises and pronelying.
(2) The maintenance and improvement of mobility and strength in all limbs and trunk.
(3) The improvement of breathing pattern.

Post-operative treatment

Medical Aspects

Although the precise timing of any particular rehabilitative procedure depends upon the condition of the patient and the convictions of the surgeon, most older amputees have approximately 2 – 5 days active bed-rest post-operatively. During this time medical care includes supervision of general health, and particular attention is paid to the state of the stump and the remaining limb, itself a potential ischaemic emergency. Adequate analgesia is mandatory, to ensure present comfort and prevent future phantom pain.

Medical emergencies such as toxic confusion, pneumonia, pulmonary embolus, cerebral thrombosis and retention with overflow may complicate the early post-operative period, and require appropriate treatment.

Some 20% of all those coming to lower limb amputation will not be referred for limb fitting. Frailty or death excludes them from referral. For the remaining 80% an active rehabilitation programme is pursued.

The regional Artificial Limb and Appliance Centre is notified on form AOF 3 that a patient with lower limb amputation requires examination for possible prosthetic fitting, once it is apparent that survival is likely. Early notification – as soon as 2 – 3 days post-operatively – ensures that the patient will be seen for the first time at the Artificial Limb and Appliance Centre about 2 weeks post-operatively, by which time a healthy amputation scar is likely to have healed.

Nursing Aspects

Post-operative nursing care includes regular preventive treatment and inspection of pressure areas, particularly those of the remaining limb, and the nursing staff combines with the physiotherapists to maintain a regular programme of thrice daily exercises and prone lying.

Regimes of stump care and times of suture removal vary considerably, but most vascular surgeons now agree that amputation wounds should be dressed with non-adherent gauze, protective wool, and a loosely woven cotton bandage of the 'Kling' variety. Micropore may usually be safely used to anchor the dressing to the skin of the stump, particularly if it is attached longitudinally and not directly to the skin, but to several 'fixture' lengths of micropore, which are left in situ until dressings are no longer needed. Elastoplast and sellotape should never be used to secure dressings as they tend to damage the ischaemic skin of the stump, producing excoriation, scarring, and sometimes permanent deformity.

Any bandaging of the amputation stump – other than with kling – is best avoided, since it is seldom done correctly, and a badly applied and overtight bandage can put back the fitting of a prosthesis by several weeks. The arterial supply to the skin may be impeded and venous and lymphatic return obstructed, both predisposing to delayed healing. Continued encirclement of a stump by constricting bandage causes terminal oedema, and this may lead to re-opening of a healed amputation wound and predispose to infection. Skin cravasses, excoriation and temporary or permanent stump distortion may complete the picture.

Below-knee amputation stumps may have plaster of paris cylinders applied over their dressings, to protect the suture line and to maintain the knee in extension. The cylinder is bi-valved to permit regular exercising. Its presence also helps to keep the dressing in situ.

When the surgeon decides that the time is appropriate, standing and then hop walking are attempted, using frame or parallel bars.

Physiotherapeutic Aspects

The post-operative objects of physiotherapy are the prevention of post-operative complications, the preparation of the patient for prosthetic walking, the assessment of his mobility potential and then

either   instruction in the intricacies of prosthetic walking

or   instruction in the most suitable way of obtaining optimal mobility and personal independence.

PROPHYLAXIS AND PREPARATION

To this end she continues chest treatment and several daily sessions of mobility and strengthening exercises for all limbs and trunk, concentrating particularly on gluteal and adductor exercises when the amputation is above knee, and adding exercises for quadriceps when amputation is below knee.

Regular intervals of prone lying are continued to prevent flexion contractures, and as soon as the patient's condition allows, balance training is introduced, followed by instruction in the techniques of transferring from bed to wheelchair or commode, and propelling a wheelchair.

ASSESSMENT OF MOBILITY POTENTIAL

Until recently the assessment of the mobility potential of any amputee was an empirical decision, except in the few hospitals where physiotherapists had the facilities and expertise to make their own early walking aids. Now, with the advent of the pneumatic pylon, the ability of an amputee to manage prosthetic walking may be accurately assessed in the early post-operative days, and his rehabilitation programme structured accordingly.

The Pneumatic Pylon,   or Pneumatic Post-Amputation Mobility Aid, is an assessment and training device, and is commercially available for purchase by individual hospitals. It consists of a rigid metal support-frame, like a short Thomas' splint, terminating in a rocker end. A plastic compartmentalized pneumatic cup in two separate parts covers the amputation stump, and cushions it from the outer frame. The cup is inflated to 40 mg Hg by the supervising physiotherapist, and the patient walks in the cushioned metal super-structure, assisted by a walking-frame or parallel bars. This device is worn for up to 2 hours a day, in several sessions lasting from 5–20 minutes each. When the patient sits to rest, between standing and walking sessions, the pneumatic cup is deflated, and is re-inflated when the vertical position is resumed.

Early trials demonstrate great physical and psychological benefits from the use of this device. Not only is the rapid loss of post-operative oedema facilitated, but the circulation and healing of the stump is apparently improved, the overall health and muscle tone of the patient benefits from early resumption of walking, and the patient himself is encouraged to find himself able to ambulate again. The device also demonstrates clearly whether or not the patient is fit enough to manage prosthetic walking, or whether he is better suited to a wheelchair existence.

At present the use of the PPAM is confined to patients with below-knee, through-knee or long above-knee amputations. A further model is being currently developed for use by amputees with short above knee stumps: for the moment the assessment of fitness for prosthetic walking of patients with above-knee amputation is therefore decided mainly on their exercise tolerance and fatigue level as demonstrated by hop walking in parallel bars or frame.

Clearly a patient who is breathless, exhausted and possibly suffering from anginoid pain after hop walking down a single length of the parallel bars is not a good candidate for walking with an artificial limb. It is generally estimated that prosthetic walking with a single below-knee amputation takes 20% more energy than walking with two legs, and walking with an above-knee amputation requires a 40% increased energy output.

Preservation of the safety and confidence of the patient at all stages of rehabilitation is crucial, and it is far wiser to avoid promoting all but the fittest patients to crutch walking until the preliminary rocker pylon has been issued and its use fully mastered. A fall in the early post-operative days may split open the amputation stump, and the resulting haematoma, tenderness, and delayed healing may set prosthetic fitting and usage back by several weeks.

Occupational Therapy Aspects

While the co-ordinated movement of the limbs and trunk of the amputee is the responsibility of the physiotherapist, his total functional efficiency is the concern of the hospital-based occupational therapist. She assesses his overall needs in making the necessary adjustment to amputation, and to this end

(1) Instructs and supervises practice in the attainment of personal independence, with the application of newly learned transfer techniques and mobility for toilet, dressing and domestic activities.
(2) Plans for return to previous work or to an alternative type of employment, contacting the personnel managers of various concerns and/or the DRO as appropriate.
(3) Advises on new leisure occupations or suggests new ways of managing customary leisure pursuits.
(4) Advises on the supply of a suitable wheelchair, when required.
(5) Liaises with the community (or domiciliary) occupational therapist as soon as it is apparent that return home is likely.

The community occupational therapist visits and assesses the amputee's home prior to discharge, and arranges for the supply of necessary aids and equipment. Many older amputees may require the provision of a raised toilet set, a free standing monkey pole and chain, a bed ladder and a sliding board, and if so, these and other essential aids should be supplied before or on discharge. One of the most dangerous periods for the older amputee is the first night home, when falls with damage to the amputation stump or fracture of the contralateral leg frequently occur. If the community OT ensures safe night toiletting by arranging for the supply of a night commode or alternatively several portable urinals, she will have gone far to preventing this. Women, as well as men, should be urged to use a urinal rather than lavatory or chamberpot, so as to avoid standing or walking in the dark when sleepy and confused.

After discharge, and depending upon his prognosis, the amputee may require structural modifications to his home. The community OT may recommend the installation of rails by the side of the lavatory seat, ramps, handrails, or alternative shallow steps if essential steps are steep, or the provision of bath aids.

She makes her recommendations to the social services department, who finance and organize any structural alterations to council-owned houses, but require private house owners to contribute to the overall cost. A member of the social services department will also visit a patient at the request of any member of the hospital or community team, if further assessment of the home situation is indicated, and will arrange, when necessary, for the supply of daily living equipment or financial aid, or for the implementation of the structural alterations recommended by the community OT.

Aspects Covered by Medical Social Worker

The acceptance of the amputation of a lower limb is never an easy one to make, particularly for the older amputee, whose functional independence may already be precarious. Wise counselling by the hospital Medical Social Worker helps him to work through his grief, resentment and depression, and allows him to express and mourn his loss without shame. By eliciting and ameliorating domestic, financial, social and emotional difficulties whenever possible, and by relieving the amputee of unnecessary worry and stress, the Medical Social Worker frees him to make a maximal effort to rehabilitate himself.

Team Aspects

Whether or not an older amputee should be referred on for limb fitting should be the combined decision of the members of the hospital team. The basic *physical* requirements for successful fitting and usage of a lower limb prosthesis are that the amputee should be able, without undue dyspnoea or pain

(1) to transfer, stand up and sit down using the appropriate aid, and
(2) to hop the length of the parallel bars or hop-walk (*circa* 4 metres) using a walking aid.

The basic *mental* requirements are that the amputee should be able to understand, remember and carry out simple instructions, and that he should be *motivated* to walk again.

Absolute age is not important, but functional age is very important indeed, and many determined old men and women in their eighties who have a home and loved partner to return to make a far better showing that many single or widowed sixty year olds.

In addition to these general requirements, a patient should not commence limb fitting until

(1) his amputation wound is healed or nearly healed (this is particularly important when the amputation is above knee)
(2) his stump is no longer unduly tender.
(3) excessive stump oedema associated with congestion, infection, haematoma or venous thrombosis has resolved.
(4) the condition of the contralateral leg permits assisted standing and walking.

As has already been said, patients are referred for limb fitting by the dispatch of form AOF3, which informs the Medical Officer in charge of the regional Artificial Limb and Appliance Centre that an amputee is considered by the hospital team to be ready for limb fitting. It is prudent, (though not required by regulations), to accompany the dispatch of this form by a telephone call to the Medical Officer himself, and so avoid the delays which postal or administrative hold-ups can impose on time of call-up.

Most older amputees are fit for attendance at ALAC by the end of the second post-operative week, and the need to have the appointment for attendance arranged for this time, together with the necessary ambulance transport, often means that the decision to refer has to be made a few days post-operatively, based on the early progress of the patient, and on the deductive expertise of the various members of the rehabilitation team. Occasionally such preliminary decisions have to be reversed in the light of the patients' condition and performance during the later part of convalescence.

Limb-fitting
Provision of Pylon
On his first visit to ALAC the amputee is examined by the medical officer, who decides whether the patient is indeed ready for limb fitting, and if so then requests a prosthetist to measure the stump and leg length. The medical officer decides with the prosthetist on the most suitable type of prosthesis for any particular amputee. In most centres this is the *rocker pylon*, an ischial-bearing, metal device, consisting of a metal or block leather socket attached by two side steels, hinged at the knee, to a foot-shaped rocker end: the device is attached by a hinged bar to a waistband, and a single shoulder strap gives additional suspension. When amputation is below-knee, the below-knee stump is enclosed in an added felt cuff or cup.

This device is usually ready for fitting and rivetting within two weeks of order, and the amputee attends for delivery for the second time usually two weeks after his first attendance.

Some centres do not fit pylons, but instead measure the amputee after a longer interval has elapsed post-operatively, and then fit him with a definitive artificial limb.

Most centres continue to supply pylons however, particularly to older patients. When the amputation is below knee, the *PTB (patella-tendon-bearing) pylon* may be used as an alternative to the more traditional ischial-bearing model. This has a split leather socket moulded to a plaster cast of the patient's below-knee stump, and attached by side steels to a rocker-foot: a single leather strap gives above-knee suspension, and the patient weightbears on a ledge on the leather socket, in the semi-kneeling position.

Advantages of Pylon Usage
The provision of a pylon for an elderly amputee has several advantages:

(1) In the first place it acts as an assessment tool. Whereas the pneumatic pylon demonstrates at an early stage post-operatively *whether* prosthetic walking is likely to be achieved, the rocker pylon demonstrates *what kind* of prosthesis is the best suited to the patient's needs and capabilities.

Some patients, even with adequate walking training, find that they can only tolerate the pylon for short intervals or not at all, and that they are better served by a wheelchair existence.

Other patients are completely satisfied by the activity which the pylon provides, and like its lightness and stability. Very old and frail people often elect to retain it as their only prosthesis: others are refused a definitive prosthesis when it is apparent that they become fatigued, distressed or dyspnoeic when using the pylon more than a minimal amount. For these patients the pylon becomes the permanent limb, and when the preliminary rocker pylon wears out, a further pylon is provided.

Most patients however become rapidly proficient on the rocker pylon and request and are apparently suitable for a definitive prosthesis. Although most of those who are supplied with a definitive prosthesis persevere with it despite the fact that it is nearly twice as heavy as the rocker pylon, a considerable number will reject it and return to pylon use.

(2) The second advantage of the pylon is that it is quickly made, easily altered for stump shrinkage or increase in size, and relatively cheaply produced.
(3) It permits walking on a personalized prosthesis (the pneumatic pylon is a piece of hospital equipment shared by many patients) at an early stage post-operatively, and so facilitates return home.
(4) Early fitting of a pylon accelerates the resolution of stump oedema, and the attainment of the 'steady state' which a stump must reach before it is ready for measurement or casting for a definitive prosthesis.

The disadvantages of pylon usage are that

(1) It is ugly and in no way aesthetically pleasing.
(2) If worn with a skirt it is disconcertingly obvious.
(3) If worn with trousers it wears out the legs of all but the baggiest creations because of its widely set knee hinges.

Synchronization of Limb Fitting with the Overall Rehabilitation Timetable
Depending on mental and physical health and on home circumstances, patients may receive their pylons while they are in hospital, convalescent ward, disabled living unit or their own homes. The advantages of inpatient walking training are so great that the majority of patients should not be discharged home until they have attained pylon independence.

Those patients who *have* been sent home before their pylons are ready must attend a selected physiotherapy department for walking training as outpatients. This form of walking training is not usually very satisfactory, since

(1) Ambulances tend to bring patients late and collect them early, so shortening each walking training session and lengthening the time for which walking training is necessary.
(2) Many patients arrive feeling upset and nauseated by the ambulance journey, or else are hypoglycaemic because they have had their morning insulin but have missed breakfast in their hurry to be ready for collection.
(3) Because of the short time actually available in the physiotherapy department during attendance as outpatients, many amputees are flustered and pressurised, and feel unable to rest as long as they would wish between walking stints. Also there may be insufficient time to discuss difficulties of daily living with the physiotherapist or occupational therapist.
(4) Since all that many physiotherapists can allow for training outpatient amputees who are unsteady on their feet, and who cannot walk without the help of parallel bars or get themselves in and out of their pylons, are constrained to leave the pylons at the department until they can use them safely, and so spend much of the week at home without any prosthesis whatsoever.

For some patients however, the wish to return home after many months in hospital is so great that it over-rides all other considerations, and it is better to treat them less efficiently as outpatients than to treat them as miserable in-patients under optimal conditions.

Long Term Care

When an amputee has had his pylon for 1—2 months he is recalled to ALAC, and his stump and prosthetic usage are assessed. If he has made good use of the pylon and his stump has shrunk to its steady state, he is measured and/or cast for a permanent or definitive artificial leg.

A patient is entitled to two definitive limbs at any one time, or else one definitive limb and one pylon. These prostheses are mended, adjusted, altered and replaced by ALAC — free — for the rest of the patient's life.

Integration of Work of ALAC with that of Hospital and Community Teams

Ideally the walking training of lower limb amputees should be carried out in a unit which is geographically and functionally a part of a limb fitting centre. In actual fact this situation is the exception rather than the rule, and most amputees have their training in hospitals which are often long ambulance journeys away from the centres which they attend.

It is therefore imperative that the walking training of these amputees should be assessed continually by the therapists concerned, and their findings and opinions communicated direct to the medical officer by note, letter or telephone. This is imperative, if the correct decision about the provision of a prosthesis is to be made, since patients are frequently unable to be objective about their progress and capabilities.

Without such communication between therapists and medical officer, many elderly but determined amputees may well be issued with complex and expensive prostheses which they are totally unfit to use.

Similarly walking training should be terminated at the discretion of the community and hospital staff involved, bearing in mind the social as well as the physical and mental state of the patient, and the progress which he has made and is likely to make in the future.

Wheelchair Provision

In addition to providing prostheses, the ALAC also provides wheelchairs to those patients who need them. Usually the type of chair best suited to the patient's shape, size and capabilities is decided by the physiotherapist or occupational therapist of the parent hospital. Whenever possible an 'amputee model' is issued, in which the rear wheels of the chair are set 3″ back from the normal position.

The supply of a chair supplements a patient's ambulatory mobility and does not discourage it. When fitted with a tray it enables the frailer amputee to carry things about the house which he may find difficult if he has to walk a walking aid to assist his progress. It also gives him a means of getting around if his stump or contralateral leg becomes painful.

Prosthetic training

Application of Pylon

The amputee is taught to put on his pylon while wearing only a vest and sitting on a plinth or low bed. He first 'dresses' the pylon in pants and trousers, and inserts his stump into a stump-sock of the correct size, pulling it up well in order to avoid wrinkles. He then pulls pants and trousers onto the contralateral leg and eases the sock-covered stump into the pylon, with the rocker end in lateral rotation. The sock is turned down over the top edge of the pylon socket, avoiding undue pressure over the end of the stump as the sock is pulled up to avoid wrinkles. As the waist band is fastened, the pylon is rotated into the neutral position. The shoulder strap is then adjusted so that it is taut when the patient stands, but not so tight that it internally rotates the pylon or makes the patient stoop. After standing to re-check the waist band, the patient completes his dressing.

Testing Fit of Pylon

Most pylons have rigid or semi-rigid sockets. The stumps which they cover fluctuate in size with posture, weather, obesity, muscular development, diuretic intake, medication for diabetes, thyroid metabolism, cardiac and renal function to mention only a few factors which will be operative throughout prosthetic life.

During the two weeks elapsing between measurement and delivery of the pylon a patient's stump may have increased by as much as 1–2 inches in circumference, if the patient has returned home to good cooking after prolonged hospitalization. Conversely and in contrast, the stump tends to shrink for many weeks after amputation, and this is accelerated by use of both the pneumatic and the rocker pylon. It is therefore essential to be able to test the fit of the pylon.

The patient puts his weight on the contralateral leg and the examiner places a finger on the top of the anteromedial lip of the pylon. When the patient then transfers his weight to the pylon, the finger should just fit comfortably between rim and adductor tendon. If the pylon is loose and the stump is slipping too far into the socket, the finger is pinched hard between rim and adductor tendon or pubic ramus: alternatively, if the pylon is too tight, a roll of flesh will be found to separate the ramus and tendon from the pylon rim. In the latter case the patient feels the pylon is too short: in the latter case he considers it too long.

The fit of the pylon at the back should also be tested, by the examiner placing his fingers on the ischial tuberosity of the patient while he weightbears on the other leg. He is asked to transfer his weight onto the pylon, when then pinches the examiner's finger between its tuber-bearing platform and the ischial tuberosity. In an overlarge socket the tuberosity slips over the platform and into the socket: in a tight socket there is a roll of fat between platform and tuberosity.

Theoretically it is therefore easy to decide whether a pylon socket is too big or too small. In actual fact it is difficult, because of the amount of muscle and fat which may obscure the bony landmarks. The wisest rule to follow is that if discomfort in the groin cannot be corrected by putting on an extra sock, the patient should be referred to ALAC for prosthetic adjustment.

Gait in Prosthetic Walking

The pylon-using amputee is taught to sit on a chair of such a height that his thighs are horizontal and his feet flat on the ground. Long chair arms assist his entry and egress from the chair, and he learns to control the knee joint mechanism so that he straightens the knee on standing, and bends it for sitting. He should sit on a cushion and not on a hard-based seat.

He learns standing and balance, followed by hip hitching on the amputation side; then weight transference in standing and forward glide positions paying particular attention to pelvic control. The latter is important to avoid a nautical roll and swaying gait when walking. He is instructed to take small even steps and to avoid turning round by swivelling on the rocker which twists the stump in the socket.

When abnormal gait patterns occur, they arise from *either* the structure of the pylon *or* the structure or function of the amputee.

Common prosthetic causes of abnormal gait are incorrect length, incorrect alignment, poorly fitting socket and inadequate or incorrectly adjusted suspension.

Common amputee derived causes are a painful weak or sensitive stump, joint contractures, poor balance, arthritic pain in any joint of the remaining limbs or spines, fear of falling and fear of pain.

The types of gait irregularity to which these conditions give rise are

(1) Abduction or circumduction gait.
(2) Vaulting gait.
(3) Uneven timing, characterised by steps of unequal duration and length.
(4) Lateral trunk bending.

The amputee at home
A fit amputee may return home as early as two weeks after amputation, often with his wound still unhealed.

His rehabilitative care is continued by the community nursing, medical and social service teams, who have been notified as soon as possible after the decision to discharge is made.

The family doctor visits and the district nurse may attend to dress the amputation stump. The health visitor, community occupational therapist and members of the social services assess and/or recommend aids, grants and equipment, as described earlier. When this is promptly implemented, the majority of patients manage to stay in their own homes. People living alone, people who are frail and people with multiple disabilities may need to move into ground floor flats or bungalows, warden supervised accommodation or Part III accommodation.

Continuing care
Even when the older amputee is walking successfully on a definitive prosthesis, his rehabilitative care is not complete. Day-to-day maintenance of stump, contralateral leg and prosthesis is vitally important, if damage to the stump or bilateral amputation is to be avoided.

Stump Care
The stump should be washed and patted dry each night, and inspected for skin damage. This is particularly important in the case of diabetics who frequently have peripheral neuritis and sensory loss. Application for surgical Most stumps do well without either, and some need the judicious use of both at different times.

The use of anti-perspirant lotion and frequent stump sock changes — at least once a day — helps to counteract the increased tendency to ulceration found in many patients who sweat copiously.

Socks should be washed by hand in warm water with a minimal quantity of liquid detergent, rinsed frequently and dried flat. Holey socks should never be worn, and if darned, should be turned so that the darns are not overlying boney prominences.

Some patients prefer to wear only woollen socks: others wear a cotton or nylon sock next to the skin in addition. In either case, all socks should be pulled on sufficiently firmly to avoid wrinkles, but not so tightly that they compress the terminal part of the stump.

Persistently sore or excoriated areas on the stump need a visit to ALAC for the limbfitters to ease or adjust the socket and/or alignment of the prosthesis.

Care of a Contra-lateral Leg

Regular inspection and preventive care can alone prevent the remaining leg of a single amputee becoming a second amputation stump.

Ischaemia is inevitable and diminished sensation likely. Therefore, as with the stump, daily washing, careful drying, regular inspection for blisters, cuts, pressure areas and ulcers are essential. The remaining foot is at maximal risk, and it is particularly important to cut the toenails regularly after a preliminary soak, avoiding cutting too deeply or leaving sharp, protruding corners.

A clean well-fitting sock in wool or cotton, without elasticated top, garters or suspenders to hold it up: a soft wide shoe or bootee, free of rough areas or protruding nails: a bedsock rather than a hotwater bottle to give night warmth: the avoidance of sitting with the foot raised above the horizontal, and/or sitting for long periods without a walkabout or a session of foot or leg exercises – the use of these measures make up the active rehabilitative care of the ischaemic foot. They are of limited use unless the amputee stops smoking and has an effective heating system in his home.

General Care of Patient

An amputee can only expect stump discomfort and frequent trips to ALAC unless he controls the size of his body and the size of his stump. By dieting to prevent the weight gain which too often follows restricted activity and compensatory eating, and by reporting oedema of the ankle and stump so that suitable diuretics may be given or medication adjusted, he can go a long way towards achieving both.

Care of Prosthesis

Prostheses need maintenance care as much as the stumps they cover. Sweat and dust should be emptied out of sockets regularly. Squeaks and rattles herald mechanical faults and should send the patient for prosthetic advice. Cracks or jagged edges and loose linings in metal parts, loose rivets and bolts, and torn or ineffective straps or other appendages all require specialist repair or replacement. Urine, sweat and faecal matter tend to remove paint and corrode underlying metal, and should be sponged away with a damp soapy cloth, and the affected surfaces rinsed and dried.

THE DOUBLE AMPUTEE

Even with every care which patient and staff can give, pain, infection or gangrene may compel the amputation of the remaining leg.

When amputation is at below-knee level, the amputee has a good chance of walking on definitive prostheses, providing he has no further disability such as hemiparesis, severe arthritis or myocardial insufficiency to impede him. He will then be fitted initially with short rocker pylons, which are usually non-hinged metal cylinders, ischial-bearing, with backward facing rockers, and then with definitive prostheses.

If, however, he has the misfortune to have bilateral above-knee amputation, there is virtually no chance of him achieving prosthetic walking except for exercise purposes. It is estimated that over 80% more energy per step is needed to walk with above-knee prostheses, and this asks far more than the myocardium of the ischaemic amputee is able to provide.

It is reasonable to provide short rocker pylons for such patients, however, so that they can at least walk about their houses and ease the discomfort of permanently sitting on short stumps. Frequently the unacceptable dyspnoea, angina and palpitations brought on by using the short rockers in the parallel bars will demonstrate to the amputee that he is incapable of managing long legs.

Even use of short rocker pylons may be denied to the elderly amputee who lives alone, since he has no one to help him to put them on and take them off, and it is extremely difficult for all but the most agile to achieve this single-handed.

Provision of a wheelchair is essential for all double amputees, and if hemiplegia, arthritis or dyspnoea makes propulsion difficult, then the chair should be a powered one.

For those amputees who cannot manage definitive prostheses, it is humane to offer cosmetic legs. These are extremely light Duralumin shells, shaped like legs with proper feet, which are usually made with the knees permanently flexed, and have soft leather upper ends to fit over the ends of the stumps. Dressed in shoes socks and trousers and kept on the wheelchair, the amputee fits these 'legs' over his stumps, and attaches them by suspenders to a lightweight belt. He looks natural, and he feels a whole person again. If relatives or friends are distressed by his legless appearance, these cosmetic, non-weightbearing legs may be a great consolation.

BIBLIOGRAPHY AND REFERENCES

Chilvers, A. S. and Browse, N. L. (1971). 'The social fate of the amputee.' *Lancet* 2, 1192

Clippinger, F. W. (1963). 'Use of temporary quadrilateral socket plaster pylon in the elderly amputee.' *Sth. med. J.* 56, 588–92

Clippinger, F. W. (1965). 'Treatment of elderly amputee by temporary quadrilateral socket pylon prosthesis.' *Geriatrics* 20, 683–7

Devas, M. B. (1971). 'Early walking of geriatric amputees.' *Br. med.J.* 1, 394

Hamilton, E. A. and Nichols, P. J. R. (1972). 'Rehabilitation of the elderly amputee.' *Br. med. J.* 2, 95

McKenzie, D. S. (1961). 'Prosthetic rehabilitation of aged in Great Britain.' In *Conference on Geriatric Amputees*. Washington; National Academy of Sciences, National Research Committee

Oxford Ischaemic Amputee Committee 'The Management of the Elderly Ischaemic Amputee.' (in press)

Redhead, R. G. and Snowdon. (1978). 'A new approach to the management of wounds of the extremities. Controlled environment treatment and with derivatives.' *Prosthetics and Orthotics* 2, 148

Report of Committee on Prosthetic and Orthotic Services (1973). London; British Orthopaedic Association

Thompson, A. (1971). 'An early walking aid for geriatric amputees.' *Physiotherapy* 57, 583

14 Rehabilitation of the Spinally Injured Patient

JOHN SILVER

HISTORICAL BACKGROUND

Patients with paraplegia and tetraplegia have been known for thousands of years, but the patients died within weeks of injury, from pressure sores and urinary tract infections. There were some excellent papers produced during the First World War mainly describing the neurological consequences and the morbidity. One of the authors of these papers, G. Riddoch, was responsible during the Second World War for organizing the Army medical services, and he instituted the setting up of spinal units throughout the United Kingdom, to deal with the large number of paraplegics injured during the land fighting in Europe. This, combined with the development of blood transfusions, antibiotics and a better understanding of the management of the renal tract, and the prevention of pressure sores, led to an integrated rehabilitation programme being developed for these ex-servicemen. It rapidly became apparent that rehabilitation commenced at the time of injury, and the early transfer of these patients to specialized units, would reduce the complications of mis-management. Soon non-servicemen were admitted to the centres, and it was found that medical cases of paraplegia could also be treated successfully.

THE NATURE AND SIZE OF THE PROBLEM

Traumatic paraplegia

Three hundred acute spinal injuries with cord involvement occur each year in the United Kingdom. This distribution is similar to that of other industrial countries. About half the injuries will be in the cervical region, of which about half will have a complete interruption of the cord. Road traffic accidents cause 50 per cent of these injuries. There are other important causes such as industrial and sporting accidents, particularly diving, horse riding, gymnastics and rugby.

Associated complications

Since these injuries are nearly always encountered as a result of a major trauma, it is very unusual to find a patient with a spinal cord lesion as the only injury, and in a personal series of one hundred consecutive cases, 75 per cent had major associated injuries. Patients with cervical injuries usually had a severe head injury

223

as well, since the force required to dislocate the spine usually knocks the patient out. Nearly all the patients with mid-thoracic fractures had a haemo or pneumo thorax. It is almost impossible to damage the spine in isolation, without causing damage to the ribs attached to the vertebrae, and by the same reasoning, fractures of the lumbar spine, are frequently associated with fractures of the pelvic rim. Many patients had fractures of their extremities.

Where will they be treated?
The practice in this country is for a patient to be removed from the scene of the accident and taken to the nearest casualty department, although it is better for a patient to travel for 20 minutes longer in an ambulance, to a properly staffed and equipped accident department. Thus, the resuscitation and immediate care of the patient falls upon the accident department, neurosurgical department or orthopaedic department into which the patient is admitted.

Should they have their immediate resuscitation in accident units and stay there for some 6 to 8 weeks, being transferred at a later stage to a rehabilitation centre? This policy leads to an inevitable fragmentation in the continuity of care, and essential psychological readjustments are not made early enough. Unfortunately, owing to lack of staff and knowledge, preventable complications occur, and patients frequently develop pressure sores and severe renal damage. Policy has been revised gradually in this country as a result of pressure from patients, and recognition by medical and para-medical staff of the superior results achieved at spinal centres, and it is now accepted that all traumatic cases should be transferred, as quickly as possible, to a spinal centre, where all the facilities for the total care of the patient are available. Gradually, this policy has been adopted throughout Europe and the world, and even in the United States of America where, owing to the insurance system, there is a reluctance of surgeons to part with patients. A relatively recent development has been for the spinal centre, particularly in Ireland and Switzerland, to be notified by the ambulancemen, who carry radios, of the nature of the injury that a patient has sustained by the roadside. A team goes out by helicopter to the scene of the accident, and institutes treatment such as putting on skull traction, and supervises the transfer of the patient immediately to a spinal centre.

Medical causes of paraplegia
There are a large number of medical conditions causing paraplegia, but not all such cases are suitable for rehabilitation. Ideal cases are patients with non-progressive conditions, such as transverse myelitis, or a tumour of the spinal cord. These patients have almost exactly the same life expectancy as paraplegic patients, and can be rehabilitated just as effectively. Unfortuately, there are many other medical causes of paraplegia, such as patients with secondary deposits from Hodgkin's disease, or multiple myeloma, in whom the primary condition may be lowering their general state of health so much, that they may not benefit from the very vigorous programme at a spinal unit. Nevertheless, these patients can still be rehabilitated to an independent life, possibly in a wheelchair, so that they can return home with the support of their family or the district nurse.

Realistic goals
The object of treatment is to help the patient help himself. He is taught to use

those parts of the body which are normal, to compensate for those that are paralysed. This demands a realistic assessment of what can be achieved, and this has to be explained to the patient at the outset, and accepted by him. How can this be achieved?

STRUCTURE OF TREATMENT

The formal structure of a grand round once a week, where everything is discussed in public, is unsatisfactory and unrewarding, nor is the daily business round the time for full discussion. There are many psychological problems worrying the patient that can only be discussed in privacy, and the practice common in psychiatry of seeing every patient weekly in private, with only the junior doctor of the ward, the head physiotherapist, occupational therapist, social worker and sister present, should be followed.

The patient is seen by his consultant in private on at least three occasions:

(1) On admission, when a discussion on the nature of the injury takes place.
(2) When first up in a wheelchair so that work, sexual function, and housing can be discussed.
(3) Prior to discharge.

It is made clear on all occasions that this interview is not a one-off meeting but a continuing exchange of information. It provides support and reassurance. At all stages the patient is taught of the dangers and complications that can occur, such as pressure sores and how to prevent them and at the final interview this is reinforced.

Psychological reactions

Patients who have sustained paraplegia of any cause, have undergone not only a severe injury to their nervous system, but will have a psychological reaction. If the patient is to be helped, these reactions must be appreciated, so that the patient and his family can be helped meaningfully through them. The family is being treated, and not just the patient alone, since it is a waste of time achieving an excellent physical rehabilitation of the patient, if his wife leaves him, and he has no home to return to.

Pre-morbid condition

Some of the patients have had an abnormal psychological situation before they were paralysed, some have attempted suicide, others have been on drugs and even the large group who are involved in car accidents have frequently been drinking at the time, exceeding the speed limit or driving stolen cars, or any combination of these. Previous history of depression or schizophrenia would produce difficulties in the rehabilitation stage, and if the patient has found life unacceptable and has attempted to commit suicide before, waking up in hospital paralysed will not enhance his condition. It should be recognized that a spinal injury in many patients is only the last of a series of disasters that has afflicted the patient.

Grieving

There is an inevitable grieving reaction, and it is understandable and only natural that a patient should be depressed at finding himself in hospital totally paralysed. He will be worried about his employment, his housing, his children and his loss of sexual function. He is also worried about all kinds of things which can be helped. For instance, many are frightened that they will never get out of bed, fearing that they will have a catheter all their life or that the paralysis may increase.

Counselling

The patients welcome a frank discussion about the future, put in unemotional terms, because they find that if you can talk about something horrible and frightening in a matter of fact way, they can accept it, whereas if you avoid the issue, they pick up all kinds of rumours from other patients, not necessarily kindly disposed, becoming more frightened. What is unknown is frightening. The doctor's own social background may prevent meaningful discussion, but because the patients do not ask questions, it should not be thought that they have received all the information they need and that they are not full of anxieties, so that efforts must be made to provide information for the patient, apart from the interviews. Information is made available to the patient and his questions about his future answered truthfully, since it is necessary to look after the patient for the rest of his life and unless he can trust you from the outset he will not believe you later on. Some information can be imparted by a booklet or by audiovisual displays, and it should be recognized that much information will be imparted by para-medical staff and other patients. The emphasis should be on stressing what is left, a positive attitude to the fact that the patient will soon be getting up, getting rid of his catheter, returning to work and going home, and in the case of a woman, having children, rather than dwelling on what is lost. However, this information can be so frightening and unwelcome that many patients and families only absorb a very small amount of it at the time and may even reject it entirely so the interview should be regarded not as a one-off occurrence but a continuing process of education. It can be safely assumed that much of the information will not be understood or just ignored because of fear.

Family

It has to be recognized with an injury of this nature, that it does not affect the patient alone, but has repercussions on the whole family. The family is seen at the outset and a much more detailed description of the problem set out than is given to the patient at the first interview since it is necessary at the earliest stage to arrange housing modifications and adjustments to so many other aspects of life. The partner must be seen and, particularly with regard to sexual problems, the partners must be seen together, so that there can be a discussion on the different techniques which can be used.

Where a patient is very disabled, support may be needed from the district nurse, and in all patients with tetraplegia, a case conference is arranged with the district nurse and the supporting social services at the hospital. The district nurses are invited to visit the hospital, so that they can learn from the nursing staff how to look after a particular patient.

Professional counselling

Counselling can be extended by arranging for a suitable disabled patient, or a professional counsellor who is a patient, to come and discuss with the new patients various aspects of, say, sexual rehabilitation or work. A useful way of imparting information is to gather all the patients together at intervals of six weeks, and then to have a group discussion in which various questions can be dealt with. Many patients who are shy welcome this chance, as other patients may raise the problems that worry them, and they are not embarrassed and can learn. This can be supplemented by having the doctors and social workers present, thus extending the scope of the discussion.

Training of staff

It is necessary to train all members of staff in an understanding of the problems, and this will be facilitated by having a joint discussion group consisting of social workers, doctors, nurses, physiotherapists, and orderlies, led by a psychiatrist, in which such aspects as reaction to injury, readjustment, and psychological problems, can be discussed. This will lead to a much greater understanding and awareness of the roles that different members of the team play in treating the patients. This counselling is a continuous on-going process.

At a later stage it is arranged for patients to go home for weekends, or where the distances are too great they can spend time in a caravan sited at the hospital which is specially modified for disabled people, so that they can learn to be with their families again.

It may be argued that immediately after injury it is too soon for the patients to appreciate the nature and prognosis of their injury. However, half-truths and evasions do not help the patient at all, and the patients welcome a frank discussion and such information.

SEQUELAE OF PARAPLEGIA

Paraplegia is a very complex subject, and it is impossible in one chapter to even superficially cover the subject comprehensively. The loss of function can best be understood by referring to the basic anatomy and physiology. Five topics will be discussed that patients find most distressing: the loss or impairment of function of the motor system and the autonomic system, bladder and sexual failure and the very distressing complication of pressure sores. Each section will be introduced by the relevant anatomical and physiological facts. It is in no way comprehensive and enormous areas such as bowel function pain, spasticity, osteoporosis and stone formation are not dealt with at all. But rather than cover many topics superficially it is hoped that those chosen will stimulate further discussion and be of help.

LOSS OF MOTOR FUNCTION

Basic anatomical facts

Phylogenetically, because of the development in vertebrates of arms and legs, the spinal cord is shorter than the spinal column that encloses it. The result is that the 8th cervical segment is located below the C.6/7 disc space and the 12th spinal segment is at the level of the 10th thoracic vertebra. The cord ends at the lower border of the first lumbar vertebra. It follows that the nerve roots pursue an oblique course downwards and so an injury to a vertebra damages the cord and roots at a different level.

Pathology

(1) *An injury of the cord* is rarely a clear cut transection; there is usually longitudinal damage to the tissues extending several segments above and below the site of maximal damage. Since no regeneration of spinal cord tissue occurs the maximal neurological deficit is usually at the time of injury and any recovery that is seen is not due to regeneration but is explained by the fact that cells have not been destroyed at the time of injury but temporarily inhibited.

(2) *Prognosis*   In general any cord lesion that is complete at the outset and shows no signs of becoming incomplete by 48 hours after injury will not recover any useful function. The prognosis in patients with cord lesions that are incomplete from the outset or which show recovery within 48 hours is completely unpredictable. The presence or absence of reflexes is of no value in determining the completeness of the cord transection or the prognosis. A distressing situation can arise when as time passes spasticity develops. This is particularly marked in incomplete lesions because the intact long descending tracts are in continuity with the reticular formation so that the partially paralysed muscles are involved in spasms. These can be initiated by the smallest voluntary effort such as trying to scratch ones nose or from a full bladder or bowel.

(3) *Cauda equina*   An injury to the cauda equina is a lower motor neurone lesion and regeneration may take place as in other peripheral nerve lesions but as the nerve roots have a great distance to travel this is usually incomplete and painful.

Combination of cord, root, plexus and peripheral nerve lesions

Spinal injury is only one manifestation of a severe accident. A blow to the head in cervical injuries can give rise to traction injuries of the roots and brachial plexus and, as there are frequently fractures of the long bones; peripheral nerve injuries also occur.

Later stages

In the later stages when the patient is up in a wheelchair the excessive use that he gives to his arms which are substituting for his legs not infrequently gives rise to ulna nerve lesions of the elbow. The presence of a spinal injury in combination with a peripheral nerve injury can give difficulty in diagnosis especially when there is a head injury, unless there is a high index of suspicion and a thorough knowledge of the root, cord and peripheral nerve distribution. This matter is very much facilitated by electromyographic and nerve conduction studies.

Special situations

Central cord lesions   This is caused by damage to the centre of the cord so that the decussating fibres of the spinothalamic tract are damaged and also the anterior horn cells, but the long tracts preserving power and sensation in the legs are spared. The result is that there is a lower motor neurone lesion at the site of the injury with a loss of useful power in the hands but preservation of power in the legs. This unfortunate injury is frequently sustained in elderly patients owing to hyperextension of the cervical spine. They are often brought to casualty confused from a head injury or alcohol, and hypothermic, having been left at the site of the accident. The fact that they cannot move their hands but yet can move their legs may lead to a diagnosis of hysteria.

Ascent of lesion

It has been observed that about 2 per cent of the patients with an established cord lesion of the thoracic or lumbar region develop an ascent of the sensory loss accompanied by some loss of power in the hands at a variable period after injury. This is often accompanied by severe pain in the affected limb and is often precipitated by a bout of coughing or straining. At operation or post mortem cyst-like cavities have been found extending from the site of the injury upwards. It is suggested that all patients have these cystic spaces but it is only a small number (2 per cent) with a valve like communication developing to the subarachnoid space which allows fluid to enter the cyst and not leave. This is analogous to a tension pneumothorax. As the cyst increases in size the adjacent spinal cord tissues are compressed.

Segmental innervation

An injury to the cord above the 4th cervical segment is not compatible with life, because the diaphragm is paralysed. At the C.5 level the trapezius, sternomastoid, levator scapulae, rhomboids, supraspinatus and infraspinatus muscles are preserved but the patient will be unable to do much for himself apart from rotating his humerus. At the C.6 level the deltoid, biceps and brachioradialis muscles are preserved and the patient can be taught to feed himself with appliances fixed to his wrists. At the C.7 level, in addition, the triceps and extensor carpi radialis muscles are preserved; these enable the patient to cock up his wrist and, because the flexor muscles are shortened, to close the fingers by a trick movement. He can thus grip effectively and develop a useful hand. Many patients with lesions at this level have achieved almost complete independence being able to feed, dress, shave, drive a car, write and manipulate equipment. Lesions at the C.8 level preserve the majority of the thenar muscles giving a useful prehensile grip. However, the loss of the intrinsic muscles of the hand (T.1) can give rise to a severe claw deformity which can impair the use of the hand.

Paralysis of the respiratory muscles

If a patient sustains a complete transection above the 5th cervical segment, it is usually immediately fatal since all the respiratory muscles, apart from the auxiliary muscles which are insufficient to maintain life, are paralysed. However, in some patients remarkably prompt first aid has kept patients with complete transections at the C.3 level alive until they could be placed on a respirator. In the early stages it is not unusual for the level to ascend one or two segments due to oedema. For example, a patient may have a lesion at C.6 on admission which rises to C.4. Daily examination and checking of the vital capacity is therefore necessary.

An injury at a lower level leaves the patient with the diaphragm intact. This is quite sufficient to sustain life, provided that there are no other complicating factors.

Paralysis of the intercostal muscles reduces the vital capacity and the patient is unable to lift the rib cage or evert it during inspiration.

Paralysis of the abdominal muscles means that there are no active muscles contracting to oppose the weight of the abdominal viscera, and consequently the abdominal wall is passively distended by their weight during inspiration. In this case the diaphragm assumes a lower position in the chest. During inspiration, the diaphragm, because of its lower position, pulls in the lower ribs paradoxically instead of everting them.

The abdominal muscles' chief function is in forced expiration, coughing and straining. Their paralysis makes it impossible for the patient to cough effectively and clear his secretions, and consequently these patients are in danger of developing aspiration pneumonia.

To compensate for this extensive paralysis, the auxilliary muscles act earlier and at lower levels of ventilation to expand the upper part of the chest. This however, is less efficient than ventilation in normal subjects. The vital capacity and the maximum breathing capacity are thus reduced and the oxygen consumption of the respiratory muscles is increased.

Immediately after injury, the vital capacity is considerably reduced, particularly in patients with injuries at the C.5 level when the diaphragm itself may be partially involved. Its efficiency may be further impaired by a paralytic ileus pushing up the diaphragm or when there is an associated head injury depressing respiration. It is hardly surprising that patients frequently succumb to respiratory failure immediately after injury. The mortality in complete cervical injuries at the Liverpool Regional Paraplegic Centre between 1947 and 1967 was 33 per cent within the first 6 weeks of injury. The mechanism of death is probably as follows.

Mechanism of death
On admission a vital capacity of under a litre is sufficient to maintain life but any subsequent chest complications, such as a pneumonia or a pulmonary embolus, rapidly proves fatal when imposed upon the diminished reserve of functioning lung tissue. The tetraplegic patient is particuarly liable to develop aspiration pneumonia in the posterior basal segments of the lung because of the paralysis of the expiratory muscles, the intercostals and abdominals. This is reflected in findings that of 50 traumatic patients admitted between 1965 and 1967, 12 of the 29 cervical cases had pneumonia on admission, and this was typically in the posterior basal segment of the lung, compared with only one out of 6 low lesions who had intact expiratory muscles. The extensive paralysis makes these patients particularly liable to deep vein thromboses and subsequent pulmonary embolism. The combination of anoxia, loss of sympathetic control with the unopposed action of the vagus leads to cardiac arrest.

Treatment
To reduce these dangers, on admission all tetraplegic patients are placed on antibiotics and inhalations to liquify secretions, postural drainage and breathing exercises are instituted, and after three or four days anticoagulants are commenced. The vital capacity and blood gases are measured daily. It is essential to measure the vital capacity in all positions in which the patient is to be treated, since if he has a high lesion at the fourth cervical segment there may be a unilateral paralysis of the diaphragm and while the vital capacity may be adequate while the patient is being turned on his side with the normally innervated side of the diaphragm uppermost, it may be quite inadequate when he is nursed on the side with the normally innervated side of the diaphragm

underneath. Chest x-rays are taken on alternate days and a neurological examination is carried out daily, with particular reference to determining whether the lesion has ascended. Should the vital capacity fall below 500 ml a tracheostomy is performed and the patient may commence positive pressure respiration.

When the stage of spinal shock has subsided there is a progressive increase in the vital capacity. After some months the risk of pulmonary embolism is considerably reduced. There is a return of tone to the paralysed respiratory muscles and the patient learns tricks to assist him coughing, the most important of which is to compress the abdominal muscles by leaning forward to cough. Even at this late stage the patient is still at risk of developing pneumonia. In this respect patients are regarded in much the same way as those suffering from chronic lung disease and as soon as they develop a mild cold they recommence postural drainage, antibiotics and inhalations. As a result of this regime there is now a very low initial mortality amongst tetraplegic patients. In a recent series of 100 consecutive unselected admissions at the National Spinal Injuries Centre between April 1971 and March 1973 there were 51 with cervical lesions. Only two of these patients died. Both were aged over 63 years with high cervical injuries and they died some two months and four months respectively after injury, one from septicaemia and the other from cardiac failure.

IMPAIRMENT OF THE AUTONOMIC NERVOUS SYSTEM

Introduction
A complete transection of the cord in the cervical region above the sympathetic outflow isolates the sympathetic from its central control but leaves the parasympathetic supply mediated by the vagus intact. Tetraplegic patients suffer from a variety of autonomic disturbances that cause them considerable disability. There is no other aspect of spinal rehabilitation in which a thorough understanding of the anatomy, physiology and pharmacology can be more valuable.

Definition
Langley in 1898 originally introduced the term and it was first regarded as the motor nerves of the sympathetic and para-sympathetic system, but today the definition has been extended to include the visceral afferents and centres which connect with the efferent pathways.

(1) Cranial autonomic — 3rd, 7th, 9th and 10th nerves.
(2) Sympathetic — T1 to L2.
(3) Sacral autonomic — S2/S3.

Sympathetic reflex arc
(1) *Sensory or receptor fibre* which begins in an internal organ and ends in the lateral horn of the spinal cord. Its nutrient cell is in the dorsal root ganglia.
(2) *Connector fibre* which begins in the cell in the lateral horn and travels out of the anterior horn as a white ramus communicans until it reaches a sympathetic ganglion.
(3) *Excitor fibre* or motor fibre begins in a ganglion and proceeds as a grey ramus communicans to a mixed spinal nerve, finally to reach an end organ such as a wall of a blood vessel.

Parasympathetic reflex also consists of three components:

(1) *Sensory fibre* which begins in the periphery. The vagus, for example, has its cell station in the nodose ganglion which corresponds to an ordinary posterior root ganglion. It terminates in the medulla around the dorsal nucleus of the vagus.
(2) *The dorsal nucleus* of the vagus forms the beginning of the connector fibre. This continues to the end organ such as the heart or blood vessel where it synapses with the excitor fibre.
(3) *Excitor fibre* — these are very short, in the wall of the organ, in contrast to the sympathetic excitor fibre.

Functions of the autonomic

Most organs receive a dual nerve supply which although they have opposite actions frequently act together synergistically. The vagus supplies from the hind brain to the hind gut. The sympathetic, because it originates between $T1 - L2$, has to send prolongations upwards to supply the face and downwards to supply the lower limbs. It follows that the somatic dermatomes are not the same as the autonomic dermatomes. Thus the upper limbs are supplied somatically from C2–T2 whereas the sympathetic fibres are from T5–T9. The hind limb somatic supply is T12–S5 but the sympathetic is from fibres T10–L2. A consequence of this dual innervation is that in a patient with a high cervical cord transection the vagal supply to the heart is intact whereas the sympathetic supply is cut off from central control.

Pharmacology

This is a very complex subject. In general, it can be said that the sympathetic nerve releases nor-adrenaline at its excitor fibre terminals and the parasympathetic releases acetyl choline. Hence the actions of the parasympathetic on the bowel and bladder may be enhanced by preventing destruction of acetyl choline or giving drugs that act like acetyl choline and the actions of the sympathetic may be reinforced by drugs such as Ephedrine. However, there are many paradoxical situations such as the presence of alpha adrenergic receptors in the urethra and those wishing to treat paraplegic patients are recommended to refer to a modern text book on pharmacology.

Central control of sympathetic and parasympathetic

The central control of the autonomic depends on the frontal lobes, the limbic system and the hypothalamus — the influence of the grain and emotions upon the heart rate, bowel function and sexual arousal is well known.

Cord transection

After a complete interruption of the cervical cord above the sympathetic outflow there is, in addition to the loss of power of the paralysed muscles, a complete isolation of the sympathetic nervous system from central control. The result is impaired control of peripheral blood vessels and abolition of sweating, which are important homeostatic mechanisms for the regulation of body temperature. In addition there are abnormal reflex phenomena found only in the isolated sympathetic system deprived of central control.

Temperature regulation

In normal people, heating the trunk and lower limbs leads to reflex vasodilation and sweating of the whole body. This reflex is probably initiated in the central nervous system and mediated via the spinal cord and sympathetic efferents, the stimulus being a rise in skin and blood temperature. As a result of these compensatory mechanisms there is no rise in central temperature. In contrast a patient with a traumatic tetraplegia when heated in identical conditions cannot increase the blood flow to the periphery or sweat so that his temperature rises.

The second consequence of this paralysis of the sympathetic system arises when a patient is cooled. In a normal person, the response to cooling is reflex vasoconstriction so that the heat loss is reduced and the body generates further heat by the muscular activity of shivering. However, when a patient with a complete cervical cord transection is cooled, because of the sympathetic paralysis there is no vasoconstriction, heat loss continues the patient's central temperature falls and hypothermia results. Shivering does not occur in the paralysed part of the body but only in the normally innervated parts, e.g. the masseter and temporalis muscles, above the cord transection. The practical implications are that a tetraplegic patient is unable to regulate his temperature independently of his environment i.e. he is poikilothermic. Environmentally induced hyperpyrexia is not a major problem in this temperate climate, but in South Africa, Australia and the United States of America it is necessary to have special air conditioned wards to prevent the patients becoming hyperpyrexial during the summer months. Of greater importance is the fact that a minor upper respiratory or urinary infection very rapidly leads to hyperpyrexia, because the tetraplegic cannot lose heat effectively. In the United Kingdom, low temperatures are much commoner and, as a result, hypothermia is much more of a danger. Tetraplegic patients are particularly in danger of developing hypothermia immediately after injury, while they are in a state of spinal shock, and this condition may be missed unless a special low recording thermometer is used. The clinical condition is similar to that seen in idiopathic hypothermia in old people. The patient is confused, has a low temperature, bradycardia, cardiac arrhythmia and a low blood pressure. He may have peripheral oedema, particularly around the eyelids. It is of interest, that terminally both old people suffering from idiopathic hypothermia and tetraplegic patients may have raised serum amylase levels, and at post mortem the pancreas is found to be necrotic.

Postural hypotension

Another result of the paralysis of the sympathetic system is defective sympathetic control of the heart and the blood vessels mediating postural vasoconstriction. As a result, when the patient is sat up for the first time, sits in a chair for prolonged periods or bends, he is liable to develop postural hypotension because of blood pooling in his abdomen and lower limbs. Venous return is diminished since the paralysis of the limb muscles abolishes the muscle pump, the patient is unable to increase the stroke volume of his heart owing to paralysis of its sympathetic supply, and therefore he faints. This is compensated by giving the patient a tight corset and elastic stockings to improve venous return. In time, with training, he is able to stand for considerable periods without fainting. The loss of sympathetic innervation and the unopposed action of the vagus on the heart makes the tetraplegic patient liable to cardiac arrest in the early stages, particularly when anoxia is present.

Abnormal reflexes

Bladder, bowel and muscle stimulation result in a marked rise in blood pressure, owing to generalized reflex sympathetic discharge from the isolated spinal cord. In a man with an intact nervous system such hypertension would be balanced by other reflexes from the vagus that would lower the heart rate, and other reflexes from the brain stem acting through the spinal cord which would inhibit vasoconstriction and cause vasodilation. If these spinal pathways are severed, the only pathway left intact is the vagus which is insufficient to control the blood pressure. This uninhibited rise in blood pressure in response to distension of the bladder is accompanied by blinding headaches and can lead to an intracerebral bleed. This reflex hypertension, bradycardia and pulmonary congestion usually appears some three months after injury, but can appear within as little as one week.

Sweating

Patients with high cord transections are liable to develop drenching sweats. These usually occur as a result of irritation by infection of the bladder or stimulation of the rectum by faeces. They may be part of the autonomic disturbance described previously but can occur alone in the absence of bradycardia and hypertension. They can be extremely difficult to treat. Usually they respond if the causative lesion in the bladder or bowel is dealt with but this is not always the case.

LOSS OF BLADDER FUNCTION

Parasympathetic — The motor supply of the bladder is derived from the intermediolateral nucleus of the sacral cord between the second and fourth segments. The parasympathetic fibres leave by the anterior nerve roots and pass by the pelvic nerve through the hypogastric ganglia without synapsing. They join the vesical plexus of nerves where the post-ganglionic fibre arises. These nerves are responsible for detrusor contractions of the bladder.

The sympathetic nerve supply to the bladder comes from the intermediolateral cell complexes between T.11 and L.2. They leave by the anterior nerve roots, pass through the sympathetic chain without synapsing and form the presacral nerve. This synapses at the hypogastric plexus. A post-ganglionic nerve there supplies the smooth muscles of the trigone and ureteral orifices and also the very important smooth muscle in the urethra and the vas. Its role is probably to shut off the bladder from the urethra during intercourse so that there is no regurgitation of semen into the bladder. Its role is controversial; it may assist in raising the tone of the bladder.

Micturition is mediated mainly by the parasympathetic nerves, but voluntary muscles comprising the urogenital diaphragm of the pelvic floor and the adductor muscles participate. Their reciprocal relaxation must take place during micturition. The urogenital diaphragm is innervated by the pudendal nerve derived from sacral roots 2 to 3 and the adductor muscles are supplied by the obturator nerve derived from L.2 to L.4.

Sensory impulses are of two forms: exteroceptive sensation from the bladder mucosa such as pain, and proprioceptive such as the sensation or the desire to void and the sensation of fullness and passage of urine. Painful impulses travel by the parasympathetic and sympathetic fibres to the posterior roots and reach consciousness by the crossed spinothalamic tract. Proprioceptive impulses from the pelvic floor are thought to take a different pathway within the cord and travel up the posterior columns on the same side.

The bladder
The bladder consists of smooth muscle, arranged in a complex manner in several layers so that when is contracts the neck of the bladder is pulled open.

The smooth muscle is made up of a multi-unit syncytium. Each cell is in close apposition to the adjacent one, leaving no extra-cellular space. There is a rich nerve supply with plentiful ganglia. It is believed that conduction can take place between each cell. This smooth muscle is sensitive to stretch and has spontaneous rhythmicity. Normally it is activated by the spinal cord under central control.

The tone of the bladder is the resistance of the cell substance to stretch. It is probably an intrinsic property of the muscle cell; it does not fatigue and is independent of the central nervous system and persists in spite of neuromuscular blockade, nerve block, spinal shock and even death. Accommodation is the ability of the muscle to maintain constant pressure with increments of volume.

Rhythmic contractions are tiny movements, barely visible by conventional means of recording, that originate in the musculature of the bladder wall. Voiding contractions are much larger, longer and stronger and result in emptying or partial emptying of the bladder. Normally, when there is a desire to void, one such voiding contraction empties the bladder. In the case of a cord transection, the threshold is lowered and they can appear when there are only small quantities of urine within the bladder.

The internal sphincter maintains continence at the bladder neck; the muscle fibres lace and interlace. There is probably no separate distinct anatomical sphincter; it is part of the bladder wall. When infection and obstruction occur the bladder hypertrophies and the bladder neck becomes thickened, oedematous and less elastic; it appears to be a distinct rigid rim because it is not taken up when the bladder contracts.

The external sphincter is composed of striped circularly orientated muscle between the two layers of the urogenital diaphragm but additional paraurethral striated muscle extends upwards to the bladder, blending with the connective tissue and smooth muscle; it is more dense anteriorly. It is under voluntary control and is normally relaxed. When the bladder fills and the subject becomes conscious of it the external sphincter tightens. The sphincter is responsible for stopping micturition in emergency but blocking the sphincter by anaesthesia of the pudendal nerve does not result in incontinence, since the tone of the elastic tissues and of the smooth muscle under sympathetic control are also responsible for continence. The external sphincter functions as an emergency stop-gap mechanism. In a patient with damage to the spinal cord resulting in spasticity of the striped muscle this can involve the pelvic floor and adductor muscles. Thus a spasm can interrupt micturition, when the legs become violently adducted resulting in incontinence.

Damage to the spinal cord and nerve roots
The main factors in classifying dysfunctions of the bladder are:

Upper motor neurone – A good guide to this is if the anal reflex and the bulbocavernosus reflex are present. These share the same reflex pathways as those for micturition and their presence indicates that detrusor contractions may return.

This can be determined by carrying out a cystometrogram or a micturating cystogram to measure the pressures and the force of the detrusor contraction. The bald account that a patient is micturating when there is severe cord damage is uninformative and can be misleading because he may have retention with overflow. If the pathways are intact and detrusor contractions present then the bladder can empty reflexly.

Lower motor neurone – If the pathways are interrupted then detrusor contractions cannot take place and the bladder must be emptied by straining or abdominal compression.

After a spinal injury
Acute – Immediately after an acute high cord transection the reflex pathways are not damaged but detrusor contractions are abolished in the stage of spinal shock. Tone and accommodation are normal.

Detrusor contractions depend upon the reflex pathways, whereas tone and accommodation depend upon the intrinsic properties of the bladder musculature. The detrusor contractions return at a variable time, usually after the plantar responses, but this depends upon the age of the patient and the method of bladder management.

Chronic – The detrusor contractions are smooth muscle contractions and their return is not related to the return of tone in striped muscle, that is spasticity in the limbs or return of tendon reflexes. Emptying of the bladder depends upon the balance between the detrusor contractions and the tone of the external sphincter. When detrusor contractions return they may at first be quite small and insufficient to overcome the tonic resistance at the external sphincter. It requires a pressure of at least 40 ml of water to overcome this. This is seen in patients with cervical lesions and early after injury in other patients. The expulsive pressure can be raised in patients with low lesions by straining or manual compression or by an attendant in the case of cervical patients.

Secondary effects
Obstruction
The bladder is composed of smooth muscle, which is easily damaged by obstruction and infection.

Obstruction prevents the complete emptying of its contents. This results in stretching of the muscle fibres. The cells become separated from adjacent ones and there is increased deposition of intercellular collagen and damage to the nerve fibres with impaired transmission of excitatory impulses from one cell to another. This damage can result from a single episode of overdistension. The outcome is a secondary paralysis of the bladder so that in a normal person after a prostatectomy an episode of retention can prevent the patient emptying the bladder. This is called secondary hypotonia.

In a patient in spinal shock the return of detrusor contractions may be delayed, or in one who has regained satisfactory micturition these contractions can be lost following an episode of overdistension. In time, the bladder may regain them if overdistension is not repeated. The practical result is that because of this impaired emptying, the bladder is more easily infected.

If the obstruction is sub-acute or partial it results in hypertrophy of the musculature including the bladder neck. This then constitutes a secondary obstruction.

Obstruction can occur in several ways. If a catheter is placed in the bladder it can become blocked or a condom drainage can become twisted. One of the most common ways for a paralysed patient is for spasms of the external sphincter to develop which occludes the urethra.

Infection

Infection has several important effects upon the bladder:

(1) It causes an outpouring of white blood cells which make the urine turbid.
(2) The bladder wall becomes hyperaemic and bleeds so that the first sign of a urinary infection can be haematuria.
(3) It has two effects upon the muscle:
   (a) In the early stages it can irritate muscle causing an increased force of contraction so that the patient presents with increased frequency and a small irritable bladder.
   (b) If the infection is very severe it can paralyse the bladder and ureter resulting in an atonic paralysis, since the B.coli produces a potent endotoxin.
(4) If the infection is very severe, and especially if accompanied by obstruction and trauma to the urethra, a highly infected part of the body is placed in contact with one with a very rich blood supply, so that organisms have access to the blood stream resulting in septicaemia.

It is a common experience for the passage of a catheter in the presence of infected urine or instrumentation of the urethra to be associated with fever. The body normally can deal with such infections of the urethra and bladder provided there is free drainage. It only becomes dangerous if there is obstruction and infection.

Preventive measures
Mechanical Washout
Bacteria multiply logarithmically; the number is reduced every time the bladder is emptied. If it empties completely it is very difficult to infect urine. Concentration is reduced by the dilution of organisms of fresh urine secreted by the kidneys.

Organisms are more easily destroyed in dilute urine, hence drinking and frequency in patients with infected urine is teleologically useful in elimination of infection. If the bladder is not emptied completely in micturition there will be a large residual urine. Once this is infected the concentration of bacteria in this sump serves to infect fresh urine. In a patient immediately after spinal injury, who cannot empty his bladder because the detrusor contractions are abolished, intervals between catheterizations are critical; the longer the interval the greater time for bacteria to multiply.

Infection can spread to the bladder wall. If the ureteric orifices are involved they become incompetent, reflux develops and allows infected urine to reach the kidneys.

The organisms originate in the patient's bowel and certain of them seem to have selective and heightened pathogenicity for the renal tract. On arrival in hospital the bowel becomes colonized by resistant hospital organisms, this being largely governed by the particular antibiotics used. These resistant organisms then spread to the perineum and colonise the anterior urethra. When a catheter is passed into the urethra the organisms are carried into the bladder (It is extremely difficult to infect the normal bladder provided there is free emptying; in a patient with a spinal injury this is impaired).

Long-term complications of pyelonephritis

The long-term complications of pyelonephritis are similar to those seen in general medical practice – hypertension and renal failure. Tribe and Silver (1969) found that 60 of 174 paraplegic patients who died at Stoke Mandeville Hospital had evidence of hypertension during life which was confirmed by the finding of an enlarged heart on post-mortem examination. There is a high incidence of hypertension in those patients with traumatic injuries of the spinal cord who survive for any length of time. The exact mechanism of the hypertension and its relationship to pyelonephritis is not clear, but once hypertension supervenes it leads to further deterioration of renal function and the patient may die of either renal failure or the complications of hypertension such as a 'stroke' or heart failure.

Another interesting complication seen in paraplegic patients is the development of amyloid disease. Amyloid disease was first described as a complication of paraplegia by Fagge (1876) and it was recorded in the First World War, but a more comprehensive study was made by Tribe (1963) and expanded by Tribe and Silver (1969). Of 174 necropsies performed at Stoke Mandeville Hospital among paraplegic patients, 65 had amyloid disease. This was caused by chronic renal and bone suppuration. It invariably involved the kidney and was also extensively distributed throughout the liver, spleen, bowel and heart. The manifestations were those of the nephrotic syndrome. The patients presented with oedema involving the face and lower limbs. They also had intractable anaemia. The most valuable investigation was the estimation of the 24 hour urinary protein: a level above 5 grams distinguished it from severe pyelonephritis. The heavy proteinuria was reflected in lowered serum-albumin values. The bowel was almost invariably involved and in order to determine the incidence of this condition in life a series of rectal biopsies was performed. This indicated that in a paraplegic population something like 5 per cent would be suffering from amyloidosis. The condition adversely affected the life expectancy and virtually half the patients were dead within three years of the first diagnosis of amyloid disease.

Management

There are about 300 acute spinal injuries per year in the United Kingdom of which some 50 to 75 per cent will be associated with other major injuries. In addition many patients have paralysis of the bladder from disease such as multiple sclerosis or spinal tumours. Except in a very few cases they will be unable to pass urine on their own because of the absence of detrusor contractions. So the bladder must be drained. There are various methods: non-intervention; manual expression; continuous drainage; and intermittent catheterization.

Non-intervention

This merely means that the bladder is allowed to fill until its elastic limit is passed. When pressure exceeds the opening pressure of the bladder-neck urine will dribble out.

This is obviously unsatisfactory, for overstretching destroys the bladder musculature and results in infection. It inhibits the return of detrusor contractions.

Manual expression

Use of a catheter introduces bacteria into the bladder but this can be avoided if the bladder can be emptied by gentle manual expression. This method was introduced during the First World War by Vellacott and Webb Johnson (1919) and was revived by Golding (1968) and Cook and Smith (1970).

In Cook and Smith's hands it produced marked hydronephrosis – no doubt from attempts to express the bladder against resistance of the closed bladder neck. They therefore abandoned the method.

It is obvious that some form of drainage is necessary but indwelling catheters during the First World War produced disastrous results. Thompson Walker (1937) found that of 339 patients with spinal injuries admitted to King George V Military Hospital during the period 1915–1916, 47.2 per cent died from ascending urinary tract infection 8 to 10 weeks later. Even today with fine plastic catheters and effective antibiotics, an indwelling catheter results in infection of the bladder within 48 to 72 hours.

The closed bladder-neck and urethra is an effective barrier to infection but the catheter breaks down this barrier. It allows infection to track both within the lumen of the catheter and alongside it. Movement of the catheter up and down the urethra helps drag organisms into the bladder.

If a Foley type catheter is used this is even more injurious, for because its oore is larger it tends to block the fine urethral glands causing urethritis. This can progress to a pressure sore of the urethra (another name for a urethral abscess) and ulcers at the external meatus. If this is allowed to continue a urethral fistula can occur. The vas can also become blocked giving rise to an orchitis. The balloon of a Foley catheter also serves as a focus for stone formation and, if it bursts, as a foreign body for egg-shell calculi.

A further disadvantage in the use of a balloon catheter is that it leaves the bladder permanently empty; there is evidence that regular distension of the bladder acts as a stimulus for return of detrusor contractions.

Intermittent catheterization

The most satisfactory form of drainage of the bladder to date is the use of intermittent catheterization. This means that the bladder is distended regularly by secretion of urine and then at regular intervals, three to four times a day, drained.

Distension serves to stimulate the return of detrusor contraction. The catheter is then removed and the barrier of the bladder-neck and the closed urethra is restored. The dangers of this method are that infection can readily be introduced by unskilled catherisation.

For this reason, at the National Spinal Injuries Centre, doctors perform all catheterizations, although Pearman and England (1973) have found that a catheter orderly can do the work satisfactorily. To prevent the urethra becoming the source of infection it is filled with ½ a per cent Hibitane to sterilize it. Every specimen of urine taken is cultured on a dip plate, so that infection is detected immediately and eliminated promptly to reduce urinary sepsis.

It has been argued that the technique can only be employed at special centres and cannot have universal application. This is not so. It has been successfully applied in Australia, France and the United States of America but it does require close monitoring, particularly with regard to infection and overdistention.

The catheter is discontinued when the bladder empties satisfactorily with a small residual urine, either reflexly or by expression.

Acceptable state of the urinary tract

The objective of urinary care is to preserve normal upper tracts as shown by the IVP, sterile urine and a residual urine of 60 ml or less. The work of O'Grady has shown that it is the absolute quantity of urine left in the bladder when the act of micturition has been completed and not the relationship of the residual urine to the total capacity of the bladder that matters. Extreme cases of an irritable, small contracted bladder may have a total capacity of 60 ml which is infected and that can also be the size of the residual. A further factor is the relationship between the pressure generated in the bladder and the resistance in the urethra. If the bladder has to generate excessively high pressures to overcome the resistance, in time this pressure will be transmitted back to the kidneys giving rise to hydronephrosis.

INDICATIONS FOR SURGERY

(1) *Inability to empty the bladder after an adequate period of bladder training* Immediately after a spinal injury irrespective of the level, unless it is very incomplete, the patient will be unable to pass urine. It takes a variable period of time, in a case of upper motor neurone lesions from 4–8 weeks, before the detrusor contractions return. They can be inhibited by over-distension and infection and are little influenced by the use of drugs at this stage, apart from antibiotics to reduce the infection. The tone of the external sphincter is present from the outset, so it is necessary to wait for a variable period to determine if the detrusor contractions will return and be sufficiently strong to pull open the bladder neck and thus empty the bladder. In the case of the lower motor neurone lesions these contractions will not return and the patient will have to learn to empty his bladder by abdominal compression. In both cases it is desirable to wait until the patient is up in a chair so that he can have the aid of gravity to assist emptying his bladder and try various tricks, that is learning forward, coughing, tapping and straining to facilitate bladder emptying.

(2) *Damage to the upper urinary tract* owing to back pressure. This indicative usually of obstruction of the urinary outflow.

(3) *Persistently large infected residual urine.* If the residual urine is infected then this will inevitably lead to ascending infection of the urinary tract.

(4) *If the residual urine is large,* that is above 60 ml and shows no growth, this is not universally accepted as indication for surgery since with training this may be reduced. However, the persistence of a large residual is always likely to give rise to infection.

(5) *Detrusor sphincter inco-ordination.* Although the upper urinary tract may be normal, the residual urine may be sterile and below 60 ml but the pressure

generated by the bladder to overcome the resistance of the bladder outflow may be excessively high and these patients have been found to be at risk of developing upper urinary tract damage over the ensuing months particularly if reflux occurs.

Contra-indications to surgery
(1) Short life expectancy, i.e. less than seven years. In this case the patient may well die of other complications before renal failure will supervene from an indwelling catheter.
(2) Gross sepsis.
(3) Fear of impotence and incontinence.
(4) Unwillingness to wear a condom. In the case of a tetraplegic patient he could have a catheter inserted in his bladder by the district nurse once a week whereas a condom may have to be put on by someone else, say his wife, once a day and some patients are resistant to this.
(5) Small penis. A very small penis which does not allow a collecting device to be applied may be a contra-indication.
(6) Allergy to skin glue.

Appliances
Male — When the patient has achieved a satisfactory pattern of bladder emptying the majority in this country prefer to use a condom collecting device rather than practice bladder training. The patient is told to empty his bladder regularly and not just let the urine trickle away. Some patients can manage without a condom collecting device but it only requires one accident in a week when the trousers or clothes are soiled for social embarassment to result.

Female — The problems in female patients are rather different. Firstly there is no satisfactory urinary collecting device so that bladder training must be aimed for, with the addition of pads. Some female patients find this too difficult and resort to an indwelling catheter. Secondly, obstruction is not a feature in female patients and it is very seldom necessary to operate upon the bladder outlet. These operations, when they are attempted, have not been successful and they subsequently result in incontinence.

Drugs
The use of drugs is a subject of great importance.

(1) Antibiotics can be used to eliminate infection but preferably in short courses. The preference is for Negram or Furadantin, or bactericidal antibiotics such as Gentamicin, rather than broad spectrum antibiotics which rapidly elicit the growth of resistant or opportunistic infections. When the urine is rendered sterile acidifying agents such as G.500 are used to make it more difficult for the patient to acquire infection. If a patient has an indwelling catheter there is no use in giving continuous antibiotics as the urine is inevitably infected.
(2) Bladder stimulants. These drugs can be given to raise the strength of the detrusor contractions but in general the emphasis is on lowering the resistance at the bladder outlet by surgery before increasing the dosage of these drugs.
(3) Relaxation of the smooth muscle. Attention has recently been drawn to

the role of the smooth muscle in the urethra causing difficulty in micturition so that lowering its tone by the use of phenoxybenzamine has proved beneficial.

SUMMARY

There is little doubt that infection and damage to the kidneys can be introduced at a very early stage of management.

Overstretching can destroy the musculature so that a satisfactory pattern of micturition cannot be established and infection can damage the kidneys, leading to pyelonephritis with the long term risk of hypertension, renal failure and amyloid disease.

IMPAIRMENT OF SEXUAL FUNCTION

Anatomy and physiology of intercourse
Erections
Erection takes place purely on a segmental reflex basis; suprasegmental connections are unnecessary. In paraplegic patients the afferent sensory impulses that initiate the reflex are caused by tactile stimuli of the glans and travel to the second, third and fourth sacral segments by way of the internal pudendal nerves. Efferent impulses leave these same segments by way of the parasympathetic supply and cause dilation of the arterioles of the penis with distention and congestion of the corpora cavernosa and spongiosum. Efferent impulses also leave these segments through the internal pudendal nerves to cause contraction of the periurethral muscles, with resultant compression of the venous drainage channels of the penis. Blood is thus trapped within the penis and an erection results.

Ejaculation
Ejaculation is a complex, spinal, segmental reflex function mediated by pathways and centres in the lower thoracic and upper lumbar segments. Suprasegmental connections are not necessary for the act. The first part of the reflex is controlled by the sympathetic nerves, which release semen from the seminal vesicles. The second stage in ejaculation is also reflex. It is initiated by sensory impulses set up by the presence of semen in the posterior urethra, which set up efferent impulses that cause contraction of the peri-urethral muscles and result in the actual ejaculation of semen from the meatus. These efferent and afferent impulses travel through the internal pudendal nerves by way of the second, third and fourth sacral segments. The final release of semen is facilitated by the contraction of striped muscles of the pelvic floor. In normal men these reflexes are under the control of the higher centres, and psychical stimuli may either inhibit or excite these reflexes.

The scrotum receives a rich nerve supply, the skin from the sacral segments and the testicles from the sympathetic system, so that in a patient with a lesion at T.12 the scrotal skin may be denervated but testicular sensation preserved.

Impaired function in diseases of the nervous system
Degree of cord damage
Though erections and ejaculations are purely spinal reflexes, they may be inhibited or stimulated by higher psychical stimuli, which are obviously

extremely important since the first symptom of cord compression may be the loss of libido. In general, even if there is only a little sparing of sensation or motor power so that the cord lesion is incomplete there is a greater likelihood that the patient will retain sexual function. Though the exact pathways within the cord for the control of the sexual act are not known they are closely related to the pathways that control micturition.

Effect of level of transection

Hence erection is a reflex phenomenon, and if the pathways serving erection in the lumbar and sacral parts of the cord are intact, erections can take place. Thus, most patients who have a clearcut transection of the spinal cord in the cervical or thoracic region will preserve the ability to have erections provided the damage has not extended longitudinally down the cord to impair the pathways in the lumbar and sacral segments. In fact, these erections are easily elicited during a spasm or during manipulation of the penis during a spasm. They are not necessarily well sustained, and they appear at inappropriate times and not in response to psychical stimuli unless the cord lesion is incomplete. On the other hand, patients with lesions in the lower part of the cord, where there is destruction of the pathways, are less likely to have erections, but they may still occur, and about half the men with low lesions may still have erections, even when the pathways to the bladder are interrupted, as shown by an autonomous bladder without reflex contractions, or when the anal reflex is absent.

Ejaculations are present in a much smaller percentage of patients with spinal cord lesions. About 10 per cent of the patients with high transections who have erections may have ejaculations, and only a very small percentage of those with low lesions can ejaculate. The intact lumbar cord and its motor connections are not necessary for the production of ejaculation. Clinical absence of such connections, as evidenced by the absence of an anal reflex and an autonomous bladder, are not necessarily a bar to erections. To have an ejaculation the periurethral muscles must be innervated at least reflexly and be activated by way of the internal pudendal nerves. Patients with cauda equina lesions, paradoxically, are unable to have an erection because of the destructive lesion of the cauda equina and yet because the testicles and seminal vesicles are innervated by the sympathetic nervous system, they may be able to have emissions.

Fertility

There is a loss of fertility in men with complete cord transections above the lumbar and sacral segments, even if they are able to ejaculate. Sperms are not mobile and there are fewer of them. The cause of these features is unknown, but it may be due to intercurrent infections of the bladder or, possibly, to the change in the temperature regulation in the scrotum seen in paraplegic patients.

Because most paraplegic patients have been men — in the first instance they were war veterans — there is much more information about sexual function in paraplegic men than in paraplegic women. The nerve supply to the female genital organs is similar to that in the male, the clitoris being innervated by the pudendal nerve and the vagina by the sacral segments, but it is doubtful whether there are reflex centres in the spinal cord that subserve sexual function in the same way as in the man. As a consequence of a spinal injury with complete denervation of the sacral centres women experience little sensation during intercourse, but in contrast to male paraplegics, their fertility and their ability to have children is usually unaffected. The denervation of the ovaries, contrary to the experience in the male, does not seem to reduce their fertility. Immediately after a cord transection there will be some change in the periods, but these will resume after a few weeks unless there is a secondary amenorrhoea owing to intercurrent toxicity.

Intercourse

Intercourse in a paraplegic patient does not revolve simply around the innervation of the sexual organs. Paraplegia, if it is complete, will cause loss of power and sensation in the bladder, bowels, and lower limb muscles, and there may also be pressure sores and severe spasticity. The denervation of the bladder may result in infection, and the patient may be incontinent of urine during intercourse or may be inhibited from having intercourse by fear of infecting his female partner. Spasms in the legs may prove a problem since the legs in the man can draw up and flex so that it is impossible to achieve satisfactory penetration, and similarly, severe spasms may occur in the woman that adduct the legs and prevent penetration. If the patient has pressure sores these too can render the act of intercourse distasteful or can be aggravated by attempting intercourse.

Operative interventions

After a spinal injury many patients have an operation in the form of a bladder neck resection to enable them to empty the bladder completely. This will destroy the sphincter of the bladder, which normally prevents semen regurgitating into the bladder during intercourse, and will thus make the patient sterile, and it is important to explain the risks involved to a patient before this operation is contemplated. It has recently been shown that an external sphincterotomy will also temporarily inhibit the ability to have an erection, probably because of local damage to the blood supply of the penis. Operative intervention such as a cordotomy or an alcohol block on the cord will also impair the power of erection.

Certain drugs that are used for the treatment of spasticity, such as diazepam and barbiturates, may well inhibit erections.

Intercourse for the patient with a normal partner

Before having intercourse the male patient should remove his catheter and empty his bladder by suprapubic compression. Many men are afraid of infecting their partner so they usually use a condom. The next thing is to achieve an erection. This can be achieved by manual stimulation, which as it is often badly sustained, may be maintained by tying a soft condom around the base of the penis to maintain the turgidity, though care must be taken to avoid damaging the penis. Paraplegic patients can achieve a superior position, but tetraplegic patients are unable to do this and the woman must take the more active part by assuming the superior position. Care must be taken to avoid pressure sores by placing a pillow beneath the buttocks. For the female paraplegic with a normal husband the problems are less difficult since there is not the necessity to achieve an erection but similar problems pertain with regard to emptying the bladder and removing the catheter and protecting the buttocks from pressure sores.

Side effects
A disturbing side effect seen in patients with high cord transection is autonomic hyperreflexia.

Marriage
Surprisingly, such severe disability resulting in impotence and sterility does not preclude the paraplegic patient from marrying. Comarr (1962) studied 858 patients with spinal injuries; 20 per cent were unmarried before and remained so after injury; 48 per cent were married before injury; and 26 per cent were unmarried before injury but married for the first time after injury. Of those who married after injury, 20 per cent were later divorced. In 1964 Guttmann analysed his experience of 1505 living paraplegics in the United Kingdom and found a small divorce rate − 57 out of 975 married patients − that was only slightly greater than that for normal people in the United Kingdom. Divorce was less likely in those already married at the time of injury than in those married subsequently because in the former group there was already the basis for a normal married life and companionship, and therefore, the loyalty of the normal partner would be greater.

Pregnancy and labour
Twenty-two babies − 13 boys and 9 girls − were born to paraplegic women studied by Guttmann. Four of the women had two children each after being paralysed. These patients were more liable to develop pressure sores and subsequent sepsis owing to the loss of sensation and mobility. The danger of anaemia and renal infection has to be guarded against since during labour patients with cervical lesions can develop severe autonomic hyperreflexia.

PRESSURE SORES

Mechanism
Pressure sores occur because the weight of the body is not evenly transmitted throughout the whole surface area of the subject but is transmitted through the feet when the subject stands, through the back of his heels and sacrum when he lies on his back, through greater trochanter, lateral malleoli and shoulder tips when he lies on his sides and through the ischial tuberosities when he sits. The tissue between these bony prominences and the surface is compressed by the weight of the body when the patient lies or sits upon them. The pressure generated by the heart is insufficient to overcome this and the tissues are rendered avascular until the subject moves and the blood supply is restored. Initially there is transient erythema and then vesiculation and oedema if the pressure continues. This stage is reversible if the pressure is relieved. If not, then the tissues become indurated. The surface may be excoriated exposing the cutis vera or again haemorrhagic blisters may be observed. If the process is not arrested at this stage, deep penetrating necrosis of the subcutaneous tissue, fascia, muscle and bone develops, leading to gangrene, osteomyelitis and septicaemia.

The appearance of such sores from the surface and even by probing can be most deceptive and x-rays of the bony parts are essential to determine the extent of the sores and the presence of osteomyelitis and possible calcification of the tissues. X-rays in the early stages will not show osteomyelitis or sequestrum formation and need to be repeated regularly.

WHY ARE PARAPLEGIC PATIENTS PARTICULARLY LIABLE TO DEVELOP PRESSURE SORES?

Acute stage
General factors lowering blood pressure
Pressure sores occur because tissues are deprived of blood, oxygen and nutrients. Thus any general factor that lowers blood pressure will lead to damage to the tissues, the sites of predilection being those places where tissues are compressed.

In acute spinal injury patients frequently have associated injuries with acute onset of spinal shock as has been pointed out earlier. In a consecutive series of 100 cases, 75 had major associated injuries.

All these injuries can give rise to blood loss, leading to surgical shock and a low blood pressure.

Nervous factors lowering blood pressure
Paralysis of the sympathetic
In the series described above 50 per cent of the patients had cervical injuries. A cervical transection results in a low blood pressure even in the absence of spinal shock. Again as has been pointed out earlier damage to the vasomotor control of the skin and impaired sweating means that the skin throughout the body cannot respond to changes in temperature or accurately alter the local blood flow. The skin does not sweat in response to environmental heating but may respond with drenching sweats to bladder distention. The combination of these factors lowers the resistance of the skin and makes it more likely to injury.

Low tissue oxygen
Patients with cervical injuries have paralysed abdominal and intercostal muscles, breathing with the diaphragm only. This results in a reduced vital capacity and decreased oxygenation of the blood.

Loss of sensation
Painful sensations are received by the peripheral receptors through nerve endings and transmitted via the sensory nerves to the spinal cord. Spinal reflex movement is thus elicited. Alternatively, they may be transmitted to the higher centres where either by reflex mechanisms or conscious efforts movements are initiated. It follows that impairment of any part of these pathways leads to a lack of appropriate protecting movements and immobility of the patient. Patients with brain stem and cerebral involvement from head injuries combined with special injuries are particularly at risk since they cannot ask for help.

Malnutrition
The first few days following spinal injury, patients suffer from ileus and are unable to tolerate food by mouth and are likely to be nourished on intravenous saline, antibiotics, steroids and analgesics. None of these drugs can improve the nutrition of the skin.

Difficulty in turning

Owing to the injuries of the long bones difficulties may be experienced in turning the patient regularly as the splintage may interfere with the turns.

Maceration of the skin

Impairement of bladder and bowel control frequently leads to incontinence in early stages and the skin is rapidly damaged if it is macerated by faeces and urine.

Iatrogenic

Doctors and nurses are justifiably afraid that injudicious movement of a patient may aggravate the spinal injury and increase damage to the cord and this combined with lack of staff and lack of proper equipment may result in a patient being left on his back throughout his stay in a receiving hospital.

Misplaced confidence in equipment

The introduction of turning beds, large cell ripple mattresses, and Stryker frames has been a considerable advance in the prevention of pressure sores. However, they are not a substitute for regular turning of a patient and the medical attendants cannot abdicate the responsibility for ensuring regular turns carried out around the clock. It is not sufficient to turn a patient since they may roll back on their backs. Turning must be supplemented by proper equipment such as a pillow and sandbag to hold the patient in the correct position.

Late stage

Patients with established spinal injuries are likely to develop pressure sores for many of the reasons mentioned previously i.e. paralysis of the sympathetic, though obviously they are not in surgical shock unless they have some intercurrent injury. The sympathetic gradually recovers some independent spinal activity so the blood pressure rises as does blood oxygen with recovery of respiratory muscles. However, the nutrition of patients in later stages may be lowered by development of uraemia and amyloid disease. An adverse factor is the development of spasms in patients with upper motor neurone lesions which makes it extremely difficult to position a patient and they easily knock themselves with an unprovoked spasm. In lower motor neurone lesions wasting of the skin makes sores much more likely to occur as the bony prominences are close to the surface.

Infection

One of the common misconceptions is that pressure sores are sterile. This is incorrect. Pressure sores are infected and serve as a potent source of infection. Connors, Nash and Kennedy (1934) noted that fully 80 per cent of United States of America army paraplegics died in the first few weeks in consequence of infection from bedsores and catheterization. Colin Tribe in a study between 1945 and 1965 of 220 postmortems on paraplegic patients found that of 97 chronic paraplegic patients three died of toxaemia from pressure sores, and another three died of septicaemia and endocarditis, one case of which was due to pressure sores. It must be remembered that sepsis in debilitated patients may not be associated with a high and swinging temperature. Gram-negative septicaemia can present as shock, a low blood pressure and hypothermia, and can be mistaken for a coronary thrombosis or a pulmonary embolus. In many cases the diagnosis is only made at post-mortem. A pressure sore can become bruised so that unless every sore is inspected every day a patient may develop a fever which may be mistaken for a urinary infection, 'flu' or a chest infection, and appropriate treatment will not be instituted. Cellutitis is fortunately rarely seen, but does occur. Perhaps the most damaging thing is to let a patient sit or lie on the pressure sore under the mistaken impression that it helps chest drainage, or that only one sore can be healed at a time.

Prevention
There is nothing magical or unique about the treatment of sores; it follows accepted principles; patients must be turned regularly every two hours. If doctors consider it beneath their dignity to concern themselves with this aspect of the patient's treatment then sores will occur inevitably as day follows night. It is not sufficient to request that the patient be turned two hourly or four hourly; correct equipment is necessary.

The simplest forms favoured are: at Sheffield, the pillow method; at the National Spinal Injuries Centre, Stoke Mandeville and at the Liverpool Regional Paraplegic Centre, an elaborate system of packs and pillows is employed. Mechanized beds of various types can produce adequate turning in the initial stages but they also require skilled supervision. Once a patient has acquired sores then they have to be treated by the method of pillows and packs. All these methods, if applied properly, can give complete protection against pressure sores. The small and large ripple cell mattresses have their advocates but unless the patient is turned regularly in addition to using the bed, sores will develop. The use of the Stryker frame can produce disability in a patient through bruising, contractures and heterotopic new bone formation. In short the equipment and the method is as good as the staff using it.

Principles

(1) Remove the pressure from the sores by suitable 'turns', including prone lying periods if the patient can tolerate it.
(2) Improve the general nutrition by high protein feeds and similar supplements.
(3) Deal with incontinence of urine and faeces. It is impossible to heal a sore macerated by urine and faeces.
(4) Deal with intercurrent infection, with awareness of the high incidence of urinary infection and renal damage. It is not appreciated that there is a high incidence of aspiration pneumonia in bedfast patients.
(5) Local treatment — all sores are composed of dead necrotic tissue that is infected. The organisms differ depending largely on the predominant organism of the ward. Necrotic tissue should be removed in a separate theatre, after the patient's general condition has been improved by blood transfusion, and with systemic antibiotic cover so that the organisms are not disseminated widely throughout the body. Closed pockets should be opened up to provide free drainage.

Sores should be inspected daily and dressing should be carried out as necessary, once or twice a day in the early stages or even more frequently. When the sores are dressed they are sealed up to prevent colonization of the skin of their own bodies with the consequent risk of the infection spreading to their own bladder and lungs, on to staff and other patients in the ward.

(6) Surgical treatment — detailing the surgical procedures for deep and extensive sores is beyond the scope of this book but there are certain fundamental points. In the first instance surgery must be carried out to remove the infected tissue and then the sore should be healed by the simplest possible means, such as split skin grafts. The simplest safest procedure is adopted since the tissues are liable to break down. If a patient is spastic with continuous flexor spasms of the hip it may be necessary to render the lesion flaccid by alcohol block or anterior rhizotomy before definite closure can be achieved since constant movement of the hip will produce pressure sores and prevent the sores healing. Any underlying bony prominence should be removed because if it is not, even if the skin is closed, the factor causing the sore is still in existence and the area will break down as soon as the patient is mobilized. Surgical treatment of the sore is a job for an expert.

(7) Psychological factors — it is hardly surprising that many patients with sores become resentful, unhappy and depressed. They are frequently regarded as psychotic. This is partly contributed to by the absorption of pus from the pressure sores, but it is also due to a very justifiable resentment at the neglect that has caused the sores. It is remarkable how treatment of the sores on the lines described cures many psychological manifestations.

It is appropriate to quote Donald Munro on the subject:

'Health Officers and nurses cannot be made to believe that failure to move a patient on schedule, failure to change a wet bed within 15 minutes of it becoming wet, failure to maintain an adequate level of serum protein causes pressure and bedsores and prevents bedsores from healing until the patient has proved it to their satisfaction by dying, and having learnt their lessons by bitter experience these trained attendants are transferred to another ward or moved to another hospital and the process has to be repeated with another untrained group. Consequently, attention to these apparently trivial details imperative on the part of the visiting staff if there is any desire to lower to mortality and shorten the hospital stay of these patients.'

BIBLIOGRAPHY AND REFERENCES

Connors, J. F. and Nash, I. E. (1934). Am. J. Surgery **26**, 159

Comarr, E. (1962). *11th Spinal Cord Injuries Conference,* American Veterans Administration; Bronx Hospital, p. 209

Fagge, C. H. (1986). *Trans. pathol. Soc. London* **27**, 324

Golding, J. S. R. (1969). *Rehabilitation* **66**, 49

Guttmann, L. (1964). *Paraplegia* **2**, 182

Kennedy, R. H. (1946). *Ann. Surgery* **124**, 1057

Munro, D. J. (1943). J. Am. Med. Assoc. **122**, 1055

O'Grady, F. and Cattell, W. R. (1966) *Br. J. Urology* **37**, 156

Pearman, J. W. and England, E. J. (1973). *Urological Management.* Springfield; Chas. Thomas

Silver, J. R. and Gibbon, N. O. K. (1968). *Br. med. J.* **4**, 79

Silver, J. R. (1974). *Internat. J. Paraplegia* **12**, No. 1, 50

Smith, P. H., Cook, J. B. and Rhind, J. R. (1972). *Paraplegia* **9**, 213

Thompson Walker, (1937). *Br. J. Urology* **9**, 217

Tribe, C. R. (1963). Internat. J. Paraplegia **1**, 19

Tribe, C. R. and Silver J. R. (1969). *Renal Failure in Paraplegia.* London; Pitman

Vellacott, P. N. and Webb Johnson, A. E. (1919). *Lancet* 733

RECOMMENDED FURTHER READING

Burn, J. H. (1975). *The Autonomic Nervous System.* 5th edn. Blackwell
Aids to the Examination of the Peripheral Nervous System. (1976). Medical Research Council, Memorandum No. 45 London; HMSO
Guttmann, L. (1976). *Spinal Cord Injuries.* 2nd edn. Blackwell

15 Rehabilitation After a Heart Attack

BRIAN HAZLEMAN

There is a high prevalence of coronary heart disease in the more developed countries; it has been estimated that 1 man in 5 in Great Britain is likely to have symptoms of coronary disease by the age of 65, and the incidence is increasing, especially in middle-aged and younger men. A reversal of attitudes to the treatment and long-term effects of heart disease has occurred in the last decade, which has resulted in more attention being given to rehabilitation of these patients.

The increasing frequency of myocardial infarction has led to the application of certain techniques already applied to the chronic, neuromuscular diseases. The World Health Organization has emphasized the complexity of cardiac rehabilitation, in their definition: 'the sum of activities required to ensure the best possible physical, mental and social conditions, so that patients may, by their own efforts, regain as normal as possible a place in the community and lead an active productive life'. Much cardiac rehabilitation is an extension of conventional clinical practice, and only in some late problem patients does it involve the special government-based rehabilitation centres.

A joint working-party of the Royal College of Physicians and the British Cardiac Society has now given guidelines for cardiac rehabilitation and also comments on the present position in Britain. It feels that insufficient attention is given to the psychological and social aspects of the illness and to the consequences for future employment; it points out that few hospitals have a rehabilitation service. Although there have been many recent advances in the management of patients with myocardial infarction, these have not always been paralleled by improvements in aftercare. Despite early mobilization in hospital a distressing number of postinfarction patients can be found leading a life of chronic invalidism not justified by their cardiac status. Whilst the overall requirement for supervised physical training remains uncertain, some cardiac patients undoubtedly need help of some kind, although much can be achieved by sensible counselling of patient and relatives.

The working-party emphasizes that cardiologists have tended to disagree on the need for rehabilitation, its value and the best means of achieving it. However, it concludes that cardiac rehabilitation is important, that conventional medical treatment is often insufficient to ensure a full active life, and that convalescence is often unduly prolonged because of ignorance and anxiety. The team feels that those that care for patients with heart attacks should have

251

rehabilitation in mind from the beginning. It points out that further work and research are required and that the logistic problems are not small as the implementation of complex programmes will require more funds and personnel than are at present available.

The present team approach should be contrasted against the negative attitudes of the past, when it was believed that after a myocardial infarction a patient was not fit for any work involving any degree of physical or mental strain. In order to reduce the patient's insecurity or prevent its development, good coordination of the team is required but of greatest importance is good communication with the patient. The family doctor still has the key position of ensuring continuity.

The rehabilitation programme for the cardiac patient is an essential part of management and in most uncomplicated patients it is the only treatment one can offer. Myocardial damage does not usually impose long-term limitations to the physical capacity of the individual and the majority of patients are able to return to their previous work with little or no change in their routine. However, it is important to realize that each patient responds differently to the stress of a severe illness, which cuts abruptly across every aspect of his life, and it is the skill with which the rehabilitation programme is adapted to the patient's individual needs that will have far-reaching consequences, as this can profoundly affect the speed and completeness of recovery.

With increasing attention being paid to the acute coronary episode there is increasing likelihood that time is not spent in planning the longterm care of patients; the long-term aims are, of course, that the patient is restored to a useful and happy life within the limits of his physical capacity. The extent of rehabilitation depends on the individual's reaction to it; above all the patient should understand that the risk of succumbing to a heart attack is not much greater for him than for others of his own age group. Anxiety and depression about the initial illness are replaced by anxiety about future employment and finance. It is important in discussing the implications of the illness that the patient be allowed freedom to express his feelings on such diverse subjects as diet, leisure activities, change of employment and retirement.

Much anxiety and avoidable invalidism is due to the patient's ignorance of the disease in general and of his own state of health in particular. A careful, sympathetic and unhurried discussion with the patient and close family about the nature and implications of the illness is one of the first and most valuable aspects of rehabilitation and this should be carried out as soon as the clinical state allows. Further advice should be given as required; in this the nurse plays a most important role in the early stages of recovery by providing knowledge, support and encouragement. Simple factual information about the possible consequences of infarction is useful, not only in relieving anxiety, but also for its sedative and analgesic affect, as stress increases heart rate and blood pressure. The wife should be reassured before she reaches her husband's bedside, so that she does not transfer her own anxiety.

It is important not only to treat the physical symptoms, but also to pay attention to the psychological and social aspects of the individual, for the ultimate purpose of rehabilitation calls for a gradual withdrawal of help as self-confidence in both patient and spouse improve. This is a continuing process and the division of care into phases such as acute, convalescent and rehabilitative is not realistic. In fact, the lack of continuity in guidance of the patient throughout the whole rehabilitation period is a definite disadvantage.

Despite the increasing emphasis on early mobilization, many patients are not subsequently followed up after discharge from hospital and there is evidence that the family doctor and friends are over-cautious in their attitude to subsequent rehabilitation and return to work. Anxiety and depression are common in both patient and spouse following infarction and the psychological advantage of early mobilization in hospital will be lost if convalescence is prolonged. It has been suggested that there is increasing lack of self-confidence and an increasing chance of permanent unemployment if the patient is away from work more than 10 weeks. Any general discussion of rehabilitation is complicated by the variety of disability encountered. Differences in age, physique and personality, or in the kind of work to which the patient will return, all have to be taken into account.

HOSPITAL CARE

Physicians have always been very cautious in their management of patients with myocardial infarction but attitudes have become more dynamic. At one time 6 weeks' absolute bed rest was advised, for it was known that this was the time required for conversion of necrotic myocardium into scar tissue and it was suggested that exercise would increase the stress on the heart and would aggravate the risks of tissue hypoxia, leading to consequent arrhythmias and cardiac rupture. In the last decade there has been a progressive tendency towards earlier ambulation and return to work, due to the realization of the dangers of excessive bed rest and the discovery that the heart has remarkable recuperative powers. Apart from the psychological advantage of early mobilization there is less risk of thrombo-embolism, muscular wasting and loss of physical performance. Bed rest leads to a loss of normal postural vasomotor reflexes, so that the systolic blood pressure may fall by as much as 50 mmHg on standing. Recent studies have shown that early mobilization after 1 week is not detrimental and there is no increase in the incidence of heart failure, cardiac rupture or aneurysm formation. It is now common practice for patients suffering from an uncomplicated myocardial infarction to be walking after 1 week of bed rest and it may be that even this is too long. During this week bed rest need not be total except for patients in severe pain, in shock or with heart failure or severe arrhythmias. Leg exercises should be carried out daily and the patient can be allowed up for a commode as the physical efforts of defaecation are less on a commode than on a bed. Patients free from hypotension and chest pain can be nursed sitting out of bed from the second hospital day onwards. Those with a small uncomplicated infarct can increase their activity during the second week: they can sit up for increasing time, walk in the ward and bath themselves. If their progress is uneventful, patients are discharged inside 2 weeks, although there are still variations in duration of stay from one hospital to another. During the first few days both physiotherapists and nurses play an important part in ensuring that patients carry out active limb movements to a scheme that has been broadly indicated by the physician in charge.

DISCHARGE FROM HOSPITAL

Despite the increasing emphasis on early mobilization many patients are not given sufficient advice whilst in hospital. It is not sufficient to give vague advice such as 'take it easy for a while', or 'avoid excitement', both of which serve only to increase natural anxiety. Anxious doctors have anxious patients. Whenever possible, both the patient and spouse should be given exact guidelines; a heart attack is an extremely traumatic experience and patients are anxious and depressed, needing reassurance and clear advice. It is important that the spouse is present as there is often descrepancy between the physician's advice and what the spouse will permit. It is important that they are both told that a return to normal life is usual. It is also important that the convalescent phase should not be prolonged, as patients become bored and worry about their ability to support their family.

During the first few weeks at home there is need for both physical and mental rest. The holiday atmosphere provides psychological benefit and graduated exercises result in improvement in exercise tolerance and an improvement in the muscular weakness which has resulted from inactivity. Walking is the best form of exercise at this stage, but at first it is advisable to avoid hills and a cold wind. A rest at lunchtime and odd jobs around the house complete the day. Competitive games are best avoided in the initial stages, although swimming, cycling, horse riding and gardening all provide suitable recretation as along as chest pain and dyspnoea do not occur. Patients tire easily at this stage and the day should be planned so that fatigue is avoided. Much depends on the home circumstances and it may be necessary to change the bedroom temporarily, so that it is on the same floor as the lavatory.

Return to work is the most important milestone on the patient's way to full recovery, as he resumes his accustomed pattern of life and role in society. A sympathetic approach is required by employers. Initially a return to part-time employment is advisable, and this can usually be attempted within 6 weeks. It is much better to return to a familiar job than to go to work in a strange environment, but sometimes the work is unsuitable and certain occupations are barred for reasons of public safety. Sometimes a decision is difficult and the prospect of loss of income complicates advice. Retraining for a new occupation often proves to be a disappointment. Particularly in winter, the stress of travelling to work may be worse than the stress of work itself, and a shortened working day to avoid rush-hour travel is initially advisable. Often there is less stress involved when driving a car to work. Probably more errors are made on the side of caution than vice versa, for most patients can return to the level of physical and intellectual activity which they enjoyed before the attack. Any patient who has not returned to normal activity after 3 months requires assessment by a cardiologist.

About 85 per cent of patients return to work after a myocardial infarction and 65 per cent of these return to previous employment. This is without the help of specialized rehabilitation centres or a formal training programme. The length of time away from work can vary, with apparently little cause, from 6 weeks to more than a year, and unnecessary delay is common and encourages invalidism. Often the decision to return is based as much on psychological and social factors as on the fitness of the patient.

Of those who do not return to work, half are close to retirement or have been persuaded to retire by doctors, employers or friends. As would be expected, the highest return to work is found in patients who have stable sedentary employment. Neither the patient's age nor the presence of angina have any overall effect on return to work, but recurrent infarction and physical signs of severe cardiac damage are associated with invalidism. In large factories a rehabilitation workshop is useful, as patients returning to work who are uncertain of their capacity for their original job can increase their workload under medical supervision until they are employed within their capabilities.

Advice to change to a lighter occupation often leads to unemployment, sometimes permanently, and is damaging to morale even in a robust personality. Return to work is one of the most important outcomes of medical care but it is often delayed through lack of precise knowledge of the nature of the work involved and through lack of communication between the patient, the hospital and the family doctor and the patient's family and employer. It is these outside factors, such as a family doctor who tends to over-protect his patient, a reluctant employer, or a factory where the firm's doctor has to give his opinion, upon which return to work depends.

Although the quality of the patient's work is unimpaired, he tires easily and allowance must be made for this. Any general discussion of rehabilitation programmes is complicated by the extreme variation of different patients' needs. Allowance must be made for differences in physique and personality and in the kind of work to which the person will return. Outside factors such as family position and the attitude of employers and partners will often have to be taken into account.

Patients will wish to know whether they can drive a car again; usually there are no restrictions, except for those who drive public transport vehicles. Fatal road accidents as a consequence of cardiac crises are rare and there is no clearcut evidence that driving heavy goods vehicles has proved hazardous to the owner or public. It is wise to avoid air travel for at least 3 months, despite the use of pressurized aircraft.

PSYCHOLOGICAL REHABILITATION

The ultimate purpose of rehabilitation calls for a gradual withdrawal of help from the patient as confidence of both the patient and his family improves. There is often marked anxiety and depression in both patient and spouse; the psychological strains are often considerable, sometimes outweighing the physical damage, and can be completely crippling. The importance of an early and detailed discussion with the patient by the medical staff has been emphasized, for the heart attack is often a terrifying experience. Often there is severe pain and a sense of impending death and the increasing role of the coronary care unit with its medical gadgetery and electronic monitoring systems only accentuates the patient's anxiety. It is important that at this stage the patient be strongly reassured. If this stage is mismanaged there can be for reaching psychological consequences. The psychological stress that is inevitable can contribute materially to the disability. It is important to protect the patient as far as possible from mental trauma and it is important that there should be no sign of anxiety or confusion among the attendants.

The initial trauma of separation from home is replaced by anxiety and uncertainty about survival and the ability to support one's family. The need for mental rest after a heart attack is often overlooked, but it often happens that the attack occurs at a time of mental stress and physical exhaustion.

The patient is often middle-aged and has a number of financial and family commitments, and uncertainty about the future, in a patient who has often previously been healthy, provides a number of unfamiliar hurdles. It if often important for a patient's spouse or business partner to visit the patient so that business affairs can be tidied up, giving the patient peace of mind. Instillation of self-confidence can be given by medical and nursing and nursing ancillaries, but the attitude of the family and friends is important. It is difficult for a patient to make progress if he is surrounded by anxious people who impede every step forward in physical activity. Self-confidence slowly increases with the patient's increasing capacity.

DIET AND LEISURE

If a patient is overweight he should be encouraged to diet. Alcohol in large quantities has a cardiac depressant effect, but is also acts as a vasodilator and it is unnecessary to interfere with previous moderate habits. All patients should be advised to stop smoking, the only exception being elderly people to whom tobacco represents life's only pleasure. It is important to advise the patient to take at least a full hour's rest at lunchtime and also to avoid large meals as this increases the cardiac output and the gastric blood flow. In particular he should not exercise immediately after eating. It has been suggested that the stress of sexual intercourse on the cardiovascular system is no greater than many activities of daily living but it can be equivalent to running up two flights of stairs. It is wise to wait for 6 weeks after the acute attack. Occasionally trinitrin might be required prophylactically. If the patient does not ask about sexual life, it is the duty of the physician to broach the subject. Impotence from fear and anxiety or as a side-effect of drug therapy is fairly common. Many wives find satisfaction in playing a more active and dominant role during the initial weeks.

Adequate leisure is of great importance and activities involving gentle exercise – walking, light gardening, swimming, riding, carpentry – provide a wide choice of suitable occupations. Pursuits to be avoided if possible are those that combine emotional stimulation with physical inactivity, such as most spectator sports. Games such as golf, tennis and squash need not be permanently rules out for patients previously accustomed to playing them, but energetic sports should not be resumed in an aggressively competitive manner. In all these activities the danger signal of excess is a sudden feeling of tiredness, dyspnoea or pain in the chest.

PHYSICAL TRAINING

Rehabilitation should not only be aimed at preventing reinfarction or death, but should be aimed at improving the quality of life by allowing more physical activity and a fuller social life. Therefore it follows that physical training is but part of the rehabilitation programme. A thorough assessment must be made prior to training and assessment of anxiety and mental attitude must be taken into account. It is important to know what the patient did before his illness and to understand what he will have to do on return to work; but it is more important to know what he wants to do, both at work and in his leisure activities.

There is increasing evidence that lack of physical activity may be a potent predisposing factor in the development of coronary artery disease. Bus conductors suffer less infarction than bus drivers and athletes who remain in training in middle age have a lower mortality from coronary disease. There is also much evidence that exercises after myocardial infarction can lead to psychological and physical improvement. Exercise programmes after myocardial infarction have been developed in many countries, particularly Europe and Scandinavia, and indeed, there are fewer facilities available in this country than in most other countries of the western world. Exercise is not a new therapy for ischaemic heart disease, for Heberden in 1802 described a patient with angina pectoris who noticed an improvement in symptoms after regular activity, and Stokes in 1854 used graduated exercise for cardiac patients.

Studies on the cardiovascular effects of physical training in healthy subjects of different ages have demonstrated the beneficial effects of exercise. There is increase in exercise tolerance and more work can be carried out for a longer time at less oxygen cost. The heart rate and blood pressure are reduced and there is an increased stroke volume and unchanged cardiac output at a submaximal work load. At maximal exercise, when oxygen uptake is higher, cardiac output and stroke volume are both increased. Training also leads to a change in the distribution of blood flow — there is an increase in splanchnic and renal blood flow and a reduction in muscle blood flow.

The physiological effects of training are not so clearly defined in patients after myocardial infarction and detailed haemodynamic studies have only been made in small groups of patients. Comparative studies have also been bedevilled by variations in the type and intensity of the physical training programmes. The considerable variations found in response to physical training probably depend on the functional state of the myocardium. With near-normal myocardial function, training can be carried out in much the same way and with similar effects as in normal subjects of the same age. However, when there is impairment of myocardial function, the stroke volume cannot increase with training and changes in the peripheral circulation predominate. Thus, training in these patients will also result in reduction of heart rate and blood pressure, but the reduction in the work of the heart is the result of an increased arteriovenous oxygen difference.

The increase of aerobic- or symptom-limited work capacity which occurs after 3 months of training is well documented. Thus patients with angina as a limiting symptom at a moderate work load are able to improve their exercise tolerance by about 50 per cent. This means that patients experiencing chest pain while walking upstairs will have no such limitation after training. Training also reduces the 'effort' of exercise and probably the reduction of fatigue and pain is the most reassuring and valuable result of these programmes.

Exercise produces changes in muscle metabolism; in particular, conditioned skeletal muscle is characterized by a higher oxidative capacity. This may be an important factor in the readjustment of the peripheral circulation. Also, regular training two or three times a week has been shown to reduce serum triglyceride and free fatty acid levels, although there is less effect on serum cholesterol. Both these effects may favourably influence pathogenetic processes in ischaemic heart disease.

Far less is known about the possible preventive effects of training regimes on reinfarction and death. This is because studies are based on randomly selected groups of patients and because many patients 'drop out' of long-term training programmes.

Thus, to summarize, exercise

(1) increases cardiovascular capacity, expressed as aerobic- or symptom-limited work capacity;

(2) lowers cost of physical activity by reduction in heart rate and blood pressure;

(3) changes muscle metabolism and reduces serum triglycerides and free fatty acids.

However, perhaps the most important gain is that of reduction in anxiety, and knowledge that physical effort does not cause harm, for patients tend to limit this once outside hospital.

An exercise programme is feasible in a district general hospital and interval training is the most suitable method of exercise. It is important that a thorough evaluation is made prior to entry into a training programme and assessment of anxiety and mental attitudes should be taken into account. Over-enthusiasm for physical training is no more to be encouraged than emotional scepticism and it should be understood that all programmes entail some risk. Therefore it should be undertaken by experienced physiotherapists under medical guidance with resuscitation equipment near at hand.

EXERCISE TESTING

Patients start an exercise course usually at about 6 weeks after discharge from hospital. A preliminary assessment of physical performance is often carried out in many European centres, although this does not have to be routine procedure. Exercise tests are usually carried out on a bicycle ergometer whilst measurements of heart rate, rhythm, blood pressure and oxygen uptake are made. Results give a good indication of the patient's capacity for work and help to determine the intensity of an individual exercise programme and to assess progress. Many patients are anxious on resuming exercise and this supervised test is a good indication of the degree of anxiety. Patients also tend to exercise to a greater extent if they are supervised and many gain confidence and are surprised at their good performance.

The risks of the test are small and well documented but facilities for resuscitation must be near at hand. There are several indications for terminating exercise, the most important being cardiac pain, ventricular extra-systoles and hypotension on increasing effort, the latter indicating impairment of left ventricular function. Patients with increasing angina or with signs and symptoms of deteriorating myocardial function should be excluded.

In most instances, it is the patient who determines termination of the test in that he develops angina or becomes dyspnoeic, or more commonly, complains of general or leg fatigue. But perhaps the commonest reason for stopping is fear.

EXERCISE PROGRAMME

Perhaps the most suitable method of supervision is to encourage attendance at hospital in the early stages of exercise training. Treatment can then take place in small groups and problems and anxieties can be discussed, if possible, with the spouse present. Although exercising in groups of about six is most suitable, it is important that the intensity of treatment is adapted to the individual and with this aim, initial training on a bicycle with medical supervision is essential, so that the intensity of treatment can be decided. Then exercise under the supervision of a physiotherapist is possible but medical and resuscitation facilities should be near at hand. The doctor must be aware and understand potential arrhythmias and have experience in dealing with these and cardiac arrest and resuscitation procedures. ECG monitoring should be limited to avoid anxiety and the physiotherapist can use the heart rate to regulate the intensity of treatment. Isometric exercises should be avoided as they cause a marked increase in blood pressure and exercise should be preceded by a period of 'warming up' and followed by a period of 'cooling down'.

Exercises should consist of progressive circuit routines or interval training which should last for about 30 minutes. A combination of six to eight different exercises, which activate large muscle groups, should include a step test, 'Indian' walking, sitting from a supine position and throwing a medicine ball. At one stage of each training session patients should exercise on a bicycle ergometer at a known work load. This allows simple objective records of changes in physical working capacity and allows adjustments accordingly to the intensity of training. In addition the patient is encouraged by seeing signs of an improvement in his working performance. It is probably best if patients attend twice or three times a week for about 6 weeks, as longer may only lead to increased dependency and long-term programmes have resulted in a high default rate. It should be pointed out that the level, frequency and duration of training are largely empirical.

The amount of exercise can be increased at each session and this should be adjusted to the patient's capacity and previous performance. A training effect may be seen if the intensity is only moderate, and a practical objective is usually an intensity which corresponds to 60–80 per cent of the maximal working capacity. In middle-aged men, physical performance, as measured by maximal oxygen uptake, can be increased by 18 per cent.

Patients should be encouraged to continue their exercise routine after discharge but probably few do so, and attention should be given in future to improving motivation. It is not known whether home exercises are as effective as those carried out under hospital supervision. If possible, return to work should occur whilst treatment continues as problems often occur at this stage and can usually be easily resolved. Exercise programmes undoubtedly help patients gain reassurance and play a part in helping patients return to work but it is psychological and social factors, rather than the fitness of the patient, that figure most in this decision.

Exercise regimes are probably of most value to those in heavy employment, those with anxiety and those with relatively sedentary jobs who have a limited working capacity. At present, it is assumed that fairly strenuous short-term bouts of exercise which increase cardiac output and work are more suitable than sustained exercise over longer periods. However, it may be that exercise which leads to the most improvement in cardiac haemodynamic performance does not have the greatest therapeutic value. It may well be that sustained exercise has more pronounced metabolic effects. There are a number of questions which still need to be resolved. For instance, it is still not known when exercise should begin; it may be that light exercise whilst the patient is still in hospital is of most benefit. It is still not know whether training influences subsequent morbidity and mortality, nor whether it influences return to work.

Emphasis is placed in many centres on detailed measurements of cardiac performance, but we still do not know which parameters are most important. Perhaps patients benefit most from a lessening of anxiety and some workers have demonstrated equal subjective improvement to exercise regimes with relaxation techniques alone. Certainly, there is a need for further studies to determine whether less ambitious programmes with more emphasis on psychological aspects are of equal benefit. This is particularly important as to many patients and their families a myocardial infarction is still regarded as a disaster that is usually fatal, and the subsequent shock and anxiety are often far-reaching.

Although most patients can enter an exercise programme, some must be excluded because of medical contra-indications or mental attitudes and others rapidly resume their former position in society without help. The remainder form a heterogeneous group and each patient must be treated individually.

About one-quarter of patients are unable to attend hospital for training, some because of cardiac limitations or because of other medical disorders or simply because of difficulty in attendance. Joint and muscle stiffness are common with training, but it seems clear that, provided case selection is careful and medical supervision adequate, patients come to no harm. Patients who should probably be excluded are those with heart failure, those with hypertension requiring treatment, and those suffering from bronchitis with dyspnoea on mild exertion.

The aims of rehabilitation can be summarized as follows:

(1) To remove the deconditioning effect of the illness.
(2) To teach the patient prudent limits of activity.
(3) To remove the fear of exertion and improve morale.
(4) To increase cardiac function.
(5) To improve or relieve angina of effort.

It is suggested that formal cardiac rehabilitation units should be set up in district hospitals, as they have well-defined physiological and psychological benefits. In particular patients gain from the support that follows discharge from hospital.

CONCLUSIONS

The major cause of persisting disability is psychological, and there is no more upsetting sight than the post-coronary patient, devoid of organic symptoms, who is too frightened to work at his job or in his home surroundings. Having a coronary is alarming, and for the first time in his life the patient is confronted with the harsh reality that he is not immortal. If sympathetically questioned, many post-infarction patients will admit that for the first year they are frequently anxious.

Rehabilitation should start concurrently with the treatment of the acute episode. Patients are being mobilized and discharged home earlier than before. The family doctor plays a key part in deciding the patient's future rate of progress and liaison between hospital and family doctor is essential. Rehabilitation should be tailored to the patient's needs, giving consideration to age, sex, marital status, level of physical fitness and the nature of previous employment. Domestic, social, psychological and economic pressures dictate that patients should return as quickly as possible to a normal way of life.

Graded physical training that requires regular attendance at a hospital gymnasium is unlikely to gain widespread acceptance in Britain, since the cost of the NHS and to the patients would be prohibitive, and supervised rehabilitation must, therefore, be reserved for selected patients who are not making satisfactory progress outside hospital.

Regular accepted exercise is safe for cardiac patients. Exercise does not necessarily hasten return to work, improve life expectancy or prevent further attacks, but the benefits to angina, morale and physical agility seem definite.

REFERENCES

Report of a Joint Working Party of the Royal College of Physicians of London and the British Cardiac Society (1975). *Cardiac Rehabilitation.*

Report of a Joint Working Party of the Royal College of Physicians of London and the British Cardiac Society (1976). 'Prevention of Coronary Heart Disease.' *J. Roy. Coll. Phys.* **10,** 213

16 Chronic Bronchitis

INTRODUCTION

The concept of a rehabilitative form of management of chronic bronchitis is one which has been developed comparatively recently, although the treatment of chronic bronchitis has challenged physicians since cigarette smoking and domestic and industrial processes provided sufficient pollution of the atmosphere to produce it.

Several forms of mainly symptomatic treatment have been traditionally employed, separately or synchronously – suppression of ineffective cough, promotion of expectoration, prevention of secondary infection and stimulation of bronchodilation. To such medical treatments, short-term because their effects last only as long as their term of employment, rehabilitative treatment attempts to graft a long-term, sustained improved in respiratory function and exercise tolerance. This it tries to effect by careful physiotherapeutic training of the bronchitic patient in:

(1) Breathing control.
(2) Postural control.
(3) Relaxation technique.
(4) Diaphragmatic dominance in the pattern of respiration.
(5) General physical fitness and the performance of regular daily exercise regimes demanding increasing effort.

When the patient can be persuaded to organize his remaining functional potential so that he aims at progressively increasing activity, instead of resigning himself to a life of progressively decreasing activity, rehabilitation is indeed taking place.

With the improvement in cardiovascular and respiratory efficiency resulting from this form of management, further intermittent improvement is effected by the occasional admission of the patient to hospital for mechanical assistance with breathing, or else by the provision of small portable respirators for use in the home.

By such measures, and by adaptations to home and place of work, and help with transport, it often becomes possible for the chronic bronchitic to plan for a resumption of gainful employment and the re-establishment of economic independence, rather than the alternative role of a chronic invalid, unemployed and housebound, maintained by Social Security, with the inevitable domestic stress and disharmony which results from such a situation.

AETIOLOGY AND PATHOLOGY

Chronic bronchitis is a disease of long chronicity, characterized by cough, sticky sputum, and gradually increasing dyspnoea. Pathologically, it is a non-infective condition of the mucosal cells lining the bronchi and bronchioles of the lungs, giving rise to progressive mucous gland hypertrophy, mucosal swelling and increased mucus secretion. This eventually produces diffuse airways obstruction and a decreased diameter of the tubes from which mucus clearance must occur. Active inspiration permits air to be drawn through narrowed airways, but during the passive deflation of expiration, the diminished diameter of these airways reduces expiratory airflow. Any active expiratory effort of coughing tends to cause increased intrathoracic, extrabronchial pressure, leading to further obstruction and collapse of the bronchi and bronchioles, and trapping of air in the periphery of the lungs.

A frequent accompaniment of this condition is the breakdown of intra-alveolar walls and the development of emphysema, although the precise nature of this process is not clearly understood. As a result, the areas of lung involved no longer take an effective part in respiration, since their component alveoli become over-distended and their mucosal lining is eventually replaced by relatively avascular fibrous tissue. Emphysematous areas produced in this manner have several adverse effects on the respiratory activity of the lungs: they reduce the volume of lung tissue in which effective gaseous exchange can occur, and they interfere with the normal mechanisms of respiration and sputum expulsion.

During the inspiratory phase of normal respiration the volume of the thoracic cage is increased by active muscular effort. Negative intrathoracic pressure is increased correspondingly, and the lungs increase in volume and draw in air. Gaseous exchange occurs in the alveoli, and expired air is extruded as the lungs passively deflate with the relaxation of the muscles of respiration and the decrease in volume of the thoracic cavity.

The extrusion of air in breathing during passive deflation of the lungs and the expulsion of sputum in coughing during active deflation of the lungs, both depend upon the effective transmission of changes in the thoracic pressure to the lungs themselves. When a significant part of the lung volume no longer reflects the pressure changes, the reaction of the lung as a whole is correspondingly diminished, the efficacy of the breathing and coughing mechanisms is reduced and the cycle of dysfunction and degeneration has been started.

It is difficult to separate physiotherapeutic from medical and social aspects of the management of chronic bronchitis, and they are all three considered as part of an integrated whole which is designed to fulfil certain specific aims.

THE AIMS OF REHABILITATION

All the various forms of treatment of chronic bronchitis are ultimately aimed at the reduction of dyspnoea and distress during rest, exercise and daily living activities, and at the overall improvement of the quality of life of the bronchitic patient.

Such treatment attempts to:

(1) Eliminate or reduce the primary causes of bronchial irritation.
(2) Reduce the degree of existing airways obstruction.
(3) Establish a more efficient respiratory pattern in a patient's everyday life by means of breathing training and a graduated exercise programme.
(4) Prevent and/or treat infective exacerbations.
(5) Integrate each patient into a scheme of management which has continuity and an understanding of the far-reaching consequences of this disease. Liaison between chest clinic, GP, family and extramural services to obtain suitable work, suitable transport, and suitable housing conditions, and the institution of regular medical check-ups form an essential part of this.

How are these aims fulfilled?

Elimination or reduction of primary causes of bronchial irritation
Smoking
Smoking is the major cause of chronic bronchitis and the major factor which ensures its perpetuation and exacerbation. Unfortunately, the basic personality of the patient who initially felt the wish and then the need to smoke has seldom radically changed with age. Furthermore, as the addiction to nicotine or simply to the smoking habit becomes established over the years, it becomes harder to break. Yet unless smoking is abstained from altogether or substantially reduced, the effect of other rehabilitative measures is reduced or even negated.

Smog
Despite the dramatic reduction of smog since the institution of smoke-free zones and the enforcement of stricter regulations on industrial and domestic air pollution, there is still enough sulphur dioxide in the atmosphere to cause considerable bronchial irritation. Avoidance of a dust-charged or fume-polluted atmosphere is essential for the chronic bronchitic, and if necessary a change of occupation or a move to a better area should be urged.

Reduction of airways obstruction
As has been stated earlier, it is difficult to separate treatment from the rehabilitation of the chronic bronchitic patient. Both seek to re-establish a more normal pattern of breathing and a more normal existence and do so by endeavouring to train the patient to incorporate disciplines which have been learnt into a permanent way of life. There is no once-and-for-all cure, and no once-and-for-all rehabilitative process for chronic bronchitis. The patient can be helped, improved, but never completely cured.

Unless he stops smoking soon enough, he is caught in a self-perpetuating system of lung destruction, in which an increasing part of his lung tissue becomes non-contributory in ventilation, and the remaining part becomes progressively more difficult to use as an effective organ of respiration. As more and more bronchioles become obstructed, first by mucus and then by collapse, expiration becomes increasingly difficult and increasing muscular effort has to be utilized to achieve it.

Bronchodilation
Treatment is directed towards keeping as many bronchi and bronchioles patent as possible. One method of assisting this is by the administration of broncho-dilator drugs, orally, parenterally and by inhalation.

Portable pocket bronchodilator inhalers are available, and inhalants are also used in conjunction with the larger respirators, such as the Bird Intermittent Positive Pressure Respirator, from which oxygen is delivered to the patient after humidification and enrichment with an appropriate bronchodilator aerosol.

The severely affected chronic bronchitic benefits greatly from periodic admissions to the chest ward of his nearest district general hospital for intensive physiotherapy and to use such a respirator. Alternatively, he is taught to use one of the several small machines now available for delivering oxygen on the Venturi principle. On these also there is a humidifier attachment by which moisture and a bronchodilator drug can be introduced into the inspired oxygen.

Bronchiolar Patency
Breathing exercises which deepen inspiration and avoid prolongation of expiration assist in maintaining bronchiolar patency by decreasing intrathoracic extrabronchial pressure and the resting respiratory level. During such exercises, patients are urged to breathe in a little more deeply, to avoid forced expiration, and to start breathing in again a little sooner than they usually do.

Establishment of a more efficient respiratory pattern
Therapists concentrate on retraining the diaphragmatic action of their patients to constitute the main muscular movement of the act of respiration. Diaphragmatic exercises are given against increased indirect resistance provided by pressure of the therapist's hand upon the abdomen, and control of rate and depth of breathing is also taught. The intercostal muscles in a bronchitic patient with an over-distended chest are working with the ribs in a position of mechanical disadvantage, and a minimum of ventilation is achieved for a maximum of effort. Thoracic respiration in this situation is inefficient. Unlike the intercostals, the diaphragm does not have to move a large mass of extraneous tissue, and small adjustments in the tone of the abdominal muscles accommodate its movements.

Advocates of this type of breathing exercise stress that diaphragmatic re-training is a part of a six-point programme involving instruction in:

(1) Breathing awareness.
(2) Increased inspiration with the diaphragm.
(3) Relaxed inspiration.
(4) Raising the respiratory level.
(5) Breathing control.
(6) Synchronization of daily activities with the breathing rhythm.

In all cases, the patient is taught to empty his chest by tipping, with or without 'clapping', before starting his exercises. Emphasis is placed on the importance of avoiding the patient's natural tendency to slow his respiratory rate while attempting to establish a new pattern. Initially, while the patient is at rest in the position of his own choice, and subsequently during exercise, always working on the inspiratory phase, the patient is taught to increase the rate and depth of breathing at will, later learning to reduce the rate and increase the depth in the same manner. By breathing in a little more deeply, and stopping breathing out a little sooner than normally, the 'level' of respiration is raised.

The greater the inflation of the lung, the greater the expiratory flow before the point of shutdown. By increasing the resting respiratory level, and so the inflation of the lung, controlled diaphragmatic breathing can produce increased lung inflation, increased intrabronchial pressure and an increased expiratory flow before bronchiolar shutdown occurs.

This patient-controlled method of increasing the resting respiratory level and bronchial patency is given an intermittent boost when the patient uses a positive pressure respirator, or when he breathes out with his lips pursed, so increasing the intrabronchial pressure and prolonging the interval of patency before extra-bronchial pressure causes shutdown of some bronchi.

There are indications that using the diaphragm as the main muscular force in respiration promotes the optimal function of normal lung tissue (accommodates the tendency of emphysematous lung to act as a space-occupying lesion) and avoids increasing the ratio of emphysematous, low-ventilating lung tissue to normal high-ventilating lung tissue in the bronchitic emphysematous patient.

How much actual improvement can occur in the bronchitic patient treated by this method must depend upon the severity and duration of the airways obstruction already present. Some improvement inevitably occurs, and further conversion of normal lung tissue to emphysematous lung tissue is slowed or prevented.

When the control of breathing and the substitution of finely adjusted diaphragmatic respiration for thoracic respiration has been taught to a patient, his exercise tolerance may further be improved by sessions of general physical training. With such training, combined with new breathing patterns, the chronic bronchitic who is initially breathless on the mildest exertion may soon learn to think in terms of walking distances of hundreds of yards and eventually of several miles. His posture and his breathing pattern are steadily improved, and fatigue and respiratory distress are averted for increasing intervals. Such functional improvement occurs even in the absence of demonstrable improvement in the levels of oxygen and carbon dioxide in the blood.

The provision of a small portable respirator for use at home and at work may be very helpful. Housebound patients may sometimes benefit from a supply of oxygen at home to use before specific tasks, such as going upstairs, and a portable oxygen cylinder may occasionally enable a patient to get to work. A portable respirator may be attached to a walking frame or carried across the patient's shoulders. Regular use of oxygen at home, other than for specific tasks, is rarely useful or advisable.

Prevention of infective exacerbations
Continuous antibiotic therapy has been shown by extensive trials to be an unnecessary and expensive method of preventing infection in the chronic bronchitic. Instead, a patient is given a small store of broad spectrum antibiotic which he is instructed to take the moment his sputum becomes purulent. In this way, although the initial virus infection is not prevented, the damaging secondary bacterial infection is quickly controlled without the otherwise unavoidable delays in obtaining an antibiotic. Further supplies of antibiotic are obtained on request from the GP and are continued until the sputum has been clear for some days.

Expectoration may be assisted by administration of mucolytic expectorant — this is particularly valuable to patients with sticky sputum.

A variety of expectorants are still widely prescribed. All are best taken in very hot water, which is probably the effective agent in promoting expectoration.

When chronic bronchitis is complicated by bronchiectasis, regular postural drainage of the appropriate segments is taught, and the spouse or parent, or person giving care, is instructed in the 'clapping' or 'shaking' which supplements this. Often lying over the side of the bed or on a pile of pillows in the correct posture is sufficient, but some patients drain better when adequately positioned over a simple frame, easily made by the patient or a local handyman.

If the patient tends to suffer from sinusitis, he is further instructed in postural sinus drainage and in the art of washing out his sinuses without recourse to the ENT department. Localized areas of bronchiectatic lung are resected as necessary. Annual inoculation with anti-influenza vaccine can provide valuable protection against the acute flare-up of respiratory infection which frequently follows an attack of influenza in a bronchitic patient. The inoculation is customarily given in the autumn.

Integrated management
The long-term rehabilitative care of the chronic bronchitic calls for the closest co-operation between the patients, their families, doctors, and paramedical workers. Conscientious attention to routine is demanded of the patient, often in vain, so that he has to be rehabilitated in spite of himself.

Abstention from smoking, regular performance of breathing exercises and regular medical supervision must be his life-long programme so that the needs occasioned by the deterioration in an inexorably progressive condition may be anticipated whenever possible.

He must accept that intermittent short admissions to hospital for boosting treatment will become necessary as his respiratory function diminishes. As an in-patient, intensive physiotherapy with intermittent positive pressure mechanical assistance to his breathing, and the exhibition of appropriate bronchodilators and antibiotics can combine to improve his respiratory status dramatically.

With a disease of such long chronicity, the social conditions of a patient's life assume a major importance, and his return home following in-patient treatment should be preluded by a visit from the domiciliary occupational therapist or social worker and the submission of a report on his home conditions to his medical advisers. Should his bronchitis be sufficiently severe, every effort is made to rehouse him in a ground-floor flat or disabled person's bungalow, rather than in a multi-storied house or a tower flat. If family or social considerations make it preferable that he remains in his present home, it may be sufficient merely for him to sleep downstairs, or he may be able to continue sleeping upstairs provided he has an electric heater for his room and has it switched on for at least half an hour before he retires to bed and then climbs the stairs very slowly. A night storage heater prevents the overall temperature of the house dropping too much during the night. Though the Social Services grant a heating allowance to patients who are financially incapable of funding the standard of heating which they require, other patients who do not qualify for a grant may obtain financial assistance from some charitable fund to enable them to purchase adequate heating equipment or to install central heating.

The place and type of work of the chronic bronchitic both need careful consideration. Indoor work, sedentary if exercise tolerance is low, and in an atmosphere which is as free from fumes of industrial, fire or tobacco origin as possible, and is well-ventilated but yet of as constant a temperature as possible, is ideal. It is also difficult to obtain. Whenever possible, a patient should attempt to remain in his old place of employment for as long as possible, preferably keeping to his specific job, unless the conditions thereof are irritant to his bronchitis and dyspnoea. Liaison with his employer, or the personnel manager or medical officer of his place of work may enable some adaptations of working conditions to be made which enable him to continue at his job. If not, he must seek re-employment, or even retraining in an alternative trade.

Application to the Disablement Resettlement Officer for the district could lead to work assessment and formal retraining for a suitable occupation.

SOCIAL PROBLEMS

Transport

If the use of public transport to get to work entails one or more long walks, long periods of standing and then probably exposure to irritant tobacco smoke and to possible infection from fellow passengers, dyspnoea and further exacerbations of acute respiratory infection may result.

In this case the patient may be advised either by his chest physician or his general practitioner to apply for the Mobility Allowance. If he is thought to be a respiratory cripple, whether or not he is at work, he becomes eligible for assistance.

The provisions of a lightweight, folding, assistant-propelled wheelchair will enable the chronic bronchitic to be taken on visits and expeditions without having to walk distances which are beyond his capacity. Such chairs are particularly suitable for stowing in the boot of a car, and further enlarge the scope of a disabled person's activities, while the power-assisted attendant-operated outdoor chair enables the large patient with a small or unfit spouse to be also taken for walks, even in hilly areas. The very severely disabled chronic bronchitic may need an electrically powered indoor chair in addition.

Family care

Patients with chronic bronchitis may become depressed, and during acute episodes of respiratory infection or during the night hours when respiratory activity is normally diminished, they may also become hypoxic and confused. Families need a maximal amount of supportive care and explanation by medical and paramedical workers and need to be reassured, yet alerted to report such conditions, so that appropriate treatment may be instituted.

The continued presence of an unemployed and unemployable bronchitic in the home can also become irksome to the spouse who must give care, run the home, support the family, and possibly do a part-time job as well, particularly as the limited exercise tolerance of the bronchitic must also limit the amount of help which he can give with the household tasks.

Subsidized holidays in suitable homes where disabled people are catered for adequately, can be of inestimable use in keeping families together by occasionally making it possible for them to be apart.

CONCLUSION

Failure of the chronic bronchitic to accept the importance of his own responsibility for the success of his rehabilitative programme must doom it inevitably to failure. Thus the bronchitic who continues to smoke in the intervals between using his bronchodilator inhalant or his portable respirator is making a nonsense of his treatment. So too is the patient who attends the physiotherapy department religiously for exercises which he never incorporates into his daily life.

The rehabilitation of the chronic bronchitic is not a once and for all form of rehabilitation, but the establishment of a more effective method of breathing and of living and the acceptance of a recurrent process of modification and regulation of home life and working life, interspaced with short hospital admissions to boost respiratory efficiency.

BIBILIOGRAPHY AND REFERENCES

Fletcher, C. M., Elms, P. C., Fairburn, A. S. and Wood, C. H. (1959). 'The significance of respiratory symptoms and the diagnosis of chronic bronchitis in a working population.' *Br. med. J.* **2**, 257

Fletcher, C. M. (1959). 'Chronic bronchitis.' *Am. Rev. resp. Dis.* **80**, 483

Fletcher, C. M. (1965). 'Some recent advances in the prevention or treatment of chronic bronchitis and related disorders with special reference to the effects of cigarette smoking.' *Proc. R. Soc. Med.* **58**, 918

Fry, D. L. and Hyatt, R. E. (1960). 'Pulmonary mechanics: a unified analysis of the relationship between pressure, volume and gas flow of the lungs of normal and diseased human subjects.' *Am. J. Med.* **29**, 672

Gough, J., Fletcher, C. M., Gilson, J. C. and Oldham, P. D. (1952). 'Discussion on diagnosis of pulmonary emphysema.' *Proc R. Soc. Med.* **45**, 576

Grant, R. (1969). 'The physiological basis for increased exercise ability in patients with emphysema after breathing and exercise training (a review of the literature).' *Physiotherapy* **52**, 541

Harris, C. S. (1972). 'Chronic bronchitis.' *Br. J. hosp. Med.* **7**, 719

Innocenti, D. (1966). 'Breathing exercises in the treatment of emphysema.' *Physiotherapy* **52**, 437

17 Aids to Mobility

INTRODUCTION

An aid to mobility assists or substitutes for lower limb function in moving a patient bodily from place to place. The optimal aid to mobility is that aid which provides maximal assistance of the required kind for movement in space of any particular patient, with minimal adverse effects on future activity and minimal inconvenience to other people. In general, simple aids are best, calling for little manipulative skill, occupying the least space and proving to be the least prone to mechanical and other failures. There is a rational progression of aids of increasing complexity which provide an increasing degree of substitution for normal movement.

Partially weight-relieving (patient manipulation) sticks, crutches, walking frames.

Completely weight-relieving patient-propelled wheelchairs; attendant-propelled wheelchairs; powered wheelchair or outdoor vehicles.

PARTIAL WEIGHT-RELIEVING AIDS

Walking-sticks

The simplest partially weight-relieving aid is the walking-stick, whether of the classical wooden variety, or of the more modern tubular metal alloy construction. The walking-stick can be used to relieve weight by patients with unilateral lower limb disease when held in the contralateral hand, but this manner of weight relief often induces an unevenly paced gait. The use of *two* sticks enables the patient more efficiently to protect one leg by weight-bearing through the sticks, from 'heel strike' to 'toe off' of the involved leg and in this way to achieve considerable weight relief and an evenly paced walk.

Walking-sticks should always be of the correct height. The handle should be level with the greater trochanter when the patient is standing erect in shoes, or alternatively it should correspond in height with the lower end of the ulna when the arm hangs loosely at the side. The handle of a walking-stick should be chosen (or even designed) to suit the shape and strength of the hand of its user. A curved handle is preferred by some with normal strong hands, but many patients prefer a straight handle. Usually the elderly or arthritic are more comfortable when the handle is enlarged by being bound with sorbo rubber, plastic foam or felt. The most generally satisfactory diameter for 'grab rails' is about 1¼ in (3 cm), and this diameter is usually preferable for walking-stick handles.

There are some patients who prefer sticks with a moulded plastic handle whereas others (particularly those with rheumatoid arthritis) can only become really efficient with handles specially moulded to their own hands. Whichever type of stick is used, it should always be fitted with a large-based removable rubber or plastic ferrule, which should be replaced as soon as its tread becomes worn.

Greater support and stability may be provided by three-legged (tripod) or four-legged (quadruped) sticks. Some designs of tripod sticks are unstable in use, since the weight tends to be transferred medial to the triangular base, and thus quadruped sticks are usually preferable. There are many different designs, and it is usually wise for the therapist to instruct the patient in their use and to provide those walking aids which the patient can use most freely and with the greatest confidence and stability.

Crutches

Crutches of various types are suitable for different diseases and thus for different patients. The traditional under-arm crutch (axillary) is suitable only for short-term use, as a weight-relieving support to be used after trauma or operation until partial weight-bearing is permitted. It is contra-indicated for long-term and short-term use in the presence of joint disease of the upper limbs, since it imposes considerable strain on the joints and muscles of the upper limbs and on the shoulder joints in particular. The long-term use of axillary crutches is also contra-indicated following spinal cord injury with paraplegia or paraparesis of both lower limbs. However, for spina bifida patients or patients with cauda equina lesions or with flail or semi-flail legs, axillary crutches do provide an acceptable aid to three-point walking, both legs being swung together. This can become an efficient and stable form of progression for patients with normal arms and is quickly learned.

If prolonged use of crutches is needed, or if patients have joint disease, then elbow crutches are indicated. This type of crutch does not put as much strain on the joints and muscles of the arm as the axillary crutch and does not predispose to the development of osteoarthrosis in the shoulder joint or to brachial neuritis.

There are several different types of this crutch, not all of which are equally satisfactory. An elbow crutch is essentially a walking-stick with an extension to the vertical component, angled at about 30 degrees to the longitudinal (vertical) axis. At the upper end of this forearm extension is an arm clip usually made of spring steel, or of rigid padded or coated metal. This clip accommodates the upper forearm. Ideally, the length of both the walking-stick part and the forearm part of the crutch should be adjustable, so that the handgrip is at the level of the greater trochanter when the crutch is held beside the body, and the upper end of the arm grip is immediately distal to the head of the radius. In practice, however, it is usually more satisfactory for the physiotherapist to choose a pair of crutches of the correct size for a particular patient, since adjustable upper components are expensive to incorporate and often unstable to use.

It is also important that the arm grip is correctly aligned and well padded to avoid pressure of the edge over the ulna where there is little muscular protection.

The handgrip is often too thin and is improved by padding with foam or leather. Some elbow crutches are now available with thicker, softer moulded plastic handgrips.

Correctly used, elbow crutches provide greater stability than walking-sticks. Not only do they stabilize the wrists, but they also spread the load of the body-weight, since the forearms as well as the hands provide some weight relief. Significant flexion deformity of the elbows and poor hand function may make the use of these crutches difficult. If elbows and wrists are painful, the use of elbow crutches cannot be tolerated. A further disadvantage is that their long-term use, by placing additional strain on elbows, wrists and hands, not only exacerbates any arthritic pain but accelerates degerative changes in the affected joints.

The alternative 'gutter crutch' demands less of the upper arm joints, as the patient rests the forearm in the gutter. This type of appliance is particularly suitable for patients with painful, weak hands and wrists. Its height should be adjustable to permit the forearm to rest comfortably in the horizontal gutter support when the patient is standing erect. The position and length of the gutter support, and the position, angle and width of the handgrip should also be adjusted to, or selected for, the patient's individual requirements. Usually some extra padding of foam or leather will be needed for the forearm gutter to overlap the metal edges. Leather or velcro straps fix the crutch to the forearm.

Walking frames

Even more support and stability can be provided by walking frames. These are usually wide based and particularly lightweight as they are commonly used for very elderly and frail patients, as well as for young ones with severe temporary disability. A great variety of walking frames exists, with different heights and widths. Some frames have two small wheels on the leading legs, or on all four legs. There are many different sorts of handgrips, or forearm gutter supports, or axillary supports. Some frames have hinged side-pieces (reciprocal walking frames). Most frames (other than the reciprocal walking frames) are rigid and take up a lot of room when standing free in the average house. However, their stability is often their most important characteristic, enabling patients to use them for getting in and out of a chair and on and off the toilet, as well as acting as an aid to ambulation.

Use of a multitiered trolley, if necessary with handgrips or forearm supports, may be a preferable solution for the disabled housewife who needs a support for walking about the house but finds herself unable to carry domestic objects from place to place while using a walking aid. The trolley provides both a walking support and a carrying surface.

The recently introduced portable parallel bars further increase the potential range of independent action of the elderly or frail patient. Designed to help the double amputee transfer from a sitting to a standing position, they are hinged to a standard walking frame and can be coupled to a standard wheelchair or to sockets fixed to an armchair, or to fitments on each side of the toilet pedestal.

WHEELCHAIRS

Historical background

In this country, the history of the design and development of wheelchairs really began with their free supply under the auspices of the Ministry of Pensions.

When this Ministry was formed in 1917 some wheelchairs were already being provided for disabled servicemen by the Lord Kitchener Memorial Fund. In 1918 the Ministry of Pensions assumed the responsibility for providing wheelchairs to:

(1) Paraplegics.
(2) Double amputees, with one amputation above the knee.
(3) Double below-knee amputees (if the patient's general condition made the supply necessary).

In the light of current supplies this disability group is interesting, as it would nowadays represent about 10 per cent of the total supply. Hand-propelled tricycles were provided for non-pensioners to go to work; and from 1920 onwards some powered attachments were made available by the Red Cross, for severely disabled pensioners in hilly districts. It was not until 1945 that the Ministry of Pensions assumed responsibility for powered tricycles.

The National Health Service was inaugurated on 1 July 1948, when the Ministry of Health had the duty to promote the establishment of a comprehensive health service, including the provision of appliances. For organizational reasons the Ministry of Pensions continued to act for the Ministry of Health for the ordering, supply and repair of wheelchairs and tricycles. The Ministry of Health did not assume *direct* responsibility for these activities until 1953. Thus, prior to 1953 the general thinking behind the supply of wheelchairs was directed towards the needs of war pensioners. In the early days of the Health Service the usual wheelchair supplied was a rigid-framed chair designed for indoor use. During the first two years of the NHS (1948–50), 9000 wheelchairs were supplied, mostly of this type.

Before the inception of the National Health Service there is little evidence of any serious work on design and development of wheelchairs; the social evolution which followed its inception had a direct and lasting effect on the production of wheelchairs and all other appliances. The wheelchairs currently available have thus evolved to fill a social need rather than as a response to a specific engineering project.

Part of the changing pattern of design has been due to the changing organization and control of supply. Before 1956 it was sufficient that a consultant informed the Medical Officer at the nearest Articifial Limb and Appliance Centre that the need for a chair existed. The patient was examined at the Centre and a chair ordered and provided. This meant that before a chair could be supplied, on each occasion the patient was seen by a general practitioner, a hospital consultant and an Appliance Medical Officer. (Such a system still exists today for the provision of powered indoor transport). After 1956 it was agreed that the hospital consultant could prescribe the particular wheelchair which he considered most suitable for his patient.

This closer involvement of the consultant with chair prescription unquestionably led to increasing interest in the design of wheelchairs, as doctors outside the DHSS's own organization could now bring more interest and influence to bear upon the type of chair supplied to their patients. As, however, there was simultaneously an increasing supply of outdoor invalid transport there grew up an increasing demand for a simple wheelchair for use in combination with these vehicles. The simple transit chair which was originally produced for this purpose weighted about 30 lb (12 kg) and could fold flat to go into an invalid tricycle. It had fixed armrests, fixed footrests and a very short backrest. Although ideal for some patients, its small size and fixed arm- and footrests rendered it unsuitable for many others. But it was this chair which gradually developed into the general purpose indoor/outdoor chair for self-propulsion. By 1963 these general-purpose wheelchairs were being supplied at a rate of over 15,000 per year. At the same time there was increasing pressure for the supply of a comfortable wheelchair for the elderly disabled. This need was for an attendant-operated pushchair which was comfortable.

Now for the first time, general practitioners are being allowed to prescribe wheelchairs. Although they are only allowed to prescribe from a small range of 'standard' chairs, it is likely that this will bring further changes in the design and contribute to the evolution of the wheelchair.

The majority of the wheelchairs on issue by the Department of Health in England and Wales are of the type of general-purpose self-propelling wheelchair (Model 8L or variant). The increasing popularity of this type of chair may be attributable to the ease with which it may be folded for car transit and the provision which it makes for occupant/attendant propulsion. It has come. to be used as an indoor/outdoor wheelchair because the disadvantages of 'tracking' castors and lack of suspension are mitigated by the obvious advantages of using only one wheelchair for both environments — namely not having to transfer the occupant unnecessarily and not having to create the extra storage space required for a second chair.

Design features and problems
In recent years there has been considerable interest in the design of the wheelchair, and several bodies have sponsored major research programmes. These programmes have been engendered by an increasingly large and loud voice of criticism coming from patients, patients' relatives, charitable organizations concerned with the welfare of the disabled, and clinicians, who note the effects of the chairs on the patients for whom they are prescribed.

The standard wheelchair is easy to criticize, particularly its appearance and its weight, but over the years, as the population of wheelchair users has grown, the Department of Health has gradually extended the range of features and alternatives available. It is the need to provide quickly and cheaply a wheelchair suitable for all patients which has led to the provision of a highly criticized chair of compromise design. Indeed the more that attempts are made to extend the range of the population accommodated by any particular type of chair, the more probable it is that irreconcilable criteria will occur and the resulting situation will be unsatisfactory to the broad mass of the population served.

The wheelchair user
A census of the physically disabled shows that there are over 3 million adults in the UK with a physical disability, and five sixths of these are of pensionable age.
The commonest disabilities are:

(1) Arthritis (rheumatoid and degenerative).
(2) Strokes.
(3) Multiple sclerosis.
(4) Amputation (of lower limb).
(5) Cerebral palsy.

(6) Spinal cord lesion (trauma and spina bifida).
(7) Muscular dystrophy.
(8) Degenerative neuromuscular disease.
(9) Cardiovascular/respiratory disease.

It is these conditions which not unnaturally feature largely among the wheelchair users. Approximately 14 per cent of wheelchair users suffer from rheumatoid arthritis, 14 per cent from osteo-arthritis, 13 per cent from cerebrovascular lesions, 9 per cent from lower limb amputations, 8 per cent from cerebral palsy, and 7 per cent from spinal injury. The wheelchair population includes rather more women than men (men 44 per cent, women 56 per cent), and 60 per cent of wheelchair users are over 50 years of age.

It is clear that wheelchair mobility is mainly required in the immediate environment of the home and its neighbourhood. Wheelchair users, according to their handicap and capabilities, can be grouped as follows:

(1) Semi-ambulant.
(2) Non-ambulant.
  (a) Chairbound accompanied.
  (b) Chairbound independent.

The semi-ambulant group, requiring the wheelchair for assistance, particularly where distances or bad surfaces are involved, is large.

The majority of wheelchair users are severely disabled. One half to two thirds are *dependent* upon the wheelchair for mobility, requiring a chair for use both indoors and out of doors (wheelchair-bound). About one half can stand long enough to transfer from chair to chair, chair to bed, but only a very few can stand or walk without support of some kind. This means that the majority of chair users are not only dependent upon the wheelchair, but are also dependent upon relatives, friends and helpers of some kind. The one third to one half of users who are semi-ambulant tend only to use a wheelchair out of doors, and most of this group are elderly and frail. Indeed, one third to one half of the semi-ambulant need their wheelchair permanently for outdoor use. If they do not have a wheelchair they never go out of doors. The majority of wheelchair users do not drive and cannot fold their chair, nor lift it into a vehicle.

Thus the general design of the wheelchair is changing to accommodate the needs of those who use them. Both the age and the diagnosis of the patients concerned are important here.

Elderly users The large and increasing number of elderly users has afffected one aspect of design. Elderly patients require chairs which are light, portable, shock absorbing, reliable, very manoeuvrable and capable of easy transport. Their attendants are often also elderly, and this too needs consideration.

Young adult users The smaller number of young adult users has influenced another aspect. Younger patients demand and are more likely to achieve a greater degree of independence than the elderly. They require chairs which are strong enough and versatile enough to permit them to undertake a wide variety of activities. Traumatic paraplegic patients fall into this category. Usually young, well motivated, extrovert and with powerful upper limbs, they are able to lead their lives almost independent of assistance. Not all young patients achieve such independence, and some severely handicapped young adults need considerable assistance to enable them to maintain even a limited degree of independence.

Handicapped children   Such users do not only need scaled-down models of adult chairs. In addition they need light, collapsible chairs in which they may be taken shopping, and which can be easily lifted on and off buses. They also need simple self-propelled chariots in which they can achieve mobility at the same stage of development as the able child.

Functional anthropometry of wheelchair occupants varies with both age and disease, age being the more important factor. It is reasonable to assume that *independent* chairbound wheelchair users are mainly young adults. The additional effects of disabilities of insidious onset and degenerative disorders are more commonly found in elderly users, who make up the majority of *accompanied* chairbound wheelchair users. But the distinction between independent and accompanied wheelchair users can never be precise, and a substantial proportion of all users suffer from weakness of grip, inco-ordination and stiffness, or other upper limb disability.

We thus see how the major types of wheelchair have arisen from these determining needs:

(1) A comfortable pushchair for the elderly and severely disabled.
(2) A strong versatile self-propelled chair for the largely independent young adult.
(3) A group of chairs to fulfil the needs of the completely dependent child who yet attempts to approximate to normal development.

Population studies indicate that the largest group of wheelchair users is made up of elderly patients, disabled by arthritis or stroke, of very limited independence, requiring help to get in and out of the chair, and needing to be pushed when out of doors. A third of all wheelchair users are incontinent, and this fact emphasizes the need for a full clinical assessment when deciding a patient's wheelchair requirements.

The care of incontinent patients places particular demands on their wheelchairs which must facilitate toileting and cleansing by the nursing staff, and resist possible recurrent wetting.

For outdoor use the increasing availability of the motor car, and the awkwardness of the average car boot, created an overriding need for wheelchairs to be light and foldable. Such is the pressure that the conventional standard chairs are rapidly giving way in popularity to similar but light-weight models with detachable armrests and legrests, reducing the main chassis and wheels to about 36 lb weight (16.4 kg). When the chair is to be attendant-pushed, the large propelling wheels can be replaced by smaller ones, thus reducing weight and overall size.

Design features of available wheelchairs

The main design features of a wheelchair are wheels (castors), footrests, seat and backrest, brakes, armrests and extras. These can be considered under three groupings:

(1) Wheels and propulsion techniques.
(2) Seat, backrest/armrests and the chair's comfort factor.
(3) General construction: materials, weight, foldability and appearance.

Methods of propulsion

Although the majority of wheelchair users propel themselves with their hands on the wheels, there are other techniques of propulsion. Two sticks can be used to 'punt' the chair along, or the patient can 'walk' the chair. Some patients with rheumatoid arthritis find such modes of propulsion particularly suitable for use with a chair on four small universal castors.

Single-arm control

Although specially designed chairs are available which can be propelled by one hand operating one wheel, these chairs are very difficult to control. Not only do they demand considerable co-ordination of thought and action from the patient attempting to use them, but they are virtually impossible to propel on sloping or rough ground. Usually they will prove unsuitable for the elderly hemiplegic.

Wheels

One of the problems with the *pram-type of pushchair* is the difficulty of man-oeuvring a four-wheeled chair in a small space when all turning must be achieved by the pusher tilting the chair on the backwheels. Some *pushchairs* are therefore fitted with one or more 'castor' wheels and this makes manoeuvring easier. There may be three wheels, with two for propulsion and one trailing castor, or there may be four wheels, with two castors in either the trailing or leading position.

In *self-propelled* chairs, the size and position of the wheels are both impor-tant. Large propelling wheels at the front of the chair allow easy manoeuvring but not easy tilting to go up kerbs; they also interfere with sideways transfers, and prevent footrests being swung out of the way or detached easily for forward standing transfers. Increasing the diameter of the wheels makes for easier pro-pulsion, but also produces chairs which are correspondingly bulkier and heavier for transit in cars. The usual compromise is to use 22 in (56 cm) propelling wheels, with 20 in (51 cm) or 24 in (61 cm) ones available as alternatives.

It is regrettable that the use of the tyres for gripping inevitably makes the hands of the patient who propels in this manner extremely dirty. Not only the size but also the surface of the tyre makes it suitable for hand propulsion. Even a weak hand with limited power can obtain a purchase on the tread of a wheel-chair tyre, the most comfortable grip size of the tube for the average patient being about 1–1¾ in (2.5–3.0 cm) diameter. Hand-rims are less easily used for propulsion. Whether wooden, chromium-plated metal or nylon-coated steel, they are less suitable than tyres both in size and surface. The use of capstans or rubber strips bound round the hand-rims at intervals to make cog-like protuber-ances may improve their manipulation in some instances. Most hand-rims now are plastic, and do not splinter, flake or feel cold to the touch; but many tetra-plegics will prefer to continue using the tyres to propel their chairs, wearing pads on their hands to protect the skin of their palms.

Castors should be as large as is practicable, in order to keep the effort required for propulsion as low as possible and to assist in negotiating thresholds, rugs and other obstacles. A reasonable compromise is to standardize on a 7 in (18 cm) diameter castor running on ball or needle roller-bearings which should be reasonably well sealed to exclude grit etc. Tyres may be solid rubber or pneumatic and should be easy to replace. Pneumatic tyres on the large wheels save about 5 lb (2 kg) of weight.

Footrests

Because of the need to maintain a high degree of manoeuvrability in the majority of wheelchairs, the footrest is usually mounted in front of the castors. This means that it becomes the limiting factor on the turning radius of the chair, and should, therefore, be kept to minimum length. To enable the user to enter the wheelchair, the footrest must fold out of the way. It is common practice to divide the footrest and fold it upwards. Another method is to swing each section outwards, which has the advantage of reducing overall length. Fixed footrests should no longer be tolerated — they add unnecessary length to the chair, they are a nuisance to helpers getting patients in and out of the chair, and they are an unnecessary hazard to the patient who stands for transferring. The swinging, detachable footrest has become a standard feature on most DHSS wheelchairs and it is designed to provide a useful hand-hold in case the occupant has to be lifted when in the wheelchair, as well as being easy to swing away and detach. Any DHSS wheelchair can be supplied with such a footrest if this is requested on the order form (AOF5G).

In children's chairs it is customary to have the castor wheels fitted in front of the footrests to give added stability. This restricts the positioning of the feet and is a feature seldom used in wheelchairs for adult usage.

Seats, backrests and cushioning

For many patients the most important feature of a wheelchair is its seating comfort. Here again there are many factors which will often necessitate compromise, for much will depend upon the amount of movement which the patient can achieve within the chair and whether he is in the chair for short or long periods.

The simplest and most commonly prescribed form of *seating* used for folding wheelchairs is of the hammock type which does not interfere with the folding action. The original material used was canvas and this has been superseded by plastic-covered canvas material that can be supplied in a wide variety of colours. Seat materials must be very strong and the rate of sag should be kept to a minimum. The aim should be to provide materials which can be easily cleaned but have an ability to 'breathe' so that they do not become too sticky in hot weather. These two requirements are difficult to achieve simultaneously, and the problem of how to do so has not been solved — even in car seats. Ideally the seat and backrest should be easily removable for cleaning. This type of hammock seat is not entirely satisfactory in providing adequate comfort for those who need to use the wheelchair over long periods. For such patients, cushions need to be provided which can be removed when the wheelchair is folded. This cannot be regarded as an entirely satisfactory solution, and, ideally, the wheelchair should be foldable without removing any of its components.

Cushions are a subject on their own. Surprisingly the softest and thickest are usually the least comfortable, for they are readily compressed and also lead to sweatiness in the perineum and anal cleft. For many patients a cushion with a hard base is the most suitable, and this type of cushion can more easily be shaped to allow for the use of a urinal in the chair.

Cushions can make or mar comfort. It is a fairly safe maxim that the more cushions a patient uses in a wheelchair the more uncomfortable it becomes, and the more likely it is that the wrong style of chair has been provided. Extra

cushions inserted behind the back will push the patient forward and create difficulties and discomfort with the knees and footrests. Extra cushions laid on the
seat will often lift the patient too high and create discomfort for back and
shoulders. Furthermore, adding cushions restricts mobility in the chair, prevents
the patient from adjusting his position and easing pressure areas and often from
achieving transfers easily.

For some patients, sheepskin covers or alternating pressure cushions are
available, or cushions which are subdivided and filled with polystyrene granules.
These cushions are usually prescribed for patients who are likely to develop
pressure sores or in whom such sores have already occurred.

Patients with severe spinal deformity may need additional side cushioning;
the use of removable side pads is often preferred by a patient with a collapsing
scoliosis to the provision of a spinal brace; a sculptured back cushion with an
appropriately sited groove may relieve the pressure on the apex of curvature of
the spine of a patient with severe kyphosis.

Occasionally, spinal deformity is so great that cushioning cannot achieve
comfort, and then it may become necessary to mould the entire seat and back of
the wheelchair to the patient, using either plaster of paris or a vacuum pack to
construct the initial negative cast.

Cushioning and support for the head may be provided by prescription of a
headrest, which is an extra and detachable fitment available for most chairs. For
such a headrest, the addition of side wings may be requested, or a carved foam
cushion may be added by the therapist giving care.

The angle or rake of the *back* of a wheelchair is vitally important to the comfort of the patient who uses it. Most chairs have their backrests angled at about
5–20 degrees to their seats. For a severely disabled patient this is often not
sufficient, and for him it may be essential to prescribe a non-standard chair with
an adjustable or fully reclining backrest.

Brakes
It is essential that brakes are provided to prevent the wheelchair 'running away'
when the patient is getting in or out. Both large wheels should be braked to
prevent the wheelchair turning during this manoeuvre.

Brakes have to be effective and they are often 'hard' to put on. Extension
pieces may make them easier to reach, and, by giving greater leverage, easier to
manipulate. In some early versions of the Model 8 chair, both brakes were
operated by one lever, but the Bowden cable and linkage always stretched
unevenly. As so many wheelchair users are elderly or arthritic, or both, it is not
surprising that many have considerable difficulty in manipulating the brakes – a
considerable hazard.

With solid tyres the brakes become ineffective as soon as the tread begins to
wear. There is sometimes a need for a unidirectional brake to prevent the chair
running backwards on a slope while the wheelchair user opens a door, or to assist
patients who cannot get enough momentum to get up a slope.

Armrests
In addition to their primary function, armrests are used to:

(1) Assist in retaining the occupant in the seat.
(2) Keep the occupant's clothes clear of the wheels.

(3) Support a feeding or working tray.
(4) Support the occupant during entry and egress.

To enable the occupant to transfer sideways from the wheelchair it is often necessary to make the armrests removable. This presents problems because attendants are inclined to lift the folded wheelchair by the armrests, and so it is the usual practice to fit locking catches. This again leads to further problems, since many wheelchair users have weak grips or difficulty in manipulating small stiff springs, and they and their companions often find the locking devices usually supplied with detachable armrests of little help, or indeed a positive nuisance.

Armrests can be made of different heights and with or without padding. Their front portions may have a cut-out to permit the wheelchair to be drawn close to a working surface — these are known as desk arms or domestic arms. The overall height and distance apart of the armrests is important to the ease with which a patient can propel, and frequently a compromise must be accepted among the optimal dimensions required for the armrests to fulfil their separate functions.

The standard chair
The following standard types of wheelchair are supplied by the DHSS:

(1) Folding pushchairs for outdoor use.
(2) Regid wheelchairs for indoor use.
(3) Folding wheelchairs for occupant or attendant propulsion.
(4) Electrically propelled wheelchairs for the severely disabled.

We have now arrived at a situation where the standard compromise indoor/outdoor chair can be provided with a series of alternatives and extras which are listed below:

(1) Propelling wheels at the front instead of at the rear.
(2) Backrest set back 20 or 25 degrees.
(3) 20 in (51 cm), 22 in (56 cm) or 24 in (61 cm) diameter wheels.
(4) Alternative seat sizes.
(5) One-arm control.
(6) Extension to footrests.
(7) Domestic armrests.
(8) Gantry for arm sling.
(9) Detachable tray.
(10) Latex foam cushions.
(11) Backrest or headrest extension.

Furthermore, the basic design of wheelchair can be provided in three sizes — child, junior and standard — and nowadays many models are available in 'light-weight' versions (overall weight of basic chair about 37 lb (15 kg) compared with 56 lb (22 kg). These versions have been achieved by gradual evolution in response to demand over 10–15 years.

The paradox of personality
'Ideally,' say the patients, 'a wheelchair should be as similar as possible in

appearance to other "normal" chairs in the user's home.' Wheelchairs are often referred to as 'clinical', thus reminding the patient that he is a 'patient'. But these attitudes, if understandable, are irrational. Who crosses a road in an arm-chair? This attitude is self-defeating. Acceptability comes from skill, skill from practice, and practice from understanding and deliberate effect to overcome disability.

Architectural and geographical constraints

It is often architectural and geographical constraints which determine our selection of an appropriate wheelchair. Living from a wheelchair restricts the ability to reach and the ability to obtain access. Critical dimensions are inter-related, and frequently it is turning area and approach rather than the width of the doorway which restricts access. Inevitably space is critical, and usually the disabled, whether semi-ambulant or wheelchair-bound, need *more* space for manoeuvring than the able-bodied.

These social factors are frequently the unyielding ones which determine whether or not rehabilitation will be successful. With modern legislation many barriers are being reduced, but many will remain with us for a number of generations yet.

Ergonomics and design

There are a number of theoretical features which should determine the design of wheelchairs for the future.

First, there are the general characteristics by which the patient (user) and the supplier should judge the design.

Comfort

Comfort is obviously of primary importance, but there will always be a compromise between the needs of the user in this and the requirements of stability, manoeuvrability, weight and foldability. The most common method of meeting all these requirements has been to provide a flexible (canvas) seat and backrest and to supply separate removable latex foam cushions for those who need a higher degree of comfort. Other approaches have been made, such as to provide a separate folding seat unit, but this has the disadvantage of requiring a separate module which has to be folded and stowed separately on each occasion that it is necessary to fold the wheelchair. The availability of new materials and techniques is likely to offer solutions to these problems in the future, but material and design research are time-consuming and expensive, and many patients are very conventional in their attitudes.

Simplicity

It is implicit in good design that it should be as simple as the functional require-ments will allow. It is likely to engender confidence in the occupant if he can see and know what his wheelchair is doing. The wheelchair should be easy to clean and to maintain. Faults and defects should be readily observed so that they can be removed before they let the user down in critical circumstances. It need hardly be mentioned that simplicity, reliability and low cost go hand-in-hand.

Reliability
Ideally wheelchairs should require no attention during their service life. Maintenance and the need for adjustments must be kept to a minimum because service instructions are often ignored. The user can rarely do the maintenance himself, and suitable labour is not often available these days. Failures can be dangerous and cases are known of users being injured as a result of breakdowns.

Stability
Manoeuvrability and overall dimensions (e.g. to enable the wheelchair to pass through doorways) limit the extent to which stability can be provided. Present-day wheelchairs are relatively stable providing the occupant knows what he is doing and appreciates the limits to which he can go. In the prescription of a wheelchair, adequate stability must always be an important consideration, although it becomes increasingly difficult to achieve as progressively more compact chairs are demanded. Where there is an increased risk of instability on slopes — as in the case of bilateral lower limb amputees who may be sitting in their chairs without wearing their prostheses — compensatory stability is achieved by setting the rear wheels back 3 in (7.6 cm) from the normal position. This may be prescribed for any standard chair which is required.

Manoeuvrability
It is essential that the wheelchair should be able to negotiate confined spaces and pass easily through doorways and around the home and workplace. There will always be a conflict between the user's personal requirements and the need to fit the wheelchair into an everyday environment. There is little object in giving him a wheelchair which cannot be taken into all the places he will want to visit.

Small bulk and weight
The overall dimensions must be as small as possible for a given seat size. The average doorway is 28 in (71.1 cm) wide. With a seat width of 17 in (43.2 cm) and an overall width of 25 in (63.5 cm) there is only a clearance of 1½ in (3.75 cm) on each side of the wheelchair. Most doors open on to narrow passsageways and so the turning radius must be kept to a minimum. For some patients the wheelchair must fold so that it can be stowed in an invalid vehicle and the DHSS specifies a maximum of 10 in (25 cm) width when folded. For others it must fit between the front and rear seats of motor cars so that a user can enter the vehicle and stow the wheelchair unaided. The height and length should also be such that they permit it to be stowed in a car luggage space. All this manhandling requires that the weight should be kept to a minimum. Probably a minimum weight of 36 lb (15 kg) can be achieved for a light-weight wheelchair without sacrificing strength.

Good appearance
It is not possible to disguise two large wheels and two castors without adding weight and complexity. A wheelchair must be functional, but appearance can be improved by the use of tube work having flowing lines rather than being a mass of straight fabrications. The use of aesthetically more attractive materials, such as plastics, is now being considered, and may effect a radical change in design.

Low cost

This is obviously an important factor, particularly where large quantities are involved, and it is worthwhile noting that the DHSS is currently spending about £1,000,000 annually on new wheelchairs. Cost is allied to production rates, and these are adversely affected if special features are specified on a bespoke basis. What may not be so readily appreciated is the value of interchangeability as a derivative of standardization. It is well worth considering that it might be better to give a user a wheelchair which does not meet his exact requirements rather than to fit him up with something which is very special and cannot be replaced at short notice if it breaks down or needs to be withdrawn for repairing. There are obviously limits to which such a policy can be taken. There will always be a small percentage of users who have special needs and require custom-built wheelchairs which cannot be used by others.

The prescription and supply of self-propelled and attendant-propelled wheelchairs will continue to be an exercise in compromise until simple, safe modular assemblies are available, all architectural barriers are eliminated, and patients and relatives understand and accept certain restrictions and limitations for wheelchair users.

Powered indoor chairs are not discussed in this book as they are a provision for the more severely disabled.

However, it must be remembered that the use of a self-propelled wheelchair, as with the use of sticks or crutches, puts a considerable load on the upper limbs. In effect any weight taken off the legs must be transferred to the arms.

People who are habitual users of wheelchairs, such as paraplegics, are more liable to develop pain around the shoulders than any other equivalent age group of the normal population. The pain may arise in the shoulder itself or in the neck. For this reason wheelchair users may need to be advised about avoiding undue strain and offered powered wheelchairs or other aids and appliances earlier than might at first sight seem necessary.

Outside transport

The whole question of transport for the disabled is a vexed one. It is clear from the steady stream of major and minor injuries incurred during the use of public transport that it is hard enough for the able-bodied to use this form of travelling from place to place, let along the disabled. If unable to use public transport then the disabled person must turn to private transport, whether this is provided for him or is of his own provision.

With physical disablement comes simultaneous loss of easy mobility, both within the home and often, more significantly, outside the home. Often a disabled man could return to work if he could get there and back, and often a family could be kept intact if the disabled mother had her own transport to do the shopping and take the children to and from school. Though the density and speed of traffic is rising, an ever-increasing number of disabled people venture on the roads. There is little evidence that, as a group, they are any more accident prone than their more able-bodied fellows. Indeed, the trend seems to be in the opposite direction. However, the combination of physical disability and inappropriate transport may well constitute a considerable danger to drivers and to road users.

For many years the DHSS provided a specially designed invalid tricycle (three-wheeler), then it introduced the added provision of specially adapted motorcars for certain categorized disabled patients.

The disadvantages of the three-wheeler vehicle itself are many. First, it further isolates the disabled driver. He is not allowed to transport a passenger, and thus can never drive out with his wife and family. Nor has he any help to hand if he should get into difficulties. As a corollary to this disadvantage many disabled drivers complain that invalid tricycles make them conspicuous, and they wish to avoid this situation, desiring to be regarded as 'normal' people. The contrary view is that disabled drivers *should* be conspicuous and that the low accident record of invalid tricycles is in part due to the fact that other road users recognize them for what they are. If disabled drivers are to be provided with faster and larger vehicles, and to be allowed to drive passengers in their cars, then it could be argued that they should accept some form of ready identification.

Second, their design has been much criticized. They are frequently said to be relatively unstable, and because of their size and power, a hazard to both driver and other road users. Their controls are also criticized as requiring considerable strength and manipulative skill to handle. Recent impartial and expert testing has given these criticisms unqualified support and has requested the complete withdrawal of both the electric and petrol driven three-wheeler vehicles from use at the earliest possible moment. Further enquiries continue.

Third, unconventional aspects of these vehicles present certain problems. Few garages are prepared to attempt emergency repairs, and a disabled driver may well be stranded because of a minor mechanical fault. The servicing of these vehicles is dependent upon an organization of 'approved repairers', but these are few and far between.

Now the standard provision is a Mobility Allowance and the invalid tricycle are being phased out. In order to be eligible for the allowance the disabled person must fall within the age limit which will eventually be 5–60 (women) and 5–65 (men) inclusive. The person must be unable, or virtually unable to walk and this inability must be likely to persist for at least 12 months and must be able to make use of the allowance (e.g. he is able to be moved and is not in a coma). Eligibility will be decided by an independent statutory authority on the basis of a medical examination.

The allowance is intended to be spent on outdoor mobility and may be used to pay for taxis, to hire a car or another vehicle, to provide holiday transport, or to buy a vehicle. The allowance (currently in 1978 – £10 per week) is taxable, but is paid *in addition* to other social security benefits.

A new charity (Motability) has been formed to facilitate car purchase and a leasing scheme is in operation. Hire purchase (and hiring) restrictions have been removed for disabled people with mobility allowance who want to buy a car. This means that they can obtain special terms – a lower deposit and longer to pay. The Royal Association for Disability and Rehabilitation (RADAR) is coordinating advice and information to help disabled people solve their mobility problems in this respect. Full details are available from the DHSS Disablement Research Branch.

Exemption from vehicles excise duty is also available to all mobility allowance beneficiaries and those nominated as the beneficiary in addition to some other categories who fall outside the mobility allowance age group.

Under this new arrangements the three-wheeler is no longer available to new applicants, but current users and certain other categories will continue to be eligible for these vehicles.

As a generalization the new regulations provide for a financial allowance to overcome the mobility of disabled people in whatever way they themselves decide to use the money. They can buy a vehicle, or hire; they can drive themselves in specially adapted vehicles or nominate someone else to secure the allowance in order to drive them. There is now a number of organizations providing advice and help for disabled people in achieving appropriate mobility.

Many disabled people might be better served by powered wheelchairs, operated by the patient, or attendant, as appropriate, and designed for outside use. As patient-operated, electrically powered wheelchairs become more freely available, some alteration of existing kerbs and crossings will be necessary and some definitive ruling as to place and manner of road crossing will need to be formulated.

BIBLIOGRAPHY AND REFERENCES

British Orthopaedic Association (1973). Report of Committee on Prosthetic and Orthotic Services. London; B.O.A.

Department of Health and Social Security (1970). *The Handbook of Invalid Chairs and Hand-propelled Tricycles* (MHM 408). London; HMSO.

Fenwick, D. (1977). *Wheelchairs and their users.* HMSO, London

Hamilton, E. A., Molden, F. R. and Nichols, P. J. R. (1973). 'Portable parallel bars.' *Rheum. Rehab.* **12,** 100

Harris, A. I. (1971). *Handicapped and Impaired in Great Britain.* London; HMSO

Jolly, D. W. (Ed.) (1964). 'A symposium on the wheelchair.' *Paraplegia* **2,** 20

Kamenetz, H. H. (1969). *The Wheelchair Book.* USA; Thomas

Nichols, P. J.R. and Mowat, A. G. (1972). 'Splints, walking aids and appliances for the arthritic patient.' In *Reports on Rheumatic Diseases, No. 48.* London; Arthritis and Rheumatism Council

Nichols, P. J. R., Morgan, R. H. and Goble, R. E. A. (1966). 'Wheelchair users – a study in variation of disability.' *Ergonomics* **9,** 131

Platts, E. A. (1974). 'Wheelchair design – a survey of users items'. *Proc. Roy. Soc. Med.* **67,** 414

Sharp, Lady (1974). *A Report on Mobility for Physically Disabled People.* London; HMSO

Wilshere, E. R., Hollings, E. M. and Nichols, P. J. R. (1977). *Equipment for the Disabled* (4th edn.). Horsham, Sussex; National Fund for Research into Crippling Diseases

18 Sexual Problems of the Disabled

ANN HAMILTON

To plan the rehabilitation of a patient without consideration of his sexuality is to condone the erroneous view that disability either brings functional castration or necessitates sexual sublimation.

In a sexually orientated society such as that of the western world of today, the ability to express sexuality fully is highly valued by the able-bodied. Far from sublimating their sexual urges, recent surveys — such as the Coventry survey conducted for the National Fund for Research into Crippling Diseases — shows that most disabled people place no less value on their sexuality and rate their sexual fulfilment as a high priority. In the achievement of this fulfilment they are discriminated against not only by the condition which disabled them, but also by society itself, which relates sexuality to body image, and discriminates against those who deviate from the ideal type.

Although disabled people see themselves as sexual beings, with sexual feelings and the ability to form sexual relationships, they frequently lack the confidence or the experience to establish their sexual identity: sheltered upbringing, isolated education and restricted mobility combine to reduce the opportunity to form sexual friendships, or to see a wide enough selection of people, places and things to develop a realistic attitude to sexual matters.

When disablement is congenital or from early childhood, parents rarely acknowledge a disabled child's sexuality or help him to form his sexual image. The medical, paramedical and teaching staff giving care likewise tend to treat him as an asexual being. The society which he longs to enter as an equal member rejects his full admission, because it cannot accept that someone with disfigurement, deformity or abnormalities of motor expression can have normal sexual feelings. Small wonder that his self esteem is low and his essays into sexual relationships are too tentative or over aggressive.

When disablement is acquired, society finds it equally difficult to realise that the wish or expectation of further sexual activity does not automatically cease with the onset of the disabling condition.

Disability results from dysfunction of any system sufficiently severe to prevent functional compensation by other systems, and disability of any derivation may lead to a sexual problem. As the incidence of disability in the community rises with our ability to avert death without the corresponding ability to restore full function, so too does the incidence of sexual problems related to physical illness.

ASPECTS OF SEXUALITY

In attempting to develop and function as a sexual being, a disabled person is constantly battling against the adverse effects which physical illness may have on various aspects of his sexuality. Sexual image, sexual drive, sexual expression, sexual competence and sexual opportunity may be diminished, distorted or destroyed by his disabling condition.

Sexual Image — or the impression created by the expression of sexuality through appearance and behaviour — may be difficult to establish or maintain when deformity, disfigurement, disordered growth or disordered function result in a real or imagined reduction in sexual attractiveness.

Sexual Drive or Libido — or the strength of the innate compulsion of an individual to behave as a sexual being — determines the frequency and intensity with which sexual attraction and arousal occur, and also the willingness to suggest or engage in sexually orientated behaviour. This drive is depressed by many diseases and by the medication which is prescribed for their treatment. Drive is also depressed by the fear, pain, anxiety, depression and insomnia which frequently accompany disablement, and may be depressed still further by the medication for these conditions.

Sexual Expression — or the ability to express sexual feelings through bodily movement — may be jeopardized by:

(1) Inability to approximate the body of the disabled partner to that of his sexual partner, because of a wheelchair, splint, brace, caliper, prosthesis, respirator or sheer bodily weakness.
(2) Inability to move the body in such a way as to convey sexual attraction or produce sexual pleasure by stimulating erogenous areas of the body, because of spasticity, ataxia, athetosis or weakness.
(3) Inability to communicate satisfactorily with a sexual partner because of disorders of sensation, sight, speech and hearing.
(4) Inability to exert sufficient control over the various functions of the body e.g. bowel activity — as in the anal faecal incontinence of spina bifida or cord damaged patients, or the stoma faecal incontinence of the colostomate or ileostomate, or the continuous drooling of the brain damaged patient; or bladder activity as in the urethral urinary incontinence from disease or dysfunction of the central nervous system or the urogenital system, or the abdominal urinary incontinence of the patient with a urinary diversion.

Sexual Competence implies the presence of the ability to experience the intact neurophysiological sequence of arousal, erection, ejaculation and orgasm in the male, and the equivalent sequence in the female. One or more stages in this sequence may be adversely affected by different disabilities. Thus *arousal* may be diminished in a patient with reduced drive from debilitating diseases such as rheumatoid arthritis or anaemia, or by the medication of these and other diseases.

Ejaculation may be lost even when erection is present, e.g. following stroke, cord or brain injury.

Orgasm is no longer experienced when the afferent tracts from pelvis to brain are damaged by trauma or disease, e.g. cord lesions.

Erection — impotence, or the persistent inability to maintain a penile erection sufficient to conclude coitus to orgasm and ejaculation, is one of the most distressing and widespread problems of sexuality associated with physical disease. The well known causes of psychogenic and behavioural impotence may operate in disabled as well as in able-bodied people, and doubt, drugs, drink and debility may supplement an organic cause, or themselves be the primary causative agents of this condition.

Organic factors causing impotence may be due to:

(1) *CNS lesions*, e.g. multiple sclerosis, Parkinson's disease, temporal lobe tumours and epilepsy, destructive hypothalmic lesions, various disorders of the spinal cord.
(2) *Local disease of the genital organs.*
(3) *Vascular conditions*, e.g. thrombosis of the aortic bifurcation, haemorrhoids.
(4) *Endocrinopathies*, e.g. diabetes (up to 25% of male diabetics may complain of impotence). Myxodoema, Cushing's disease, acromegaly.
(5) *Ageing.*
(6) *Post surgical conditions*, e.g. post prostatectomy, post-cystectomy.
(7) *Drugs*, e.g. analgesics, anti-inflammatory and anti-hypertensive drugs, anxiolytics, anti-depressives, β — blockers, sedatives, steroids, hallucinogens, cytotoxics, have all been quoted as depressing drive and potency in some individuals.

Sexual Opportunity — or the chance to meet members of the opposite or same sex and to establish a sexual relationship with them — is directly proportional to the mobility and privacy which a disabled person can command. Those who are totally dependent for daily care and transport, are limited by the goodwill and attitudes of parents or nursing staff as to whom they meet and what they can do when they meet them.

ASPECTS OF DISABILITY: GENERAL PROBLEMS

What then are the sexual problems of disabled people? How are they caused and how may they be helped?

The problems for the single disabled patient are:

(1) How to establish a sexual image.
(2) How to find a sexual partner and express sexuality to the satisfaction of both members of the partnership.
(3) How to satisfy sexuality if a partner is not forthcoming.

The problems of the married disabled are:

(1) *either* how to achieve a pattern of sexual activity as like as possible to the chosen premorbid pattern,
(2) *or* how to establish a new pattern as satisfying as possible to both partners.

The precise nature of the problems of the single and married patient will depend upon the extent to which the various aspects of sexuality are affected — sexual opportunity, sexual image, sexual drive, sexual competence and sexual expression — and also on:

(1) Nature, severity and duration of the causative illness.
(2) Age.
(3) Sex.
(4) Age at onset of illness.
(5) Domestic, marital and family status.
(6) Conditions of the society and country of residence.

The sexual problems of all disabled people eventually result in difficulty with partner acquisition, pleasuring, potency, partner satisfaction, and procreation.

A further problem common to all disabled people is the difficulty they experience in finding out the information necessary to help them to solve their sexual dilemmas. They are reluctant to mention a subject which may bring ridicule, disapproval or suspicion of perversion upon them, and there is a great need for all those giving medical and paramedical care to be alert for the presence of such problems, and to be ready either to supply information or counselling as required.

In any one person the problems may be related to difficulties present before the onset of the disease, to the disease process itself, or to the treatment of the disease. The exact delineation of the sexual problems and their causes for each individual is often extremely complicated.

Thus the problems may be:

(1) Directly due to disabling disease, e.g. painful hips of rheumatoid arthritis; painful back due to prolapsed intervertebral disc.
(2) Treatment related, e.g. reduced drive caused by some anti-inflammatory drugs.
(3) Premorbid, e.g. hypertension treated by anti-hypertensive drugs with autonomic effect prejudicing erection.
(4) Disease related, e.g. depression, which diminishes sexual drive, and anti-depressive therapy, which may further diminish drive and potency.
(5) Disease unrelated, e.g. anaemia from heavy periods, reduced drive from contraceptive pill.

The problem complex of a patient may be even further complicated by the physical problems of the able partner (who may also have sexual problems due to disease or its treatment), and by the psychological problems which the disabling condition may have upon the sexuality of both partners.

NEUROLOGICAL ASPECTS

Normal sexual function depends on the integrated action of various centres in the brain with two closely related centres in the cord. A parasympathetic centre in the sacral cord (S2/3) mediates erection by the vasodilator action of its efferent nerves on the penile arterioles: a sympathetic centre in the L1/2 area causes ejaculation to take place when its efferents cause a contraction of the smooth muscle surrounding the epididyimis, vesiculae seminales, vasa deferentia and prostate with consequent ejaculation of semen into the prostatic urethra. Somatic nerves control the bulbo and ischio cavernosus muscles which eject semen by rhythmic contractions from the posterior urethra and penile urethra.

A sensory centre in the brain interprets as orgasm the pleasurable sensation produced by the involuntary contraction of pelvic and penile musculature during ejaculation. Cord and brain damage transecting the afferent tracts which transmit these impulses from pelvis to brain will therefore prevent orgasm.

Within the brain itself, the thalamus, the pituitary/hypophyseal complex, the limbic areas (the amygdala in particular), and the parietal and temporal lobes are thought to be particularly concerned in the sexuality of the individual. But the visual, auditory and speech centres also initiate inhibitory or stimulatory impulses to these and to other sexuomotor centres in the brain, and to the autonomic centres of erection and ejaculation in the cord. Interruption of the psychic or sensory input to the sexuomotor centres in the brain will affect the barrage of efferent impulses modifying the action of the sex centres of the cord. This barrage may be stimulatory, or inhibitory in its effect, since although erection may occur entirely from visual, auditory or psychic stimulation, for the most part the brain exerts an inhibitory influence on the natural tendency of the penis to erect to pleasurable repetitive stimulation of the erogenous areas of the body.

In many cultures, the brain appears to exert this inhibitory effect on erection and ejaculation as a learned behavioural characteristic gradually developing during the progression of each individual from infancy to adult life. This reduces the occurrence of erection and ejaculation as automatic responses to erotic visual, auditory and peripheral stimulatory sensory input, unless its occurrence is deliberately permitted as appropriate for the given circumstances. Disease or dysfunction of the nervous system may lead to severe impairment of sexual function. Not only may sexual drive and sexual image be adversely affected by damage to the brain or cord, but sexual competence is frequently compromised and sexual expression is also jeopardized when neurological dysfunction leads to disturbances of sensation and of muscle tone, power and co-ordination. Whether the onset of dysfunction is *acute* following trauma or a vascular accident, or *gradual* following the progressive degeneration of nerve cells and tracts occurring in many neurological diseases, the likely outcome is that the conventional view of sexual satisfaction culminating in orgasm will not be obtainable for many disabled people.

Brain injury
When acute brain injury occurs, whether from cardiovascular accident (CVA) or trauma, sexual drive and sexual competence are initially lost in the majority of cases.

After a CVA both sexual drive and competence usually return within approximately three months provided brain damage is unilateral. If the damage is bilateral and sufficiently severe, they may never return.

During the early days of recovering sexual response, the normal sequence of arousal, erection, ejaculation and orgasm may be desynchronized and premature ejaculation and difficulty in sustaining erection may be exasperatingly combined with increased sexual desire.

The mechanical difficulties of sexual expression experienced by a hemiplegic hampered by spasticity and weakness of voluntary movement, and possibly also by hemianopia, hemianaesthesia and diminished perceptual ability as well, combine with these disorders of sexual function to create severe sexual problems.

The sexual partner may be fearful of precipitating further strokes by requesting or permitting sexual intercourse, or be repelled by the physical changes caused by the stroke: dysphasia or dysarthria may complicate communication and thus enhance sexual difficulties yet further.

Administration of β — blockers and/or anti-hypertensive drugs may drastically reduce sexual competence in some patients. Careful enquiry for the presence of sexual difficulty is therefore essential after a CVA, which frequently occurs in early middle age when sexual drive is still strong. With counselling and possible revision of medication and/or technique, most couples can achieve a mutually satisfying pattern of sexual activity. Some couples, with a low premorbid sexual drive, are content to live in loving companionship without making the effort to establish a new sexual relationship with each other. But it is an unwise and unkind assumption to make that any couple is 'beyond it' since the more restrained sexual intercourse employed by elderly couples can be productive of a comfort and joy which is as important to their happiness as the more athletic activities preferred by those who are younger and more agile.

In the early recovery phase after *brain injury of traumatic origin* sexual activity is initially decreased. With recovery, the resultant level of sexual activity depends upon the location and severity of areas of irreversible damage. Frequently, however, there is an interval of disinhibited sexual behaviour of variable duration, when any remotely erotic sensation causes unrestrained erection. This erection tends to persist for long periods, since the further persistent stimulation necessary for ejaculation does not necessarily occur, and the young brain-damaged patient is left with an erect penis, often unable to masturbate sufficiently to effect relief, or to find a surrogate with whom to have the intercourse he desires. Such sexual dysfunction leads to considerable distress both for the patient and those giving care. The patient may be found in the lavatory, ward, or gymnasium, desperately trying to masturbate an already erect and engorged penis, and may experience great difficulty in micturating in a socially acceptable manner when the penis is in this state.

Careful explanation of the existence and cause of this disinhibited sexual behaviour goes far to reconcile those concerned to the occurrence of frequent and prolonged erections, and to unconcealed masturbation in public places. Avoidance of unnecessary peripheral stimulation — such as tight jeans and pants — and the use of deliberately non-provocative behaviour on the part of those giving care will also be of assistance.

When the severity of brain damage is such that a patient's chances of marriage and a normal sexual life are minimal, it is merciful to advise the patient and those who care for him that the use of manual or mechanical self-stimulation and phantasizing are acceptable alternatives which are neither perverted nor dangerous.

Two of the most important factors in determining whether or not the marriage of a brain-damaged patient will survive when marriage precedes injury, are the nature of the *personality* change which that injury may produce, and the alternation in *premorbid sexual activity* which it necessitates. A woman will care for and be faithful to a man she loves and who loves her and can express his love: she finds it difficult to remain with someone who has changed not only in body, but in mind and spirit.

Cord lesions

The impairment of sexual function following cord injury or disease is determined by the level, site and nature of the resultant lesion. In the male paraplegic or tetraplegic patient *sexual drive* may not be disturbed; *sexual competence* is seriously affected. Thus although *erection* is still experienced in the majority of cord damaged patients, it may be erratic in cause and duration, and no longer forms a part of the normal sequence of arousal, erection, ejaculation and orgasm. Patients with upper motor neurone lesions have the more favourable prognosis, and one survey quotes 92% of such patients as having reflex erections and 22% psychogenic. Patients with lower motor neorone disease are less fortunate, the same survey quotes 26% of these patients with psychogenic and none with reflex erections.

An ancillary pathway coming down through the sympathetic system from the mid-thoracic cord may be activated in some paraplegic patients, and may enable erection to occur even in patients with cauda equina severance.

Ejaculation tends to be retrograde into the bladder, and external ejaculation tends to be dribbling in character on the rare instances when it does occur.

Orgasm does not occur, but a sensation known as para-orgasm or quasi-orgasm is experienced simultaneously with the orgasm which the sexual partner experiences during intercourse, followed by a sensation of wellbeing and decline of sexual arousal.

Fertility is reduced or absent when cord damage leads to atrophy of the seminiferous tubules secondary to a disordered autonomic efferent nerve supply to the testicles or to ascending infection from the urethra. This is thought to be productive of a raised testicular temperature which predisposes to atrophy of the germinal epithelium.

Sexual expression is frequently complicated by the presence of spasticity and weakness of voluntary movement, limiting the duration and nature of foreplay, and the ability to achieve genital intercourse in the superior/inferior position.

In the female patient, once again sexual image and drive need not be disturbed by cord damage; normal menstruation returns after initial cessation immediately after injury; sexual competence is present inasmuch as most female patients remain able to have coitus in a passive role. However, orgasm is not experienced; fertility remains unchanged in the majority of patients and delivery by the vaginal route with possible help in the second stage is usual. Ascending urinary infection and hypertension may complicate pregnancy.

The effect of cord damage on sexuality is one of the earliest questions raised by the recovering paraplegic or tetraplegic, and early counselling, film shows, and access to informative literature are essential. Social mixing between the sexes is encouraged in Spinal Injury Centres to help the re-establishment of sexual image, and mutual discussion on sexual expression. Visits home for weekends are arranged as early as possible for married patients, so that they may determine the particular difficulties in sexual activity with which they need help.

Investigation of fertility entails examination of the semen produced by masturbation or sexual intercourse, to detect the presence of abnormal forms or abnormal motility. Intrathecal injection of neostigmine or electrical stimulation of the rectum will enable some patients to produce semen who are unable to produce it otherwise. Semen produced in either of these ways has been used for the artificial insemination of the marital partner, but unless it has been produced naturally during intercourse it is unlikely to be fertile and to result in pregnancy.

Many patients with incomplete paraplegia are able to have active erection and ejaculation of living spermatozoa and to fertilize their partners without assistance, but there are few, if any, proven cases of a woman fertilized by a man with a complete cord lesion. Some Spinal Injury Centres now take a specimen of the spermatozoa of their male patients as soon as possible after admission and store it in a sperm bank for possible future use. Artificial insemination of the wife of a paraplegic patient may then be made using her husband's sperm.

The importance of adequate counselling cannot be overstressed for patients with spinal injury. They are usually young, physically and sexually active, anxious to recreate as normal a pattern of sexual activity as possible, and avid for any information which will help them do so.

In such counselling, the marital or sexual partner should be included, so that a basis for mutual discussion and experiment may be provided based on accurate knowledge. Penovaginal intervourse is the ultimate goal of many couples, even though transient and irregular erections, absence of true ejaculation and orgasm, and fear of erratic bladder and bowel function make this difficult to achieve. Such patients usually attempt intercourse in the inferior/superior position with the paraplegic patient lying on his back and his wife kneeling astride him. After emptying the bladder, removing the catheter or condom, or doubling back and taping the indwelling catheter to the penis, the lubricated penis is massaged into an erection, or else milked into the vagina while still flaccid. Vigorous pelvis thrusts and vaginal contractions frequently serve to sustain or induce erection after penile entry has been affected and the female partner then brings herself to a climax and her husband to a state of quasi-climax or paraorgasm, which has been described as a feeling of deep physical 'well being'.

When the female partner is paraplegic, the unaffected male experiences the usual arousal—erection—ejaculation—orgasm sequence during genital intercourse. This is most conveniently attempted in the side-lying position with posterior entry of the vagina, permitting an indwelling catheter to be left *in situ* without mechanical difficulty ensuing. If however the male enters from the front in the superior/inferior position he risks the occurrence of precipitating involuntary micturition if an indwelling catheter is first removed, or else tangling with the catheter if it is left *in situ*. In either case, the female experiences no orgasm but can reach the state of quasi-climax or paraorgasm.

Counselling stresses the enhanced sensitivity of those parts of the body above the level of the spinal lesion, particularly the skin immediately proximal to the anaesthetic area, and the pleasure which may be obtained from their stimulation. It stresses also the need to experiment with various techniques and positions, and the necessity of accepting the fact that any one technique is unlikely to pleasure both partners equally, because of the profound differences in sexual expression and the sexual sensation which may exist between the normal and the cord-damaged partner. Simultaneous sexual satisfaction frequently cannot be achieved; orgasm may take longer to develop; quasi-orgasm is difficult to delineate. Indeed, both partners are not always able to obtain satisfaction during the same episode of lovemaking, and mutual agreement determines the technique which is used to pleasure one or other of them maximally during any one episode. As one patient remarked 'When you are disabled, your sexual satisfaction may need to be experienced in sequence with that of your partner, rather than in parallel'.

Multiple sclerosis
The irregular progression of events by which disablement is established makes

the sexual problems of the multiple sclerosis patient difficult to enumerate, since their severity and duration are as variable as the order of their occurrence.

Depending on the sites of neurological involvement, certain general patterns of dysfunction are common. Sexual image may be jeopardized when the depressive or euphoric phases of the disease cause an unacceptable character change in the patient, or exhausting loquaciousness discourages verbal, let alone sexual, intercourse. Poor sight, diminished sensation and co-ordination, weakness and spasticity may all make self-care difficult and further reduce sexual attraction and the ability to continue established patterns of sexual expression.

Despite a sexual drive which is often increased, there is frequently reduced sexual competence in the male. Depending on the levels of cord damage, erection may be reflex or in response to persistent masturbation, rather than a part of the usual sequence of arousal, erection, ejaculation and orgasm, and ejaculation and orgasm may be infrequent or absent.

Fertility is apparently usually unimpaired in the female but there is often an exacerbation of the disease after a pregnancy, and the fatigue of caring for a family can depress her sexual drive. Fertility may however be depressed or destroyed in the male if testicular atrophy occurs secondary to degeneration of the testicular afferent nerve supply, and/or to the presence of ascending infection from the urinary tract. It may also be destroyed when neurological dysfunction prevents normal ejaculation of spermatozoa and retrograde emission into the bladder occurs.

Disorders of the special senses

So much of sexual behaviour is influenced by feedback from the reactions of those to whom it is directed. When these reactions are distorted, invisible or inaudible, the appropriate behaviour modifications are harder to achieve. Speech affected by dysarthria, dysphasia or deafness cannot adequately convey desired emotions or meaning. For these reasons those with disorders of the special senses or speech may find it difficult to learn enough about sex, to achieve a satisfactory sexual image, to attract a sexual partner and to form and maintain a stable and happy relationship. Particular care is needed during the education and upbringing of such children to prevent the sexuality and their concept of sex being unduly coloured by their disability.

NON-NEUROLOGICAL ASPECTS

Cardiovascular diseases

Patients with cardiovascular disease sufficiently severe to restrict their normal activity are likely to have sexual problems, and frequently refrain from the more active forms of sexual expression. Many people who have had a coronary thrombosis either completely stop or drastically curtail genital intercourse through fear of precipitating a further heart attack. This is hardly surprising when it is recalled that a rise of heart rate, respiratory rate and blood pressure, and angina of effort, may be symptomatic of either condition. Therefore it is particularly important that detailed advice on sexual activity should routinely be given to patients with cardiovascular disease.

Many authorities advise sexual abstinence until 8—12 weeks post infarction.

After this time, sexual intercourse usually may be attempted with the accustomed sexual partner, in a warm room, in a warm bed, and in familiar surroundings.

The able partner takes the more active part, and postures and movements likely to precipitate dyspnoea or angina are avoided. Unacceptable rise of pulse rate, the occurrence of angina, dyspnoea or palpitations are indications for the cessation of sexual activity on the occasion of their occurence, and sexual technique is modified to avoid these on subsequent occasions. A 10 mg tablet of isosorbide dinitrate may be advised for some patients ten minutes before lovemaking is started and a box of glyceryl trinitrate tablets should be at hand, under the pillow or on the bed table.

Elementary precautions should be followed, such as avoiding sexual intercourse under stressful conditions. Illicit affairs, heavy meals, and times when exertion, anger or worry have given rise to frequent attacks of angina are unwise preludes for sexual intercourse.

Respiratory disease
Patients with severe chronic respiratory disease are frequently sufficiently disabled to find it difficult or even impossible to have sexual intercourse in the usual superior/inferior position, whether lying above or beneath their partner. Thoracic and abdominal compression for someone with reduced thoracic excursion from obstructive or restrictive airways disease can rapidly produce intolerable dyspnoea, when intercostal, diaphragmatic and abdominal respiratory movements are still further curtailed.

The use of alternative postures for intercourse, such as the able partner kneeling astride the disabled, of the use of posterior entry with both partners side-lying, or intercourse in the standing, sitting or kneeling position may be sufficient to prevent the onset of dyspnoea. Sexual techniques may need to be adjusted so that the able partner takes the more active part, employing penovaginal, manual or oral intercourse as indicated. The use of a bronchodilator prior to intercourse may be helpful, and lovemaking should only take place in a room which is warm and airy.

Urogenital disease
Patients with structural or functional abnormality of the genito-urinary tract, whether acquired or congenital, may find it difficult or impossible to achieve normal penovaginal intercourse. *Incontinence* of urine from any cause constitutes a major problem to sexual expression and frequently leads to abstinence from intercourse. When the incontinence is untreated, fluids should be limited and the time of administration of diuretic tablets adjusted to avoid a diuresis during lovemaking, and the bladder should be emptied immediately before this is attempted. The superior/inferior position should be avoided to minimize pressure on the bladder.

From female patients in whom incontinence is treated by use of an indwelling catheter, this should ideally be removed before intercourse, but is usually merely taped securely to the abdomen.

If the incontinent male wears a drainage condom and portable reservoir, the condom and reservoir should be removed prior to intercourse and the penis cleaned and lubricated, following manual expression of the bladder. If an indwelling catheter is worn many urologists and neurologists advise its removal prior to intercourse and the insertion of a new catheter immediately afterwards. Many patients however elect to double the catheter back along the penis and tape it to the body of the penis and the abdominal wall to avoid traction. Intercourse is then attempted after lubrication of the penis and catheter with KY jelly, with or without prior enclosure of the penis and catheter in a contraceptive sheath.

The presence of an ileal conduit may require an adjustment of sexual technique, since the reservoir bag is likely to be detached from the abdominal wall during unrestrained sexual activity in the superior/inferior position.

If the conduit is in the male partner, the female partner may kneel astride him. If it is in the female partner, posterior entry in the side-lying position may be used. In both cases the bag should be emptied immediately before intercourse, and supported by a closely fitting garment or belt.

Women who have a colpoperineorrhaphy involving anterior and posterior repair for uterine prolapse and vaginal laxity may be left with a small rigid vagina which defies penile penetration. For these patients, and for others for whom correction of their structural or functional disability is not possible, counselling on the use of orogenital and manuogenital stimulation acquaints them with alternative forms of sexual satisfaction.

Vaginitis, Vulvitis, Cervicitis, Balanitis, Urethritis may sometimes complicate certain sero-negative arthritides and painful ulceration, lack of lubrication, or offensive discharge may temporarily prevent genital intercourse. During such times the affected partner may employ oral or manual stimulation to satisfy the unaffected partner, unless prevented by ulceration of the mouth, or arthritis of the upper limbs, from using such methods.

Gastrointestinal disease

When gastrointestinal disease causes conditions of the mouth, abdomen, or anus which are painful or distasteful, sexual difficulties are likely to result.

One particularly distressing problem is the presence of an ostomy, whether it is an ileostomy or colostomy. 5000 new permanent colostomies are created each year and about 50 per cent of these patients refrain from sexual intercourse following creation of their ostomies.

In some centres colostomies are now being created which are continent, owing to the construction of an artificial rectum deep to the stoma, or to the insertion of a magnetic, cobalt alloy, peristomal ring subcutaneously, and the use of an obturator. These techniques should go far to reduce problems of sexual expression for many future colostomates.

Even for those with established conventional colostomies, sexual intercourse may still be enjoyed in the majority of cases. A colonic washout will usually prevent effluent for 12–16 hours. Timing of intercourse to occur before or several hours after a meal; avoidance of intercourse on a day when the bowel is overactive from infection or unwise diet; use of a well fitting colostomy bag and an effective deodorant and belt; employment of firm, lightweight, supportive underwear; alteration of technique to avoid direct pressure over the stoma or bag — such as one partner kneeling astride the other, or the use of the sidelying position with posterior entry if the affected partner is a female, or the use of the sitting position for the male with the female sitting astride him — can all be helpful for those who prefer conventional genital intercourse.

Others may prefer to use orogenital or manuogenital stimulation as alternative forms of sexual expression.

In some unfortunate patients it is not merely distaste and discomfort which the presence of a colostomy invokes, but frank impotence, when the nervi erigentes are damaged during preceding abdominal operation.

Arthritis and other locomotor dysfunction

Whether occurring as a mechanical affliction of the joints or as part of a systemic disease, arthritis may lead to the development of a wide range of sexual problems. Sexual image, drive, competence and expression may each or all be adversely affected by its presence. When locomotor disability takes the form of fixed hips, it is generally accepted that sexual difficulties are likely to ensue, but pain and stiffness in any joint can impede sexual expression, and the sexual disability-equivalent of an arthritic joint is often far greater than the apparent locomotor disability it incurs.

Thus the painful neck of the patient with severe cervical spondylosis can act as a potent deterrent to foreplay. The inflamed metacarpophalangeal and interphalangeal joints of the rheumatoid patient can reduce the ability to hold or caress and may limit foreplay sufficiently to jeopardize the attainment of a satisfactory climax. Painful and possibly unstable joints of the upper limbs restrict the ability to hold a partner or take part of the body weight. The stiff painful spine of the patient with lumbar spondylosis or ankylosing spondylitis reduces the scope of tolerable body postures and prejudices both the ability of the affected partner to approximate the genital organs to those of the sexual partner and also the ability to make rhythmical pelvic movements. Stiff painful hips of any derivation, although not constituting an absolute bar, can provide a formidable deterrent to intercourse in the super/inferior position. Arthritic knees, ankles and feet, when tender to touch and painful to move, may also limit the variety of postures which can be tolerated, and inhibit the free movement of both partners during lovemaking.

Depression, chronic pain, insomnia, fatigue, malaise, coupled with the frustration of the progressive restriction of sexual, familial, domestic and social activity, and with the fear of the future and rejection which arthritis too often produces, may combine to reduce sexual drive further.

Adequate medication to control pain and the disease process of which arthritis is a part must be the initial aim of the treatment of the sexual problems of the arthritic. Medication to control the sequelae of the arthritis, such as insomnia, anxiety and depression, and inflammation and ulceration of the oral and genital tracts, may also be needed.

Surgical repair or replacement of painful and disorganized joints which impede the physical expression of sexual love,

Physiotherapeutic measures to ease painful joints and muscles prior to lovemaking, such as hot or cold packs, warm baths, massage or vibration,

Orthotic aid in the shape of appropriate splintage to stabilize, support, protect or ease painful and unstable joints may, at some stage in the disease process, produce amelioration or solution of the sexual problems at issue.

The presence of marked bodily deformity which results from many *diseases of the locomotor system and the central nervous system* such as spastic cerebral palsy, osteogenesis imperfecta, severe poliomyelitis, muscular dystrophy, scoliosis, collapsing kyphos, amelia or phocomelia, has its maximal effect on sexual image, but may also reduce competence and expression.

Restricted mobility and reduced strength impede sexual expression. Wheelchairs, calipers, artificial limbs, and spinal supports, impede approximation and contact of hands, faces and trunks. Kissing, caressing, and genital intercourse may be impossible for the seriously disabled to achieve without assistance from someone giving care.

Surgical procedures

Mutilating operations of any kind, particularly those involving the genitourinary system, or the parts of the body particularly concerned with sexuality, may cause sexual problems.

Thus prostatectomy and cystectomy may cause frank impotence. Amputation of one or more limbs may lead to a depreciation of sexual image and difficulty with sexual impression. Mastectomy may cause loss of sexual confidence for the female partner and revulsion amounting to complete rejection by the male.

For all these procedures, pre- and post-operative counselling is mandatory.

IMPOTENCE

Patients who are impotent as the result of a disabling condition may find that the use of oral sex, or manual or instrumental stimulation with a vibrator, may provide a satisfactory alternative.

For some couples however, the actual penetration of the vagina by the penis is such an integral part of their concept of sexual expression that no alternative forms of pleasuring are acceptable and for them the use of a penile shell, made in the shape of an erect penis and worn over the flaccid organ, provides physical satisfaction for the female partner and psychological satisfaction for the male. This psychological satisfaction may be very important to the maintenance of the man's sexual image, and the knowledge that he can still satisfy his wife by an adapted form of genital intercourse can go far to compensate him for his own lack of full sexual expression.

Alternative devices to simulate erection and permit vaginal penetration are the penile ring, energizer, and various forms of penile splintage.

The penile ring is a rigid ebonite structure which fits over the base of the penis and scrotum; the energizer is an ebonite ring in which several galvanic plates are incorporated; the simplest splint is a soft cylinder of rubber which fits over the basal half of the penis. All three devices produce erection of the penis by obstructing its venous return. In addition, the energizer assists this by producing small stimulant electrical impulses. Internal splintage of the penis may be achieved by surgical implantation of silastic rods into the corpora cavernosa; these rods may be solid or hollow, in which case they are filled from a reservoir by a manually controlled valve.

When a man is intermittently impotent, or has erections which are slow to occur, erratic in duration, and quick to subside, stimulation by vibrator, tongue or lips, or by manual caressing following penile lubrication may encourage the flaccid penis to erect.

GENERAL EFFECTS ON MARITAL AND FAMILY RELATIONSHIPS

The sexual problems derived from disability are not only those of the disabled patient, but also those of the sexual partner. Both resent the restrictions which pain, fatigue, weakness or motor or sensory dysfunction place on the patterns of lovemaking. Spontaneity is replaced by expediency, and the natural expression of sexual desire, excitement and pleasure, is curtailed by the mechanical difficulty of relating movement complexes and body postures productive of the minimal amount of discomfort and maximal pleasure from the restricted range available. This frequently leads to a curtailment of the duration and variety of foreplay and after play, and to the adoption of the most direct and rapid techniques conducive to the production of orgasm. To the distress of both partners, the mechanical aspect of sexual intercourse becomes obtrusive, while the expression of tenderness and caring for which it can form the focal activity is overshadowed or omitted.

A diminished satisfaction in lovemaking may result. The affected partner may fear to compensate for the emphasis on the mechanics of sexual expression which disability induces by being more caring and loving in overall behaviour, lest this be interpreted as an invitation for further unsatisfactory lovemaking. Feelings of guilt, inadequacy, and distress for diminished physical attractiveness and reduced prowess combine with dread of rejection and desertion by the able partner, to produce emotional chaos for the disabled partner.

When the disabled partner is a woman she is torn between the need to maintain her three roles of mother, housekeeper and wife, when fatigue and disability make it difficult to support even one role adequately. She frequently becomes depressed, with further sexual problems, since depression itself reduces sexual drive, and anti-depressant medication can reduce both drive and competence.

As for the able-bodied husband, apart from the sympathy he feels for his disabled wife, frustration and annoyance at her inability to respond to his wish for lovemaking cannot but lead to resentment of her behaviour. He may also have to cope with the extra work in the house and a greater share in the care of the children, while living with a wife whose personality, appearance, and activity have been drastically altered by disablement and its treatment. Understandably, unless the premorbid marital situation was a good one, the husband may well be tempted to find sexual satisfaction outside his marriage, or to walk out of what he feels is an intolerable situation.

When the roles are reversed, and the disabled patient is male, further factors may adversely affect his sexuality. His earning capacity may be reduced, likewise his prowess as a husband and his capability as a father. He feels threatened as a person, and his male self-image suffers because of the more active part which his wife may have to take during lovemaking. All these factors serve to increase his irritation with himself, his illness, his children, and above all, his wife.

She on the other hand, may have to adopt increasing responsibility for maintenance of the house, garden, car, and family, and may have to seek employment to supplement a reduced income. Her sexual drive may be reduced by sheer fatigue, and she may be disinclined for lovemaking unless she feels it is worth the effort; she may find the switchover from nurse to lover a difficult one to accomplish.

Marriage between an able and a disabled person possibly stands a greater chance of success when disablement precedes the marriage, provided both partners have realistic expectations and accurate knowledge on which to base their sexual and day-to-day relationships. When disablement occurs after marriage, comparison with premorbid sexual behaviour and resentment at the inevitable changes incurred by disablement must prejudice the relationship's success. Some disabled people go so far as to say that the happiest marriages of all are between two disabled people, who are able to understand each other's problems, and to appreciate more fully the various aspects of marriage other than the purely sexual one. Companionship, caring, belonging, and the chance to give and receive compassion, understanding and love form the nucleus of any happy marriage, but to these are added a priceless relief from isolation and loneliness when the marital partners are disabled.

Within a marriage in which one or both partners are disabled, infinite courtesy and consideration are essential in day-to-day behaviour to each other, so that the continual frustrations and limitations which disability produces shall not erode their relationship. Within this conscious effort to express love as a continuous act of living, sexual intercourse can then be integrated as a jump-lead recharge of the batteries of sexual love. But sexual intercourse can only occupy a minute fraction of the lives of most couples, and during the remaining time, sexual love can be communicated by touch, voice or expression of face and eyes.

SEXUAL COUNSELLING

What is being done
The acceptance by those giving care of the existence of the sequence:

Chronic disease → Disablement → Sexual Problems

would lead to the routine enquiry for such problems, and to their solution or amelioration in a large number of cases.

Already, the organization called SPOD — The Committee on Sexual and Personal Relationships of the Disabled, launched by the National Fund for Research into Crippling Diseases, is setting up a counselling service in many areas. The Family Planning Association and the Disabled Living Foundation and many individual societies have published numerous books on sexual subjects. Courses and symposia are being held in many districts on the sexual problems of the disabled, both to outline some of the more pressing problems and to alert staff to their presence, and possible means of solution. Many Family Planning Association doctors are skilled in psychosexual counselling, and offer domiciliary visits to disabled people who are unable to attend formal clinics.

What remains to be done
The realization that everyone has the need to love and be loved, and has a further need to express sexuality, could be a useful starting platform from which to assist the amelioration of the sexual problems of the disabled. These needs are not identical. Many disabled people feel both needs and cannot fulfil either one of them. With foresight and organization the freer meeting of able and disabled people should be promoted, so that hopefully they could establish friendly relationships with each other. From these may develop sexual relationships with people of the same or opposite sex, sometimes resulting in marriage or other permanent couple-bonding.

The cultivation of a less reproduction-orientated attitude towards sexual activity would also be helpful. Disablement may cause absent or abnormal function of the sexual apparatus of reproduction or a physical dysfunction of one or other system which positions and activates the body to use this sexual apparatus. If arousal and pleasure remain, however, it does not prevent sexual fulfilment or the giving and receiving of love. Potency and pleasuring are fortunately not synonymous. The erogenous areas of the body are widespread, and those areas with intact central connections may become hypersensitive when disease has rendered others ineffective. Reproduction may be undesirable genetically or impossible mechanically for many disabled people, but the joy of expressing their sexuality with a loved partner is not.

When two people are lucky enough to find each other, fall in love, and marry, their sexual problems may be many but they will at least — or perhaps at most — have love. The marriage of disabled people should therefore be encouraged whenever possible, and every facility which is economically possible should be extended to enable them to live together as independently as possible. Whether disability dictates that they share a room in an institution, a disabled person's flat or bungalow, warden-assisted accommodation or a normal flat or house, the quality of their lives will be greatly improved because they are no longer isolated units, but married people. Accurate assessment of the ability of a couple to manage to live outside an institution may be made during their admission to the assessment flat of a disabled living unit immediately before or shortly after their marriage. Sexual counselling during such admission will solve or ameliorate the problems whenever possible.

When people do *not* find a permanent partner — what then? They may be deprived of love but they need not necessarily be deprived of an outlet for their sexual feelings. Attitude training, not only for the staff of long-stay hospitals and institutions, but for all those giving care to disabled people should teach that self-stimulation manually, or by mechanical or electrical device, is *not* perversion, and that aids to phantasy such as books and pictures which contrive to give pleasure through showing the human body need not be pornographic but can be beautiful. Who accuses Michael Angelo or Leonardo de Vinci of being porn merchants? Or the visitors to art galleries displaying nude paintings and sculptures as being perverted?

Many disabled people cannot get to galleries or museums but they *can* buy and read books showing them the 'body beautiful' and they can phantasize more satisfactorily as a result.

Many homes and institutions frown upon marriage between their inmates, and discourage even the most innocent sexual relationships. But 'the disabled' are not a race apart. They are ourselves as we should have been had disability struck yesterday, or ourselves as we shall be if it strikes tomorrow. Disability does not alter the need to love and to express sexuality. At its highest level, the encouragement of love and marriage between disabled people brings untold joy and satisfaction; at its lowest level, it is much more economical to care for a married couple determined to help each other, than for two single individuals.

In homes, in the waiting rooms of family doctors, and in the outpatient departments of hospitals, it would be helpful if notices could be displayed giving addresses which could be written to for information, i.e. SPOD, the FPA, (which in turn will advise on counselling), literature, the existence of clinics in the vicinity, or the addresses of reputable retailers of apparatus to help those who have sexual problems.

A greater awareness among those giving medical and paramedical care would lead to readier enquiry for the presence of sexual problems from patients disabled for any reason, and to the amelioration by explanation, change of medication, education, or appropriate referral. More clinics, more courses, more interest and routine counselling for newly disabled patients are needed.

Love and marriage for physically handicapped people can be as desirable and wonderful as for the able bodied. Sexual experience can be richly rewarding in the giving and receiving. The right of our disabled patients to experience both demands our recognition and help.

BIBLIOGRAPHY AND REFERENCES

Camplin, J. (1979). *Better Lives for Disabled Women.* London; Virago
Enby, P. (1975). *Let There be Love.* Elek/Pemberton
Greengross, W. (1976). *Entitled to Love.* Mallaby Press, NFRCD
Heslinga, K. (1974). *Not made of stone – the sexual problems of handicapped people.* Staphen Nordquist. Int. Leyden. Thomas, III
Miller, E. J. and Gwynne, G. V. (1972). *A Life Apart.* London; Tavistock
Nordquist, I. (1972). *Life Together.* Swedish Central Committee on Rehabilitation
Shifier, E. (1975). 'Rehabilitating the young paraplegic'. *Brit. J. Sex. Med.* **2**, 21–26
Stewart, W. F. R. (1975). *Sex and the Physically Handicapped.* National Fund for Research into Crippling Diseases, Vincent House, 1 Springfield Road, Horsham

19 Psychological Aspects of Physical Disability

PAUL MARTIN

The importance of psychological factors in the rehabilitation process is well accepted. Clinicians have for many years grappled with such difficult concepts as motivation, attitudes and personality, believing them to be important determinants of the success of rehabilitation programmes. In addition, counselling patients and relatives has always been one of the roles of the rehabilitation team. The interest in psychological aspects of physical disability, however, has grown exponentially in recent years to the extent that a new branch of psychology known as *rehabilitation psychology* is emerging, as evidenced by the formation of a section of the American Psychological Association under this name. The trend is apparent in terms of the increasing scale with which the principles of psychology are being taught to the professions involved in rehabilitation. More research is being carried out resulting in the subject gaining a more sound empirical base. New assessment and treatment techniques are being developed, or adapted from other health-care areas, to come to terms with the complex behavioural problems associated with physical disability.

This chapter on the psychological aspects of physical disability will be divided into three sections. The first will consider the possible relationships between behaviour and physical disability, thereby providing a framework for the subsequent sections — the assessment and treatment of behavioural problems in rehabilitation. Of course, the distinction between assessment and treatment is rather arbitrary, but is convenient for the purposes of presentation.

RELATIONSHIP BETWEEN BEHAVIOUR AND PHYSICAL DISABILITY

An in-depth discussion of the interaction between behaviour and physical disability is well beyond the scope of this book — it would verge on the mind-body problem which has teased the imagination of philosophers for many centuries. It is possible, however, to list some of the factors that must be considered in trying to understand this interaction.

(1) An association between behaviour and physical disability may or may not be a causal one; and causal relationships can be in either of two directions. Hence, behaviour may be a cause, concomitant or consequence of physical disability. Whilst this statement is obvious it is frequently ignored in practice.

In particular, correlations are interpreted as demonstrating causal relationships.

(2) If impairment and disability are differentiated on the grounds of impairment being the medical condition and disability the loss of functional ability resulting from impairment, it becomes clear that behaviour and disability can interact directly at the level of disability or indirectly via impairment.

Diagrammatically the possible inter-relationships can be represented as below.

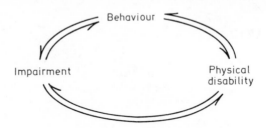

(3) In addition to simple relationships between behaviour and physical, disability, more complex ones are possible in which secondary factors operate. For example, disability may lead to depression which further increases the level of disability.

(4) The behaviour relevant to the relationship between behaviour and physical disability could be that of the patient or of others. For example, physical disability will have consequences for the behaviour of the individual and all those who come into contact with him, (particularly his family).

(5) It is sometimes relevant to distinguish between factors that are important in the onset of a problem, and those that are important during the course of the disorder. For example, behavioural variables are often of no significance in the development of physical disability, but play a major role in determining the level of disability during the subsequent years.

Behavioural factors in the aetiology of physical disability

As physical disability can be caused by such an enormous range of variables (genetic, disease, accident, etc.), the role of behavioural factors in the aetiology of physical disability will clearly vary. This problem has been approached from several perspectives. One such approach is to look for events associated with the onset of impairment and disability. For certain types of disability the events are usually very clear (e.g. those associated with brain damage or amputation), but in others, the situation is more controversial. A good example of the latter is rheumatoid arthritis for which there is some evidence from studies of monozygotic twins discordant for rheumatoid arthritis that onset of this disease is preceded by a period of psychological stress (e.g. serious illness or death in the family, accident, marital discord) with no comparable experience of stress in the unaffected twin. However, this type of hypothesis is usually tested in retrospective studies where reports of such events are very subject to memory distortions by the patients, and bias by both patients and investigators.

An alternative approach is to suggest that certain types of disability are associated with particular personality characteristics. Sometimes authors go further and suggest that these personality characteristics predispose the individual to the disease or illness. Again this type of hypothesis has typically been tested in retrospective studies so that where associations between personality and physical disability have been found the nature of the relationship (i.e. cause, concomitant or consequence) is never clear. However, the current concensus of opinion is that there is no clear evidence of an association between types of physical disability and particular personality characteristics. The almost universal finding from studies in which personality tests have been applied to cases of physical impairment or chronic illness is that the patients are more neurotic in personality (i.e. emotionally labile and possibly predisposed to suffer from psychiatric disturbances), than 'normal' controls.

Finally, the role of behaviour in the aetiology of disability can be analysed in terms of learning theory. This is a complex theoretical area and can only be discussed superficially here. The most fundamental learning principles are that a behaviour increases in frequency if it is followed by positive reinforcement (reward), or results in escape from or avoidance of negative reinforcement (punishment). Conversely, a behaviour decreases in frequency if it is not followed by a reward, or is followed by punishment. Viewed from this perspective it can be seen that much of the behaviour towards the disabled of relatives in the home setting and staff in the hospital setting is inappropriate. For example, if a patient produces 'pain behaviour' (e.g. complaints, grimaces) in the presence of friends and relatives he is likely to receive attention and sympathy (i.e. positive reinforcement), and perhaps will be excused from carrying out tasks he considers undesirable such as digging the garden, or doing the washing up (i.e. avoid negative reinforcement). In this situation, the learning model would predict that the frequency of pain behaviour will increase. An example from the hospital setting is that independent behaviours (e.g. a patient finding his own way to the toilet) are often met with disapproval (i.e. negative reinforcement) whilst passive, dependent behaviours (e.g. asking for a bedpan) are followed by approval (i.e. positive reinforcement), so encouraging dependent rather than independent behaviour. Clearly this may be convenient to staff whilst the patient is hospitalized, but is unlikely to be in the long-term interests of the patient or his relatives.

In some cases, learning processes may largely be responsible for a disabled patient's behaviour, even if the original disability was the result of organic impairment. Wilbert Fordyce has written extensively on this subject with reference to problems of chronic pain. He suggests that patients may initially report pain as a result of some physical stimulus (e.g. low back pain caused by a prolapsed intervertebral disc). Over a period of time the physical problem may be resolved but the patient continues to produce pain behaviour because such behaviour has been rewarded, and has enabled him to avoid carrying out undesirable activities.

One of the advantages of viewing behavioural problems and disability in this way is that it has immediate implications for management — it suggests that the behavioural problems can be remedied by changing the patient's 'environment' (the rewards and punishments consequent on behaviour). The techniques for achieving behaviour change will be discussed in the final section.

Behavioural concomitants of physical disability
Situations in which behavioural variables and physical disability are non-causally related typically arise when behavioural deficits and physical disability are the product of the same organic impairment. The most striking examples are

cases in which the patients have sustained brain damage (e.g. cerebrovascular accident, head injury, cerebral palsy). The behavioural deficits that arise from damage are related to the site and extent of the lesion but the relationship is not perfect — the behaviour of two persons who have the same lesion in a particular area of the brain may vary widely, and there may be similarity in symptoms shown by people with different brain dysfunction.

One of the possible psychological consequences of brain damage is impaired intellectual functioning. For most individuals (approximately 96 per cent of right handers, and 53 per cent of left handers), the left cerebral hemisphere is primarily concerned with language and related skills, and the right cerebral hemisphere is primarily concerned with visuo-spatial and perceptual abilities. Hence, damage to the left hemisphere results in impairment of verbal abilities (e.g. asphasia), whilst damage to the right hemisphere results in visuo-spatial impairment and perceptual difficulties (e.g. visuo-spatial neglect).

Memory impairment is a frequent consequence of brain damage. The impairment is most marked for learning new material — memory for events that took place earlier in life is much less affected. As for intellectual functioning, there is a tendency for left versus right hemisphere damage to correlate with verbal versus visual memory deficits.

Brain damage may lead to impairment of orientation — an individual may not know who he is or where he is, and lose all track of time. Emotional expression can be affected — emotion may become labile (e.g. outbursts of crying or laughter with little or no provocation from the external environment), or all affect blunted. These disturbances are more likely in cases where damage involves the frontal lobes or limbic system.

Investigation of the psychological sequelae of brain damage is one of the major areas for assessment in rehabilitation.

Behavioural consequences of physical disability

Serious physical disability affects a wide range of the individual's life activities — his work, recreational and social activities. It also can have dramatic effects on his family. For example, onset of a severe disability for an individual who is a husband and father is likely to result in his wife assuming greater responsibility for home management and perhaps having to take on extra employment; the children carrying out more household activities and possibly finishing their education earlier than planned; and all the penalties associated with decreased financial circumstances (inferior accommodation, food, clothing, etc.).

The individual will also have to face negative attitudes from most people with whom he comes into contact. Many positive attitudes toward the disabled are expressed publicly but are far outweighed by a generally negative view. The practical disadvantages of most forms of disability are obvious to everyone, although often exaggerated, and knowledge of these disadvantages creates a relatively strong negative attitude, even if this is accompanied by expressions of tolerance, sympathy and understanding. The point is well illustrated by the behaviour of relatives and friends of a girl who expresses interest in marrying a physically disabled man, for example, one who is confined to a wheelchair. Many parents 'understanding' attitude toward the disabled does not extend to support for their daughter's intention to marry such a person.

In cases of sudden onset of severe disability these factors combine to produce an emotional crisis. Individuals experience fears and doubts about survival, and about the competence of those around them to deal with the problem. They do not know what will be possible in the way of functional alternatives given their disabilities, so they tend to underestimate what they will be able to accomplish. They expect to be devalued by others because they themselves have had negative attitudes towards disability. Confusion and disorganization are accompanied by grieving and depression. Depressive reactions may be transitory in traumatic disabilities such as paraplegia but may persist for years in cases of chronic illness. Suicide and other self-destructive behaviours appear to be conserably more common for the disabled than the general population.

PSYCHOLOGICAL ASSESSMENT IN REHABILITATION

A vast range of psychological tests are available — one of the well known books on the subject makes no claim to comprehensiveness and yet lists over three hundred tests under eleven main headings (Anastasi, cited in reference list). Although there is a trend in clinical psychology away from giving tests (particularly those for assessing personality) towards more active involvement in treatment and management, new tests continue to be developed. The Mental Measurements Year Book is a cumulative index of tests which is published every 5 years. Some of the ways in which these tests vary are listed below as they are important in selecting which tests are given:

(1) Purpose of the test. The psychological variables for which tests and scales are available include those for assessing intelligence, memory, aptitudes, creativity, achievements, interests, attitudes, personality and mood. The tests for each of these variables can be categorized under more specific headings. For example, achievement tests for children include those for reading, writing and arithmetic. Tests can also be used for diagnostic purposes such as differentiating between depressive and organic syndromes, or locating cerebral lesions.

(2) Technical aspects of the test. Tests vary in terms of reliability (whether the results are repeatable from one occasion to another, and from one assessor to another), and validity (whether they measure what they purport to measure). Tests also vary as to the standardisation data available (tables of scores obtained by various defined populations on the test). This particular aspect of tests frequently presents a problem in assessing the physically disabled — tests do not have normative data for the physically disabled so that it can be difficult interpreting whether results reflect what the test is supposed to be measuring or the patients disability.

(3) Reception and response systems required by the test. Tests may involve visual or auditory perception, and verbal or motor responses. These factors are particularly important in selecting the most appropriate tests for the physically disabled as there is a need for the reception and response systems to be unimpaired. For example, a test requiring complex motor behaviour (e.g drawing) would not be suitable for a patient suffering from athetoid cerebral palsy, or a test involving understanding the spoken word for a patient suffering from receptive aphasia. When patients have multiple disabilities, it can be very difficult finding an appropriate test.

(4) Practical aspects of the test. Administration of some tests requires specially trained personnel whilst others do not. The same can be said with respect to

scoring and interpreting test results. Tests vary in how long they take to complete – from a few minutes to one of two hours. Some tests can be administered to a large group of individuals whilst others require a one-to-one situation. Group testing is usually not appropriate for assessing patients (as distinct from, say, screening job applicants), so is rarely used with the disabled.

Some of the questions for which psychological testing is most appropriate are as follows. Assessment can play a useful role in determining whether a patient is suffering from any impairment which may affect his ability to benefit from the rehabilitation programme. For example, memory deficits are common in patients with multiple sclerosis, and visuo-spatial difficulties in left-sided hemiplegics; and these problems can interfere with a patient's ability to learn new skills. Determining the exact nature of the disabilities is important as it has implications for management. For example, a right-sided hemiplegic (with disordered language skills) is likely to profit more from pantomime and demonstration instructions than by oral or written instructions, whilst the reverse is true for left-sided hemiplegics (with disordered visuo-spatial abilities). Patients with memory deficits can be taught to minimise the effects of their impairment by using cue cards with printed directions or diagrams (depending on the exact nature of their deficits).

Another important area to which psychological testing can contribute is making predictions and plans for the individual's future. In the case of children, assessments will usually concentrate on the child's abilities on the one hand, and achievements on the other. Where discrepancies exist (i.e. the child is underachieving) it becomes important to first identify and then remove any barriers to progress. For adults assessments are more likely to concentrate on abilities and interests (vocational and recreational). As many physically disabled individuals are going to have to rely on their intellectual abilities, it is particularly important to establish their levels of competence.

A rather different use of psychological tests is to carry out *serial testing* (repeated assessments over a period of time). This is a useful technique for monitoring changes in a patient's condition, whether the changes are for the better or worse. For example, serial testing can be used for assessing the hopefully beneficial effects of spontaneous recovery or treatment; or for monitoring cases where deterioration is anticipated. Serial testing can raise problems of interpretation owing to *practice effects* – superior performance on a test may reflect increasing familiarity with test procedures rather than improvement in the patient's condition. The reverse can also happen – a patient may lose interest with a corresponding drop in performance as a consequence of repeated testing.

Although there are a very large number of tests available a much smaller number are in common usage. The most popular ones come from the areas of assessing intelligence, memory, personality and vocational opportunities and these will be discussed below for illustrative purposes.

Tests of intelligence

Tests of intellectual functioning divide into those for children and those for adults. The two intelligence tests which have been used most extensively are the Wechsler Intelligence Scale for Children (WISC), and the Wechsler Adult Intelligence Scale (WAIS); and both require special training to administer, score and interpret. The WISC is appropriate for children from ages 5 to 15 years, and consists of 12 subtests, six of a verbal or numerical character and six of a performance nature. The verbal subtests yield a verbal IQ, the performance subtests yield a performance IQ, whilst all the results can be combined together to provide a Full Scale IQ. The IQ values show performance relative to age peers, and ordinarily relative position shifts little across the years after the first few years of life.

The profile of scores provides opportunities for assessing the presence or absence of learning deficits relating to brain damage. By observing individuals carrying out a wide variety of standardised tasks, the experienced examiner can gain a great deal of information beyond the actual test scores (e.g. willingness to follow instructions, and ability to concentrate).

In recent years the WISC has largely been replaced by a revised version – WISC–R. All the points made about the WISC apply equally to WISC–R, the latter test merely being an updated version (in terms of questions and norms).

The WAIS is appropriate for ages 16 years and older, and is very similar in format to the WISC. Hence, it too yields measures of Verbal, Performance and Full Scale IQ on the basis of 11 subtest scores. Predictions from the Full Scale IQ are rarely useful as they can usually be made more accurately from other information. Academic performance, for example, is better predicted by examination of class room test results than by IQ estimates. Patient performance in rehabilitation is rarely correlated with overall intelligence, except as regards specific vocational planning or when brain damage is extensive. When brain damage has been largely limited to one cerebral hemisphere, tasks performed by the other hemisphere provide an estimate of premorbid functioning.

One disadvantage of the WISC and WAIS is that they take between one and two hours to administer. More rapid estimates of general intelligence can be gained by either giving a shortened version of the WISC or WAIS, or a briefer test such as the Shipley-Hartford or Quick Test. Another disadvantage to using the WISC and WAIS in Britain is that the norms are extensive but collected on American subjects. With respect to children this problem should be solved when the British Ability Scales are finally published in 1979. This test has 24 scales and is appropriate for children aged 2½ to 17 years.

A problem that sometimes occurs in using the WISC and WAIS with the physically disabled is that the subtests require a complex range of verbal and motor responses. For this reason, Progressive Matrices and Mill Hill vocabulary may be used for assessing intelligence. Progressive Matrices is a perceptual reasoning task and comes in three forms – Coloured Progressive Matrices for children, subnormals and old people; Progressive Matrices for adults in the normal range; and Advanced Progressive Matrices for adults of superior intelligence. Mill Hill vocabulary is a test of verbal ability. Both tests have multiple choice forms so that they only require individuals to be able to signal their choice.

There are intelligence tests for use with children below the age of 5 years. The Stanford–Binet has a lower age limit of 3 years. Developmental scales such as the Bayley and Griffiths can be used from birth. However, performance on these scales does not correlate highly with results of testing later in childhood let alone in adulthood.

Some intelligence tests have been developed for use with special groups. For example, there is a version of the Stanford–Binet appropriate for blind people, and AH6 is a test of intelligence suitable for very intelligent individuals (between whom the WAIS provides little discrimination).

Tests of memory

Assessment of memory functioning should take into account the distinction between immediate, short-term and long-term memory; and between memory for verbal versus visual or perceptual material. As no test measures all these aspects of memory, psychologists often use a 'rag-bag' selection of scales. The most commonly used psychological test of memory is the Wechsler Memory Scale (WMS). It has two forms to reduce interference from practice effects during retesting. The scale consists of seven subtests, six of which deal with language and numbers. All the scores can be combined and used to calculate a Memory Quotient (MQ), but this single score is rarely of any predictive value.

There are several rather similar tests for assessing perceptual memory. The Benton Visual Retention test utilises 10 cards, each containing one or more simple geometric figures. In the standard administration, each card is exposed for 10 seconds and the subject is told to draw what was on the card immediately after its removal. The test thus requires spatial perception, immediate recall, and visuomotor reproduction of drawings. Variations of this test include using a shorter exposure (5 seconds), a 15 second delay, or asking subjects to copy the designs. Detailed instructions are given for scoring subject's performance. The Bender—Gestalt test consists of exposing nine simple designs one at a time, and asking subjects to copy them, or reproduce them from memory. The Graham—Kendall Memory-for-Designs test utilises a series of 15 designs presented briefly one at a time, and subjects are asked to draw each design as soon as it is removed.

Personality assessment

Personality tests can be divided into projective and objective tests. Projective techniques involve presenting subjects with an ambiguous stimulus which they are asked to interpret in some manner or other, and examples include the Rorschach, Draw-A-Person (D-A-P) and Thematic Apperception Test (TAT). Objective tests consist of questionnaires on which subjects have a choice for each question of two or three responses and examples include the Minnesota Multiphasic Personality Inventory (MMPI), Cattell's Sixteen Personality Factor Questionnaire (16 PF), and the Eysenck Personality Inventory (EPI). The rationale of projective techniques is that the stimulus ambiguity promotes projection of inner thought into test behaviour. The proponents of projective techniques argue that this is a more subtle approach to assessing personality functioning than directly asking questions, and consequently it is more difficult for subjects to falsify their responses. The major problem with projective techniques is how to devise reliable, valid scoring systems for the diverse material these techniques yield. Projective techniques also have the disadvantage that trained personnel are required for administration and interpretation, and this can take as long as three to four hours (objective tests can be given by receptionists and interpretation takes only a few minutes).

The Rorschach is the most popular projective technique and is used extensively in America (less so in Britain). It utilizes 10 cards on each of which is printed a symmetrical inkblot, and subjects are asked to tell the examiner what they see (i.e. what the blob could represent). Responses are classified and related to personality traits and diagnostic categories. The D-A-P and TAT use slightly different approaches, the former technique requiring subjects to draw two people of opposite sex, and the latter calling for subjects to make up stories to fit each of 19 pictures.

As with the Rorschach, the MMPI is very widely used in America, and has stimulated an enormous amount of research. It consists of 550 statements to which the examinee answers 'true', 'false' or 'cannot say'. In its regular administration, the MMPI provides scores on ten clinical scales (e.g. 'depression', 'hysteria', 'paranoia'), although research has lead to the development of over 200 new scales some of which are of interest to rehabilitation (e.g. 'low back pain' scale).

The EPI and 16PF are much shorter scales. The EPI provides scores of two clinical scales, 'neuroticism' and 'extraversion'; and the 16PF provides scores of 16 independent factors (e.g. 'assertiveness', 'suspiciousness', 'shyness') as well as two second order factors ('anxiety' and 'extraversion') which are virtually identical to the EPI scales. The latest version of the EPI – the Eysenck Personality Questionnaire has one additional clinical scale ('psychoticism').

There are parallel forms of personality inventories for retesting, and versions for children down to age six years. However, personality tests have never achieved the high levels of reliability of some intelligence tests, and this is one of the reasons for their decline in popularity. Another reason concerns doubts as to their practical utility, particularly with the individual patient as distinct from applications to groups of subjects in research projects.

Vocational tests
Assessment for vocational guidance concentrates on two main areas – what the patient is capable of doing (i.e. his abilities), and what he wants to do (i.e. his interests). With respect to the former, many of the tests described previously could be considered appropriate, particularly those for assessing intellectual functioning. However, it has been appreciated for many years that intelligence tests cover a limited range of abilities (essentially those involved in academic performance), so that aptitude tests have been developed to fill the gaps. The best known test that measures a variety of aptitudes is the General Aptitude Test Battery (GATB), which comprises two tests yielding scores on nine factors (e.g. 'clerical perception', 'motor co-ordination', 'finger dexterity'). Other tests have been designed for measuring specific aptitudes such as mechanical, clerical, artistic and musical aptitudes.

The tests of vocational interests that have been used most extensively are the Strong Vocational Interest Blank and Kuder Preference Record (Vocational). The Interest Bank has 399 items and subjects record their preferences for activities in one of two ways. For items in the first five parts of the test they circle one of the letters L, I or D. (signifying 'like', 'indifferent' or 'dislike'), while for items in the latter three parts of the test they rank given activities in order of preference. Scores are calculated so that the performance of examinees can be compared with criterion groups from 54 different occupations.

A scale which has been developed more recently in Britain is the Applied Psychology Unit (APU) Occupational Interests Guide. This scale is shorter (112 items) than its American counterparts, and simply involves subjects indicating which of pairs of activities they would prefer to do. Results are given in terms of a ranking of eight interest areas (e.g. 'outdoor', 'scientific', 'literary') and jobs appropriate to the different orderings are suggested.

Other psychological tests

One area that has so far not been discussed is assessment of the language and related disorders that can arise as a consequence of brain damage. There are a large number of tests for aphasia available two of the most widely used being Eisenson's Examining for Aphasia, and Schuell's Minnesota Test for Differential Diagnosis of Aphasia. Both consist of large batteries of tests (16 in Eisenson and 47 in Schuell), and assess a wide range of aphasic disorders. A more recently developed set of tests which is superior to the Eisenson and Schuell by virtue of including a scoring system and normative data, and having a more standardised administration, is the Porch Index of Communicative Ability (PICA). The PICA has 18 subtests assessing a narrower range of aphasic disorders, and the results yield scores on three scales (verbal, gestural and graphic), plus an overall score.

Another area in which psychological testing may prove valuable is that of assessing psychiatric disturbance or problems of mood that may interfere with the rehabilitation process. Goldberg's General Health Questionnaire is a test of non-psychotic psychiatric disturbance and has the advantage that shortened versions are available which are suitable for the physically disabled (in the abbreviated versions, items that could reflect physical problems rather than psychiatric disturbance have been removed). Many scales are available for assessing mood such as the Zung Self-rating Depression Scale and Beck Inventory, for depression; and the Taylor Manifest Anxiety Scale and Spielberger State-Trait Anxiety Inventory, for anxiety. Alternatively, the Multiple Affect Adjective Check List gives scores for depression, anxiety and hostility.

Finally, psychological techniques can be used for the assessment of attitudes (attitudes of the disabled, and attitudes towards the disabled). These techniques are likely to be of most interest to those carrying out research into the psychological aspects of disability but are of relevance to the everyday management of patients as research has shown that for some groups of patients (e.g. chronic bronchitics) attitudes are a better predictor of return to work than physical illness variables such as severity of disorder. The technique which has been used most extensively for assessing attitudes is the Semantic Differential which involves patients being asked to rate various concepts on a number of rating scales. An example would be rating the concept 'My work is . . .' on scales such as 'hard — easy', 'pleasant — unpleasant', 'satisfying — unsatisfying'. With respect to assessing attitudes to disability, a scale has been specifically developed for this purpose called the Attitudes towards Disabled Persons scale.

BEHAVIOURAL TREATMENT IN REHABILITATION

This section will concentrate on describing some of the behavioural techniques developed by psychologists and psychiatrists which are particularly relevant to problems of the physically disabled.

Crisis management following onset of disability

As described earlier, sudden onset of severe disability is likely to result in an emotional crisis characterised by confusion, disorganization, anxiety and depression. Wilbert Fordyce has suggested three steps which can be taken to help the newly disabled individual and his family.

(1) Buy time until the patient's coping mechanisms can become more effectively operative. Patients should be encouraged to engage in tasks that are sufficiently simple for them to practise in their distressed state, but are as demanding of their attention as possible. Activities should be selected which are relevant to the aims of the rehabilitation programme, rather than merely diversionary. For example, a paraplegic patient could be taught to weave on an overhead loom as a prelude to a programme for arm strengthening, whilst a hemiplegic with perceptual problems could be given matching tasks to carry out as a prelude to retraining in dressing skills.
(2) Break down problem into workable pieces. The attention of patients should be focussed on elements of their problem that they are capable of solving. For example, a patient could be encouraged to try and sort out with the social worker simple family problems such as transport difficulties arising out of hospitalisation. Successful completion of tasks can give patients a sense of mastery, and the opportunity for receiving the reward of attention and approval from staff and relatives for having engaged in effective performance.
(3) Provide calm, stable models. Individuals in a state of crisis arousal tend to be more susceptible to influence by others than at times of stable functioning, and are consequently more likely to emulate the behaviour of those around them. Hence, it is important for staff to maintain a calm, confident, problem-solving style in the presence of patients. Similarly, visits by relatives and friends should be discouraged or limited until they are able to behave with self control.

As members of the patient's family will also be in a crisis state, the same principles of encouraging individuals to carry out specific, manageable tasks, and providing stable models, can be used to help them.

Behaviour modification
In an earlier section reference was made to the possible role of learning processes in determining the behaviour of the disabled. The same principles of learning can be used to systematically change patients' behaviour, the therapeutic techniques based on these principles being referred to as behaviour modification or behaviour therapy. Hence, the term behaviour modification is used to describe an approach to problems of human behaviour rather than a single specific procedure.

One of the characteristics of behaviour modification that differentiates it from many other approaches to human problems (such as psychotherapy) is that the emphasis is on behaviour rather than inferred, underlying psychic mechanisms. The behaviour itself is considered to be the problem rather than a symptom of a more fundamental disturbance. Consequently, the first step in any behaviour modification programme is to observe and accurately record the patient's behaviour (what he does and does not do). *'Desirable'* versus *'undesirable'* behaviour is distinguished on the grounds of whether the staff, patient and relatives consider the bahaviour should be encouraged or discouraged. The key question in deciding whether a behaviour is desirable or undesirable is whether it will help or hinder a patient's life outside the hospital. *'Deficits of behaviour'* refer to behaviours that would aid a patient's function but are absent, as in cases of lack of speech or domestic skills. The term *'target behaviour'* is used for the behaviour specified as the goal of a behaviour modification programme. *'Frequency'* refers to the rate at which a behaviour occurs, and a *'baseline'* is a record of behaviour frequency taken before training begins. Hence, a measure of a programme's effectiveness can be gained by comparing the frequency after training with the baseline.

Behaviour modification approaches the problem of changing the frequency of behaviour by manipulating the consequences of behaviour. A *'positive reinforcer'* (or reward) is any stimulus which increases or maintains the frequency of a behaviour when it occurs immediately after the behaviour. A *'negative reinforcer'* (or punisher) is any stimulus which decreases the frequency of a behaviour when it occurs immediately after the behaviour. Stimuli accompanying or just preceding any positive reinforcers come to function as positive reinforcers themselves and are referred to as *'conditioned reinforcers'* (similarly stimuli can become *'conditioned punishers'*) For example, a mother who provides warmth and food for her baby becomes a conditioned reinforcer.

Reinforcers have to be identified for each person being trained and this can be done in several ways. One is to ask the patient what he likes to do (e.g. go for a walk, sleep), or to have (e.g. cigarettes, sweets). Another way is to observe how the patient spends his time when given the opportunity (e.g. watching television, eating, sitting in a particular chair). These are called *'high probability behaviours'* and may be used to reinforce desirable behaviours of lower probability. For a stimulus to be used as a reinforcer it must be under the control of the staff so that it can be presented immediately after the occurrence of desirable behaviour (delay decreases reinforcer effectiveness). This is not possible for many potential reinforcers such as home visits or going swimming. A solution to this problem is to give tokens or points immediately following the desirable behaviour which can later be exchanged for any of a range of reinforcers.

There are three main techniques for reducing the frequency of a behaviour. One method is to present negative reinforcement after undesirable behaviour, sometimes referred to as *'aversive conditioning'*. As technical and ethical objections can be raised against this procedure, it is preferable to use the other two methods if possible. A second approach is to withdraw the positive reinforcers which are maintaining the behaviour, a process known as *'extinction'*. Finally, it is sometimes possible to reduce the frequency of a behaviour by rewarding an incompatible behaviour. For example, if the objective of a programme is to reduce the time a patient spends sitting down, he could be rewarded for standing up.

A variety of *schedules of reinforcement* (programmes according to which reinforcement is delivered) can be used for changing the frequency of a behaviour. Each occurence of the desired response can be followed by a reward (*continuous reinforcement,*) or only a proportion of the desired responses followed by a reward (*intermittent* or *partial reinforcement*). Continuous reinforcement more quickly produces an increase in the frequency of the bahaviour it follows than intermittent reinforcement, but this increase will extinguish more rapidly if reinforcement is not maintained. Consequently, a common strategy is to begin reinforcing on a continuous schedule, and then change to an intermittent schedule as the behaviour becomes established.

If a desired behaviour does not occur at all, it can be established by initially reinforcing approximations to it. Gradually reinforcement is restricted to behaviour which is increasingly similar to that desired. The process of rewarding successive approximations to the target behaviour is known as *shaping.*

To help ensure that desired behaviour occurs, *prompting* can be used. Prompts can take many forms such as verbal comments and suggestions, gestures and signals, or written instructions and diagrams. *Fading* is a training procedure in which a prompt is gradually withdrawn so that the behaviour can continue without the supporting stimulus. An example of fading would be gradually reducing the number of words in a verbal instruction, or reducing its loudness.

A final technique which can be used for establishing a behaviour is *modelling* — the therapist provides a model for the patient to imitate. For example, a therapist might demonstrate to a patient how he should use a dressing aid. Modelling can itself be developed by first demonstrating a simple component of the desired skill. The patient is then reinforced for any approximation to the model. Gradually more complex demonstrations are arranged as the patient succeeds at each progressive imitation.

Behaviour modification techniques have been increasingly applied to the problems of the physically disabled since the mid-1960s. Laurence Ince has comprehensively reviewed this area and his book is cited in the reference list. Applications in physiotherapy and occupational therapy include those to problems of ambulation, wheelchair propulsion, posture, muscle weakness, spasticity, movement, co-ordination, typing, writing and use of orthotic devices. Behavioural techniques have also been used for treating speech and language problems (e.g. dysarthria, aphasia); and in the assessment of auditory impairments. Other areas of application include motivational problems, disruptive behaviour, pressure sores, bladder control and chronic pain.

The application of behaviour modification techniques becomes clearer by considering concrete examples. Two case studies will be briefly mentioned here, both described by Ince, the first carried out by Goodkin and the second by Sand and his colleagues. Goodkin's patient was a woman with Parkinsons Disease who was considered physically able to propel her wheelchair but who refused to do so. She said that there was no point in trying to propel the wheelchair as even small children could do so faster than she could. Goodkin prepared for the treatment sessions by marking the floor with red tape at five foot intervals for a distance of 20 feet. Sessions were divided into trials during which the patient had to propel her wheelchair forward for a distance of five feet. On the first day, a baseline measure was obtained of the time taken to do this. One minute rest periods followed each trial.

Treatment began on the second day. The patient was reinforced for faster times by telling her that she was doing well, and telling her the number of seconds it took her to travel 5 ft. At the end of the sessions, the patient was informed of her average time for the session, and this was compared with that of the previous session. The patient was seen for just 3 days before discharge from hospital during which her mean times per trial were 24.8, 18.9 and 17.8 seconds, and the numbers of trials she completed were 6, 8 and 11.

The patient of Sand was a 7 year-old boy who had sustained brain damage at age 4½ years. After an initial rehabilitation programme, the boy had learned to ambulate with a wheeled walkerette and use a few words but he had been re-admitted to hospital as a result of making little progress since being discharged.

In hospital he appeared to understand his need for rehabilitation but progress was severely hampered by frequent temper tantrums characterized by spitting, kicking, biting and loud screaming. The tantrums occurred most frequently when he was asked to do something which was mildly uncomfortable such as physiotherapy exercises, or when he was requested to try a new activity e.g. self-feeding.

The investigators observed that the attention received by the patient following his maladaptive behaviour appeared to be maintaining its frequency. In addition, they thought that signs of progress would not be as clear or as meaningful to a child as they were for adults. The nurses and therapists were instructed to put the child in his room for 15 minutes as soon as he began a tantrum, thus removing the opportunity for paying attention to the tantrum behaviour (a procedure referred to as *time-out*). They were also asked to give him tokens when he did as he was instructed, or when he worked on new or difficult tasks. At the end of each day these tokens could be exchanged for small toys, sweets, a picnic lunch or other tangible rewards.

The introduction of these contingencies led to a marked reduction in disruptive behaviours. During the fifth week, an eight day period was introduced during which neither tokens nor time-out periods were used, but praise was given for good performance. As disruptive behaviour increased during physiotherpy but not occupational therapy sessions, the token and time-out procedures were reinstated during the former but not the latter. The reinstatement resulted in the problem behaviours significantly declining. At the end of the rehabilitation programme, the child had made excellent progress in terms of independent ambulation and self-feeding, as well as being more well-behaved.

Biofeedback training

Biofeedback training consists of using instrumentation to provide subjects with moment to moment information concerning some biological process as an aid to their learning to control the process. The 'information' referred to can be presented in three modalities — auditory (e.g. tone varying in frequency), visual (e.g. needle deflections on a scale), or tactile (e.g. vibrations varying in rate.). The range of 'biological processes' that biofeedback has utilised is enormous and includes electromyographic activity, electroencephalographic activity, heart rate, blood pressure, galvanic skin response, skin temperature and stomach acid pH. The word 'control' is potentially deceptive as biofeedback training is usually aimed at simply producing increases or decreases in the variable monitored. Occasionally the treatment goal has required a more sophisticated form of control as in instances where subjects have been instructed to use the biofeedback to perform a tracking task (cause the monitored process to track a stimulus).

Just as a wide range of biological processes have been utilized for biofeedback training, so the technique has been applied to a diversity of clinical problems. These include epilepsy, migraine, cardiac arrhythmias, hypertension, encopresis, tension headaches, insomnia, anxiety, athetoid cerebral palsy, spasmodic torticollis, bronchial asthma, stuttering, hemiplegia, Bell's palsy, Huntington's chorea and poliomyelitis. Clinical applications of biofeedback training have usually involved patients attending a hospital facility for two or three sessions per week over several weeks. In addition, *home trainers* (simple, portable versions of biofeedback instrumentation) have sometimes been lent to patients so that training can be continued at home. The strategy of giving patients *homework assignments* (and asking patients to keep records of their achievements) is common in behaviour therapy. Written instructions pertaining to the assignments are often given to patients (and relatives too if they can be of any assistance), and this technique is sometimes elevated to providing comprehensive, self-help manuals.

Of the various areas to which biofeedback training has been applied, the use of electromyographic (EMG) feedback training with neuromuscular problems appears most relevant to rehabilitation (the literature in this area has been comprehensively reviewed in an article by Inglis which is cited in the reference list). Treatment of hemiplegia following stroke has been reported by a number of authors. John Basmajian, for example, used a combination of EMG feedback training and therapeutic exercises with patients suffering from chronic foot drop. Surface electrodes were attached over the tibialis anterior muscle and patients were given visual and auditory EMG feedback to help them learn to increase the EMG activity in this muscle. Results were impressive in terms of increased strength of dorsiflexion, increased range of movements, and improved gait.

An application calling for the opposite response — a decrease in EMG activity — was reported by Swaan. His patients showed undesirable contractions of the peroneus longus muscle whilst stretching the knee joint (they were hemiplegic or had suffered from poliomyelitis). The patients were taught to inhibit this motor activity with the aid of auditory EMG feedback. A novel use of EMG feedback which appears to have potential is training subjects to control prosthetic devices by the firing of single motor units. Some promising results were reported in the literature during the early 1970s, but this application has received little attention since.

Whilst biofeedback training appears to be a useful adjunct treatment for a variety of clinical disorders, there is still a shortage of hard evidence pertaining to its efficacy. Most of the literature consists of case studies which suffer from lack of experimental control and poor outcome measures. However, single case experiments and controlled group designs are being used with increased frequency so that the advantages and limitations of biofeedback training should become much clearer in the ensuing decade.

Other behavioural treatments

Many behavioural treatments which have largely been developed in psychiatric settings can be used to advantage in rehabilitation. It is beyond the scope of this chapter to do more than briefly mention some of the techniques that are most relevant to treatment of the physically disabled. This will inevitably fail to do justice to the behaviour therapies by making the approach sound oversimplistic but will hopefully enlighten the reader as to the potential areas of application and the types of procedures currently available.

As has been stressed previously, physical disability (particularly its onset) is often associated with disturbances of mood such as excessive depression and anxiety. A large number of behavioural treatments for anxiety have been developed, the best known of which is *systematic desensitization.* This technique involves three main procedures. Initially a list of anxiety evoking items is organized into a hierarchy (ranging from situations or objects which arouse very slight anxiety, to those which cause high levels of anxiety). The second stage consists of relaxation training which can be done in a number of different ways (e.g. progressive relaxation, autogenic training). The final stage is to gradually progress up the hierarchy with the patient relaxing in the presence of the anxiety evoking items. Hence, the patient imagines the first item on the hierarchy (or is confronted with it *in-vivo*), and then uses his newly acquired skills to relax. When he is able to successfully do this the next item from the hierarchy is presented.

The behavioural treatment of depression has received less attention. Most authors on this subject suggest the use of a variety of procedures. An example of one such procedure is termed *self-reinforcement* which involves four steps. First the person establishes standards for what he considers to be an acceptable performance. Then the person performs the task and evaluates his performance according to these standards. Finally, the person administers a positive or negative reinforcer to, or withholds a postive reinforcer from, himself.

Another area to which behavioural techniques have been applied, which is very relevant to the problems of the physically disabled, is that of marital discord and sexual dysfunctioning. Masters and Johnson have formulated therapeutic techniques for the whole range of sexual disorders (e.g. impotence, premature ejaculation, orgasmic dysfunction) and their approach has two main elements — counselling and directed practice. The aims of counselling include discussion of factors that might have contributed to the presenting problem; education with regards pelvic anatomy and sexual response; encouragement of more communication between partners; and discussion of feelings, attitudes, and expectancies associated with the relationship. The directed practice involves a period of *sensate focus* for all couples during which they are encouraged to explore sensate rather than sexual sensation (by stroking and massaging each other). This prelude is followed by a series of procedures which are specific to the presenting problem.

Simultaneous use of several techniques is usually advocated for treating marital discord one of which is *behavioural or contingency contracting*. As the name implies, this technique refers to specification in writing of behaviour expected from one or more individuals and the ways in which they will provide reinforcement for the emission of desired behaviour. Contracts can be between therapist and patient, or between two patients.

A third area in which behavioural techniques can be utilised with the disabled is that of social skills. Onset of physical disability results in the individual having to learn to cope with people behaving differently towards them (e.g. reluctance to allow them to do certain activities, staring, looks of disgust). Social skills training is usually conducted in groups and includes *modelling* and *role-playing*. Modelling refers to demonstrations for the patient to imitate and can be given by the therapist or another patient. In role-playing, patients are encouraged to practise handling the situations they find difficult, and this typically followed by feedback from the therapist, and sometimes, other patients.

Finally, behavioural treatments can be applied to the problem of 'addictive' behaviours, the two most relevant to physical disability being over-eating and smoking cigarettes. Reducing weight is an important part of the management of patients suffering from disorders such as heart disease and back pain; whilst reducing smoking is important for those suffering from chest disorders such as chronic bronchitis. The behavioural treatment of obesity has emphasized the development of self-control skills featuring techniques such as self-reinforcement, and contingency contracting. Contingency contracting to reduce weight in obese patients usually involves returning sums of their money contingent upon weight loss. A wide variety of different behavioural techniques have been employed in attempts to reduce cigarette smoking including systematic desensitization, role-playing, contingency contracting and aversive conditioning procedures.

BIBLIOGRAPHY AND REFERENCES

Anastasi, A. (1971). *Psychological testing.* 3rd edn. London; Macmillan

Cobb, B. (Ed.) (1973). *Medical and Psychological Aspects of Disability.* Springfield Illinois; Chas. Thomas

Fordyce, W. E. (1968). 'Psychology and rehabilitation'. In Licht S. (Ed.) *Rehabilitation and Medicine.*

Fordyce, W. E. (1971). 'Psychological assessment and management'. In Krusen, F. M., Kottke, F. J. and Ellwood, P. M. (Eds). *Handbook of Physical Medicine and Rehabilitation.* 2nd edn. Saunders

Fordyce, W. E. (1976). *Behavioural methods in chronic pain and illness.* Mosby

Ince, L. P. (1976). *Behaviour Modification in Rehabilitation Medicine.* Springfield Illinois; Chas. Thomas

Inglis, J. Campbell, D. and Donald, H. W. (1976). 'Electromyographic biofeedback and neuromuscular rehabilitation'. *Canad. J. Behav. Sci./Rev. Canad Sci. Comp.* 8, 299–323

Kazdin, A. E. and Wilson, G. T. (1978). *Evaluation of Behaviour Therapy: Issues, Evidence and Research Strategies.* Ballinger

McDaniel, J. W. (1976). *Physical Disability and Human Behaviour.* 2nd edn. Oxford; Pergamon

Michael, J. L. (1970). 'Rehabilitation'. In Neuringer and Michael (Eds). *Behaviour Modification in Clinical Psychology.* Appleton Century Crofts

Neff, W. (1971) (Ed). *Rehabilitation Psychology.* Washington, D.C.; American Psychological Association

Rutter, B. M. (in press). 'The prognostic significance of psychological factors in the management of chronic bronchitis'. *Psychological Medicine*

20 Research in Rehabilitation

PAUL MARTIN

PRINCIPLES OF RESEARCH

There is a considerable and continuing demand for research into all aspects of rehabilitation medicine. In spite of the fact that research is a prerequisite for advance in medical treatment adequate research in rehabilitation is singularly lacking. Most physical treatment regimes and rehabilitation programmes are a blunderbuss compendium of treatment, quite unevaluated.

The effects of conventional rehabilitation derive from a variety of people (doctors, therapists, nurses, social workers, counsellors, etc.) in a variety of situations.

The outcomes sought, in the clinical situation, are a behavioural response — return home from hospital, return to work, independence in activities of daily living.

Research in rehabilitation is needed in order to evaluate the effectiveness of the various components and to establish features enabling prediction of response to the various components. The complexity of the situations in rehabilitation makes research difficult.

It is hoped that this chapter will help those intending to carry out research in this field. However, even for those with no such intentions, there are advantages to becoming familiar with research principles; such knowledge is of value in situations where the clinician comes into contact with research and it can directly benefit clinical practice. A deeper understanding of all aspects of research aids critical reading of books and journals, and is useful when help is solicited by those wishing to carry out research. The potential for directly benefitting clinical practice results from the fact that, to a large extent, the principles of good research and good clinical practice are the same, since approaching problems in a logical systematic manner, stating the aims clearly, critically evaluating assumptions, and comprehensive assessment are as appropriate to clinical work as research.

Classification in research

Three ways of classifying different types of research will be considered here: descriptive versus manipulative; retrospective versus prospective; and cross-sectional versus longitudinal. Manipulative research differs from descriptive in that it involves an attempt at influencing the situation being studied. A treatment trial would be an example of the former, whilst a survey would be an example of the latter. Prospective studies are forward looking whilst retrospective studies look to the past. For example: if the aetiology of a disorder was the focus of interest, some light might be thrown on the problem by studying the records of all patients with this disorder. Such an investigation would be a retrospective one. The prospective approach would be to study a large population at two points in time — before and after some members of the population developed the disorder. Cross-sectional studies involve measurements on each individual at one moment in time, whilst longitudinal studies involve repeated measurements on each individual over a period of time. For a cross-sectional study of the relationship between age and intelligence, intelligence would be measured across a wide age range. To investigate the same problem longitudinally intelligence would be measured repeatedly on a number of individuals as they aged.

Classifying into these dichotomies is not always appropriate as some research studies fall into both categories of the dichotomies. In the examples given above of studying the relationship between age and intelligence, the problem could be tackled with a combined cross-sectional and longitudinal approach. Hence, intelligence could be measured across a wide age range at a particular moment in time, and then subsequent measures carried out as the population aged.

The main advantage of considering classifications in research is that it stresses the wide variety of forms that research can take. This is important as clinicians often believe that their circumstances make research impossible, when in fact they only limit the *type* of research that is feasible.

Stages in research

The stages typically involved in a research project can be represented diagrammatically:

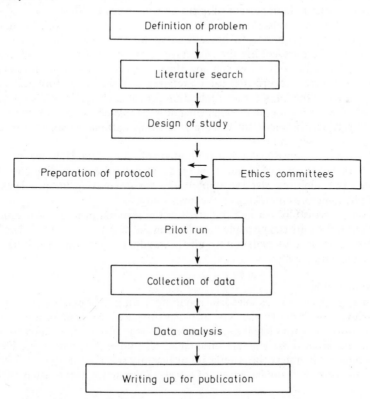

These stages are interactive rather than independent and no one stage can be completed in isolation. In addition, the stages may proceed out of sequence. For example, the literature search could lead to re-defining the problem, or the results of the pilot run might necessitate a change in design.

The first stage — definition of the problem — refers to transforming the original ideas for the research into the form of testable hypotheses. The ideas may come from clinical experience, reading an article or book, a previous experiment, or discussion with a colleague. Time must be spent thinking about the ideas, the implications and possible alternatives. The thinking process inevitably needs to be accompanied by further reading and discussion.

Literature searches necessitate the availability of a library although extensive facilities are not necessary as librarians can usually borrow books and journals or obtain photocopies. For those unfamiliar with using medical libraries books are available on this subject. The two main approaches to searching the literature are use of Abstracts Journals (e.g. Index Medicus and Excerpta Medica) or computer retrieval systems (e.g. Medlars and Medline). The former approach requires scanning the subject indexes whilst the latter involves feeding key words into the system. As papers are accumulated the cited references provide an additional source of material. Also, other workers in the field can be contacted for suggestions. In literature searches it is important to remember that information must be sought on all aspects of the proposed research. For example, it is often necessary to seek papers on outcome measures as well as the central theme of the study.

The design of the study refers to the proposed plan and will not be discussed further here as it is an important subject that will be dealt with separately.

As plans are formulated they should be recorded as a protocol. In addition to allowing the proposals to be scrutinised by the local ethics committee, preparation of a protocol has the advantage of encouraging the research worker to be explicit about objectives and how they are to be achieved. A protocol also serves as a concrete record that can be referred to if details are forgotten and it may be used as the basis for an application for research funds. It also provides the basis for writing up the research when it is completed. A comprehensive protocol is particularly important when participating staff may change before completion of the research project.

The pilot run consists of a first attempt at collecting data. How ever carefully plans have been formulated, practical problems will arise when they are implemented. The pilot run gives an opportunity for discovering the problems and solving them before embarking on the main study.

Having successfully reached this stage in the research process, preparation is complete and a start can be made on collecting the data to be analysed. The final stages of data analysis and writing up the results for publication will be dealt with in separate sections.

Selection of subjects

The first problem to be solved in acquiring a subject population for clinical research is how to define the type of patient required. To achieve this, a set of criteria must be formulated which *unambiguously* differentiates those suitable for the trial from those who are unsuitable. All studies should be replicable and this is impossible unless the criteria are sufficiently specific for other researchers to be able to collect similar groups of subjects. In practice, this is often difficult to achieve but there is never any excuse for such vague criteria as *patients suitable for this form of therapy*, without further elaborating how this is to be interpreted.

Having decided on the criteria, the next question is how to get the patients. Any *single* source will be a 'biased sample'. It will reflect such factors as the interests of the clinician referring the patient, and the geographical area in which the study is being conducted. This is important in determining the implications of the results – the findings will only be applicable to patient populations that are similar to the one in the study. For this reason it is important to seek referrals from a number of clinicians, and replicate the research in other centres.

It is often difficult to decide how many subjects should be included. A simple 'rule of thumb' is to have a minimum of 10 patients in each group but often many more are needed. The first factor to be considered is the homogeneity of the subject population – the more variable the patient problems the more patients will be required. The second factor concerns the objectivity of the outcome measures – the more subjective the measures the more patients will be needed. The final factor is the amount of variance in the data. The more variability the more patients will be required. Of course, it is unlikely that such information will be available on these factors until some pilot data has been collected, so that the estimates of numbers of subjects usually has to await this stage.

Some patients who are initially included in a research project will not remain in it (sometimes referred to as 'subject attrition'). The usual procedure is to replace these 'drop-outs' but it is essential to record and report all such instances. Ignoring the potential biasing effect of subject attrition can lead to very erroneous conclusions being drawn.

RESEARCH DESIGN

Although most designs more or less conform to one of a few well established patterns, the number of variations are infinite. There is no such thing as the correct design – plans are formulated with many considerations in mind and merely vary in terms of how well they come to terms with the problems.

The major factor involved in selecting the most appropriate design is the degree to which it will enable the data unambiguously to test the experimental hypotheses. For example, when interested in evaluating the efficacy of a physiotherapy technique it is of little value simply to give this form of treatment to a group of patients and assess the results. If the group improved two major questions remain unanswered: would they have recovered spontaneously (i.e. without treatment), and were they responding to the non-specific elements of treatment (e.g. receiving attention) rather than anything specific (e.g. effect of exercises on muscle strength)? A more sophisticated design would be that in which one group received the treatment of interest, another received a 'placebo' treatment (i.e. *were given the same amount of therapist attention but no actual treatment)*, and another received no treatment (a 'waiting list' control condition). This design would enable separate evaluation of the specific and non-specific (placebo) benefits of treatment over and above what might be expected on the grounds of spontaneous recovery. Most research projects generate more questions, or can be criticised. For example, it might be claimed that observed differences between the effectiveness of a treatment and a control procedure were due to differences in the plausibility of the procedures rather than a specific action of the treatment (i.e. the patient's response to the treatment was superior because it was more plausible, and therefore led to higher expectations of success). This claim could be evaluated by describing the treatment and control procedures to a group of subjects and asking them to rate the expectations of success they would have if they received these 'treatment' procedures.

In choosing the most appropriate research design there are also a whole host of practical factors that need to be taken into account. Some designs will require more time to complete than others. Availability of apparatus for assessment and treatment must be considered, and the personnel who are prepared to participate (e.g. it is impossible to evaluate a treatment without practitioners skilled in its use, or conduct research requiring sophisticated data analysis without the services of someone competent in statistics).

Ethical considerations

Most professional societies have produced their own guidelines (one such set appears in the reference list). Some ethical principles pertain to the way in which individuals should be approached – information should be given as to what participation in the research would involve, and the experimenter should give his name and occupation. Individuals (or parents in the case of children) should then be asked whether they wish to participate (i.e. the research worker is seeking 'informed consent'), and their right to withdraw at any stage emphasized. Other ethical guidelines concern the wellbeing of the patient during and after the research project. Clearly, there is an obligation to avoid assessments or treatments that are potentially harmful, and confidentiality must be respected. Patients in control groups should be offered treatment if they fail to improve during the control period. Provision should always be made for patients to be withdrawn from the research project if there is any suggestion that this is in their best interests (e.g. a deterioration in their condition). Submitting detailed research proposals to an ethics committee acts as a safeguard and some journals require proof that this stage was carried out before they will accept reports of the research. It should also be remembered that ethics committees can be approached for advice at the beginning of the planning research rather than simply being used as a means of vetting finalized proposals.

In designing research there are certain principles that are always worth bearing in mind. It is essential, for example, to think the whole research process through before starting. Hence, questions should be considered such as: what data is to be collected; how will it be analysed; what sort of conclusions may be drawn; and what implications might these conclusions have? Although this strategy may sound obvious all too often data are collected because they are considered 'interesting' and problems of analysis and potential implications are only considered afterwards.

It is also important to keep the research simple. It is difficult enough to answer convincingly one or two questions in a research project let alone more. Research always takes longer than anticipated. In estimating the time to complete projects it is wise to try to anticipate all the problems that could arise. A realistic estimate can then be gained by assuming all these problems will occur and then doubling the time period calculated on this basis!

Other factors to be considered in designing research can best be illustrated by considering some of the basic designs available. Research designs can be divided into *group designs* and *single case experiments,* although some combination of these methodologies is possible. In group designs data from a number of subjects are pooled together whilst in single case experiments the focus of attention is on the individual.

Before discussing these different types of design it is necessary to define some terms. The variables in an experiment can be divided into independent and dependent. Independent variables (IV) are those which the experimenter manipulates or decides the value of in advance of the study. Dependent variables (DV) are those whose values are observed in the course of the study. For example, in a trial investigating the effectiveness of three physiotherapy regimes on pain ratings, the different treatments would constitute the IV and the ratings of pain the DV. The different values of the IV are referred to as levels, so that in the example just given the IV had three levels (corresponding to the three different treatments). An alternative name for an IV is a factor, so that experiments involving only one IV are called single factor experiments, and those involving more than one IV are called multi-factorial experiments. An example of a multi-factorial experiment would be a comparison of two drugs each given in one of four doses. This experiment would have two IV ('drugs' and 'doses'), having two and four levels.

Group designs

There are essentially two types of group designs. Subjects can be divided into several groups and each group can receive a different treatment. In this type of design the problem is in determining whether any differences between the results of the groups are due to differences between the subjects in the groups or to the differential effectiveness of the treatments. This problem can be overcome by using the second type of design – giving all subjects all the treatments. Of course, if two treatments are being compared it is inappropriate to give all subjects one treatment followed by the other. Using this design any apparent superiority of one treatment over the other could merely reflect the fact that it was given first or last (i.e. an 'order effect'). This problem can be overcome by giving half the subjects treatment A followed by treatment B and the remaining subjects treatment B followed by treatment A (i.e. using the cross-over design). Unfortunately the strategy of giving all the subjects all treatments cannnot always be adopted (as in the case of comparing two forms of operation!)

There are two main methods of assigning subjects to groups – random allocation and matching. The name of the first method speaks for itself and is typically carried out using a random numbers table (lists of numbers bearing no relation to each other). If subjects are to be allocated to three groups the random numbers table is scanned for numbers 1 to 3 and a list made. This list determines which treatment each subject will receive. Hence, if the number 2 was the first to appear in the table the first subject would receive treatment 2. Other random procedures can be utilised such as tossing a coin or rolling a dice.

In practice, a pseudo-random procedure is often used. For example, if two treatments are to be compared, alternate referrals could be assigned to one group then the other. This procedure has many practical advantages arising from the fact that whenever an even number of patients have been entered into the trial the treatment groups contain equal numbers. However, if for any reason alternate referrals could systematically differ (e.g. as a result of coming from different clinics) this method of allocation would bias the results.

Allocating subjects to groups by matching is sometimes used when a variable (X) is believed to have an important influence on the dependent variable (Y). If subjects are to be split into two groups matching proceeds by dividing the subjects into pairs, each member of which is equivalent in terms of variable X, and randomly allocating one member of each pair to each group. For example, in an investigation of the effects of two exercise regimes (the IV) on strength (the DV) it might be anticipated that age (variable X) would have an important influence on the results. In this case subjects could be 'matched' for age (i.e. patients of approximately the same age could be paired together).

The purpose of matching is to ensure that the results are not the product of the variable X rather than the independent variable Y (in the example above, differences in strength occur as a consequence of the exercise regimes adopted rather than because one group has younger subjects than the other). The acceptability of matching is a matter of some controversy as it is argued that researchers typically do not really know what variables to match for, and by systematically allocating subjects to groups in this way they create the possibility of biasing their results. If matching is not adopted a check should be made after completing the study that the groups are not significantly different in terms of the variables that could have been matched for. Should such differences be found, the data could prove very difficult to interpret.

Single case experimental designs
Group designs have many disadvantages both technical and practical. This approach involves pooling the data and calculating means which can obscure individual patterns of response. Group designs require large numbers of relatively homogenous subjects which are often not available. They also typically involve a large investment of time and as such are not usually practical for those who are not full time researchers. A recently developed approach to research is the use of single case experiments. In essence, the basis of this approach is to plan treatment for individual patients so that they can act as their own controls. The notion is that each treatment of a patient is an experiment in its own right. Of course, results have to be replicated for generalizations to be made, so ideally single case experiments are carried out in series (i.e. several patients are treated).

There are two main types of single case experiments — reversal designs and multiple baseline designs. The rationale for reversal designs is to study the effects of treatment by looking at what happens when treatment is started and when it is withdrawn (the 'reversal'). If a patient is treated and improves it is not clear whether this is a specific effect of treatment (as distinct from a nonspecific effect or spontaneous recovery). A better test of treatment effectiveness is obtained if patients are monitored for a period prior to treatment — should patients only improve after the introduction of treatment, it is less likely that this can be explained as spontaneous recovery. Pre-treatment assessments of this nature are usually referred to as 'baseline' assessments. A more powerful design would be to monitor the patient before, during and after treatment. If some deterioration followed withdrawal of treatment this would suggest that treatment was important to the patient's improvement. The process of adding and subtracting treatment can be carried on indefinitely. Hence, a baseline period can be followed by treatment which is then withdrawn prior to reinstatement. If no-treatment periods are denoted by A and treatment periods by B then this design would be referred to as an A-B-A-B design. An illustration of the pattern of results that would be expected evaluating an effective treatment with this design is produced below.

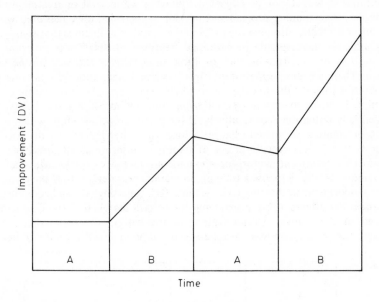

Figure 1. Reversal design

Hence, in this example, the patient's condition did not change during the baseline period, but improved as soon as treatment was started. Some deterioration took place when treatment was withdrawn and further improvement occurred when treatment was restarted.

More sophisticated reversal designs can be used. For example, in assessing a drug the objective might be to estimate the 'placebo' effect and 'active ingredient' effect independently. If the effects of 'no drug', 'placebo drug' and 'active drug' were labelled, A, B and C, respectively, an A-B-BC-B-BC design could be used. In a similar way, elements of a treatment package can be evaluated by withdrawing and reinstating them.

There are certain rules pertaining to reversal designs. Firstly, the baseline phase should be continued until the patient's condition is steady or deteriorating. If there is a trend towards improvement during the baseline phase it is very difficult to evaluate whether any additional improvement during treatment is really a function of the treatment. In plotting the data it is essential to have at least three data points for each phase of the design as three is the minimum number necessary for discerning a trend. Ideally, each phase should have far more data points. Only one variable should be changed at a time as contravening this rule results in difficulties of interpretation. For example, if an A-BC design was used it would not be clear whether improvement during the second phase was due to the introduction of B or C. Finally, each phase of the design should be the same length. The reason for this rule is that if treatment is conducted over periods of 10 days but only withdrawn for periods of 3 days it is difficult to decide whether improvement occurred during treatment phases as a function of time or treatment.

One of the main problems with reversal designs is that in certain situations, deterioration would not be expected following withdrawal of treatment. For example, some training programmes develop skills which once mastered would not suffer from discontinuing the programme. Another problem is that sometimes it is ethically unacceptable to withdraw treatment. A single case experimental design that suffers from neither of these drawbacks is the *multiple baseline design*. There are three types of multiple baseline designs although only one will be described here — the so-called 'across behaviours' type. With this approach an attempt is made to change several behaviours by modifying the behaviours sequentially rather than consecutively. If the particular behaviour to which treatment or training is applied changes whilst the other behaviours do not this suggests that it is a specific effect of treatment bringing about the change, as non-specific treatment factors or spontaneous recovery should affect all the behaviours equally. Suppose a training programme was devised to make a patient more independent in dressing (A), cleaning (B), toiletting (C), and cooking (D). To assess the effects of the programme the behaviours (A, B, C and D) could be trained in that order. An illustration of the pattern of results that would indicate the programme was having a specific training effect is produced below.

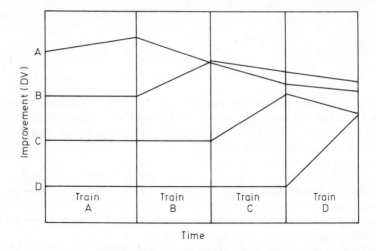

Figure 2. Multiple baseline design

For the multiple baseline design to be used there is a need for at least three to four 'baselines' (behaviours). In addition, the behaviours must be independent because in some situations training effects will generalise from the target behaviours to other behaviours. For example, training in handicraft skills might increase the patient's ability to feed themselves. Two types of research for which single case experiments are *not* very appropriate are comparing two treatments (although this can be achieved using a third type of design known as 'multiple schedule'), and answering actuarial questions such as what percentage of the population improve with a particular technique.

OUTCOME MEASURES

Research in rehabilitation uses a great variety of outcome measures, e.g. activities of daily living indices, pain ratings, range of movements, electromyographic activity, grading of spasticity, gait analysis, questionnaires, psychometric tests. It is in this area of assessment however that rehabilitation research projects are most open to criticism.

In assessing outcome it is usually necessary to have a number of different measures. One advantage of multiple measures is that it results in more information being gathered. In most clinical research we are ultimately interested in how the patient functions so that measures at this level are desirable. However, there is also usually a case for assessing the more direct effects of treatment. For example, in an investigation of lower limb exercises, physiological measures of muscle strength and joint range as well as functional levels (e.g. gait) would be desirable. Another advantage of multiple measures is that they can be used for corroborating one another. For example, if the same questionnaire about activities of daily living was given independently to a patient and his spouse, and the answers agreed, one would have more confidence in the data than if the questionnaire had only been given to the patient.

Some phenomena are, of course, more difficult to measure than others. Unfortunately, all too often the phenomena of most interest are also the most difficult to measure (e.g. pain). However, there are relatively good and bad measures even of subjective states so that the emphasis is on selecting or designing the *best measures possible*. Ideally, measures should have known reliability and validity and appropriate normative data should be available. The reliability of a measure refers to its repeatability and can be assessed in various ways. Test-retest reliability is the extent to which a measure produces the same results on different occasions, whilst inter-rater reliability is the extent to which different observers obtain the same results. The validity of a measure is the degree to which it measures what it purports to measure. Normative data refer to tables of test results obtained with populations that are defined in certain ways (e.g. with and without disorders, and according to age, sex and socio-economic status), and serves as a standard for comparative purposes. Where the reliability and validity of measures is not known they can always be calculated prior to carrying out the research. Similarly, normative data may have to be collected when either none is available, or it is inappropriate.

Another important concept in measurement is that of 'blind' assessment — the assessor in a clinical trial being unaware of which treatment the patient receives. Blind assessment can be very difficult to set up as patients often make comments from which the assessor can deduce which treatment they have received. As the purpose of the assessor being 'blind' is to avoid him biasing the results, its importance depends on the degree of subjectivity present in the assessment. Hence, where the assessor is merely carrying out electromyographic recordings there is less opportunity for bias and 'blindness' is therefore less important than if he were estimating recovery on a rating scale. Other important principles of measurement include minimizing the memory component, and the use of direct observation rather than verbal report whenever possible. The former principle applies whether a clinician or patient is providing the measure. For example, if a clinician is making a rating he should do so as soon as all the information relevant to the rating has been collected. If a patient is to rate his mood, he should be asked to make *regular* ratings of his mood as it is at the moment of rating rather than try to estimate how it has been in the past. The value of direct observation derives from the fact that what *people say they do and what they actually do is often different.* Questionnaires are frequently adopted in preference to direct observation as the latter is more time consuming. In this situation there is a case for at least carrying out direct observation for some of the items on the questionnaire for all subjects, or all the items on the questionnaire for some subjects. Using direct observation in this way enables a check to be made on the validity of the questionnaire. One technique which incorporates some of these principles and is being used with increasing frequency, is instructing the patients to keep records usually referred to as 'home diaries'. The two most common forms of home diaries are patients keeping records of activities they have carried out, or recording ratings made at specified times. An example of the former would be a housewife recording all household activities she accomplishes, whilst an example of the latter would be rating pain hourly and recording the ratings. Such a system has the advantage of minimizing the memory factor in measurement — it seems likely that a more accurate picture of activities will be gained by asking the patients to record them than by asking the patients what they have done the previous week. It also results in much more detailed information being collected so that additional hypotheses can be tested. For example, hourly pain ratings enable hypotheses concerning pain cycles (e.g. daily, weekly, and monthly cycles) to be examined and the immediate effects of drugs to be assessed. Of course, such records are open to falsification, but steps can be taken to minimize the likelihood of this occurring, and also to check whether this does occur. In this respect one important factor is to keep the records simple — patients are much less likely to complete them if this involves much time or trouble. Hence, systems should be devised that enable patients merely to place a cross or a number in the appropriate place, and it should be possible for the patients to carry the records around with them (small cards are often the answer). Careful attention must be paid to how patients are instructed — they must be convinced of the value of keeping the records (to themselves as well as others), whilst every effort should be made to avoid influencing the content of the records. Some system for checking the records is obviously desirable and in the case of hourly ratings spot checks on whether the patients are uptodate with their records is one way of assessing whether patients are complying with instructions or completing the records at less regular intervals. Checks are much easier to organize when dealing with inpatients than outpatients and the help of relatives may have to be solicited when the patients are spending little time at the hospital.

Another technique which often provides a useful source of data is direct observation. One of the first questions to be considered with this approach concerns the setting in which to observe the patient. A common choice in rehabilitation is between a hospital and home setting. Both have advantages — the hospital setting can be standardized so that it is easier to compare patients' performances. However, the home setting may be adapted to the patient's needs and he will probably feel more relaxed there so that observation in this situation may result in a more realistic appraisal of functional capacities. In cases where patients' problems are influenced by the environment the procedure of choice may be to observe them in a variety of situations. For example, in an investigation concerned with gait, patients could be asked to walk a route incorporating a number of different surfaces and obstacles.

Videotape equipment can greatly assist observational assessment. The facility it provides for allowing behaviour to be shown over and over again, and run at slow speeds, makes the task of estimating the reliability and validity of measures greatly simplified. By reducing behaviour to two dimensions it also enables specialist assessment techniques to be devised. For example, a measure of the number of spasms that occur for a patient with spasmodic torticollis can be obtained by videotaping head movements and placing a grid over the television screen so that a count can be made of the number of times the patient's nose crosses one of the lines.

Two observational techniques that are particularly worthy of mention are time-sampling and event-sampling. Time-sampling proceeds by first formulating a list of behaviours that are of interest to the investigation. A time interval is then defined such that at the end of each interval the observer records which behaviour (from the check list) the subject is carrying out at that moment in time. The frequency of time-sampling and duration of observation period are determined by how long the activities being observed typically last — long lasting activities are sampled less frequently (perhaps every 60 seconds) over longer periods than brief activities (perhaps sampled every 15 seconds). The behaviours on the check list need to be clearly defined (which often requires quite considerable pilot work) for this technique to prove reliable.

Event-sampling is typically used when the behaviours to be recorded are relatively brief. Again behaviours have to be defined unambiguously and each occurrence of the behaviour is recorded. There are a number of automated event-recording devices commercially available which facilitate this technique.

DATA PRESENTATION AND ANALYSIS

Statistics tend to arouse fear and suspicion. This is unfortunate as they are a crucial part of research. The subject of statistics is typically poorly taught; courses often devote time not only to teaching endless formulae but also their mathematical derivations. Such mathematical sophistication is quite unnecessary for the majority of researchers, particularly as calculators and computers are now readily available which are capable of producing answers for anyone who can follow 'cook-book type' instructions, and most researchers can secure the assistance of a statistician. The areas in which researchers do need some knowledge are those of selection and interpretation of statistics.

It is important to point out that whilst statistics are usually mandatory with group designs they are rarely used with single case experiments. When statistics are employed in the latter type of methodology they typically are of a complexity well beyond the scope of this chapter.

All researchers are strongly advised to consult with experienced research workers and statisticians during the *planning* stages of their work.

Data presentation
The two main ways of presenting data are constructing tables and drawing graphs or diagrams. Appropriate use of these methods can save many words of text but because they are expensive to publish they should be used sparingly. In constructing tables there are several rules to follow. Most imporantly they should be kept simple and the temptation to include all available data must be

resisted. Tables should have short explanatory headings, and units of measurements indicated. Avoid spurious accuracy in the data (e.g. using numbers correct to several decimal places when the method of measurement does not justify such precision), and do not include columns of data that can easily be calculated from other columns (e.g. a column of numbers followed by a column in which the numbers have been converted to percentages).

Graphs are a particularly useful form of presentation for demonstrating the relationship between two variables. In general, the independent variable should be plotted as the abscissa (horizontal axis) and the dependent variable as the ordinate (vertical axis). The points of a graph should normally be joined by straight lines (rather than free hand). Most of the rules pertaining to tables — keeping them simple, using a self-explanatory title, including units of measurement — apply equally to graphs and diagrams generally.

Like a graph, the histogram is a diagram with a horizontal scale representing the independent variable. The scale is divided into intervals and the number of people falling into each interval noted. Rectangles are then drawn above each interval, the area being made proportional to the number of people.

A frequency distribution describes the frequency of occurrence in a population of the values of a variable. Imagine that a large sample of people is drawn from the population and the histogram constructed. If the number of people in the same sample is increased and the interval size of the histogram reduced then eventually the outline of the histogram will become a smooth curve. This will represent the frequency distribution of the population. A scatter diagram is used when pairs of observations have been obtained from a number of people and simply consists of plotting one against the other. Examples of histogram and scatter diagram appear below.

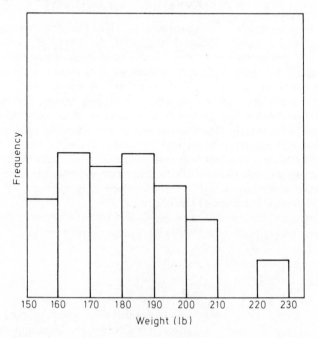

Figure 3. Histogram

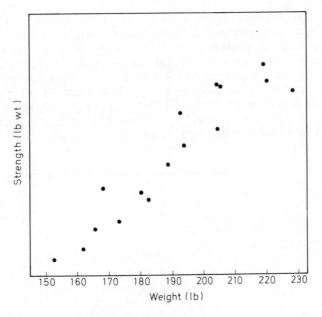

Figure 4. Scatter diagram

Other forms of data presentation include the bar chart, pie diagram, ogive and ideogram, and examples of these can be found in most textbooks.

Descriptive statistics

As their name implies, descriptive statistics are used for describing data — given that one cannot publish all the data collected they provide means of summarizing it. For any set of numbers the two main characteristics are the average value, and the variation, or scatter, about the average value. Statistics pertaining to the former are referred to as measures of central tendency and include the *mean, mode* and *median* whilst those pertaining to the latter are referred to as measures of dispersion and include the *variance, standard deviation* and *range*. The mean is the arithmetic average of the values, the mode is the most frequently occurring value, and the median is the value that divides the population into two equal parts. The standard deviation and variance can be calculated using simple formulae (or calculators) whilst the range refers to the difference between the largest and smallest values.

To explain the standard deviation more fully it is helpful to introduce the concept of the Gaussian or normal distribution. The *normal distribution* is a type of frequency distribution — one that conforms to a particular mathematical expression. Many variables in nature tend to be normally distributed (e.g. height, weight and intelligence), and much of statistical theory is based on the normal distribution. Graphically the normal distribution is a symmetrical bell-shaped curve, which shows that the most frequently occurring values are those near the mean. Returning to the standard deviation — if the data on which it is calculated are from a normal distribution then approximately 68 per cent of the population will be within one *standard deviation* of the mean, and 95 per cent will be within two standard deviations of the mean. For example: suppose the intelligence quotients (IQ) of a large number of people were tested and the frequencies of obtaining each score calculated. If these frequencies were plotted as a frequency distribution the result would be a normal distribution. One of the properties of a normal distribution is that in this special case the mean, mode and median will coincide – the value of each will be 100 for IQ. As the standard deviation for IQ is 15 the above definition leads to the conclusion that 68 per cent of the population will have an IQ between 85 (100–15) and 115 (100+15) and 95 per cent will have an IQ between 70 (100–2x15) and 130 (100+2x15). Alternatively 16 per cent will have an IQ above 115, and 2.5 per cent will have an IQ above 130.

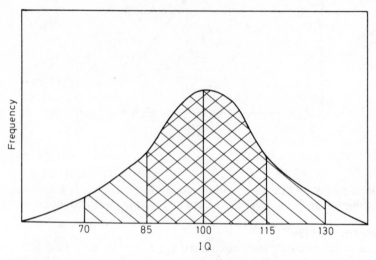

Figure 5. Normal distribution. The doubled hatched area represents 68% of the population and the total hatched area represents 95% of the population

Statistical tests
Statistical tests are used for inferring facts about a population from facts about a sample. For example, suppose treatment A is given to one group of patients and treatment B to another, and the outcome measure is ratings of improvement. It is most unlikely the average rating will be exactly the same for each group, but "are any observed differences due to chance or the fact that one treatment is 'better' than the other?" – this is the sort of question to which the statistical test is addressed.

The first stage in a test is the setting up of a *'null hypothesis'* which is always of the form that there is 'no difference' or 'no association'. This is the hypothesis the research is trying to disprove. The 'alternative hypothesis' is the converse – that the null hypothesis is false. For example, the null hypothesis might be that there is no difference between the effects of two treatments. The alternative hypothesis could be that there was a difference (without specifying the direction of the difference), or that one particular treatment was superior to the other.

Having decided upon the null and alternative hypotheses the next stage is to calculate the probability of the observed values or more extreme ones, given that the null hypothesis is true. If this probability is very low (below an arbitrary criterion) the null hypothesis is rejected in favour of the alternative hypothesis. The arbitrary criteria are referred to as 'significance levels' and the ones most commonly used are the 5 per cent and 1 per cent levels (corresponding to probability values of 0.05 and 0.01, respectively). Hence if the probability of the observed values or more extreme ones is less than 0.01 we can reject the null hypothesis at the 1 per cent level of significance (or confidence) in favour of the alternative hypothesis.

In selecting the most appropriate statistical test one of the factors to be considered is the type of measurement used. Four levels of measurement can be distinguished:

(1) *Nominal or classificatory scale* Nominal measurement consists of classification where no relation between the categories exists. Examples would be classifying objects according to colour or patients according to diagnostic group.

(2) *Ordinal or ranking scale* Ordinal measurement occurs when the categories stand in relation to one another (relations such as 'greater than', 'higher than', 'more difficult than'). Examples would be classifying according to grades in the military services or socioeconomic status.

(3) *Interval scale* An interval scale has all the characteristics of an ordinal scale but in addition the distances between any two numbers on the scale are of known size. Examples would be the centigrade and Fahrenheit scales of measuring temperature.

(4) *Ratio scale* A ratio scale has all the characteristics of an interval scale and in addition has a true zero point as its origin. Examples would be the scales we use for measuring weight or length.

The statistical tests available can be divided into *parametric* and *nonparametric* tests. Parametric tests require that the scores under analysis result from measurement on an interval or ratio scale, and make various assumptions about the parameters of the population from which the research sample was drawn. For example, the observations must be independent and drawn from normally distributed populations and the populations must have an equal variance. Nonparametric tests can be used on scores resulting from measurement on any type of scale and do not specify conditions about the parameters of the populations from which the sample was drawn. Common examples of parametric tests include Student's t-test and analysis of variance, whilst examples of nonparametric tests include Chi-square and the sign test.

Correlation and regression methods
Correlation and regression methods have been developed for describing the association between variables and providing a basis for prediction of one variable, given the value of another. The degree of association or correlation between two variables is described in terms of a scale ranging from −1 through zero to +1. Values of −1 and +1 are the maximum correlations theoretically possible in which variation in one variable is accompanied by exactly corresponding variation in the other. The sign of the values indicates the direction of the relationship – a negative correlation indicates one variable increases whilst the other decreases, and a positive correlation indicates both increase or decrease

together. Zero correlation signifies absolute unpredictability of variation in one variable from the other. A rough idea of the correlation between two variables can be gained by plotting a scatter diagram as described previously.

There are various types of correlation and the appropriate one to use is determined by similar factors to those involved in the selection of statistical tests. For example, calculation of a Pearson product-moment correlation coefficient requires data from an interval or ratio scale, but calculation of a Spearman's rank correlation coefficient only requires data from an ordinal scale.

Having calculated a correlation coefficient it may then be of interest to assess its significance by a statistical test. The purpose of such a test is to estimate to what extent the correlation reflects a real relationship, taking into account the degree to which it is expected to vary because of chance factors.

Predictions of the value of one variable from the values of another variable is usually accomplished by calculating a regression equation which can be done once a correlation has been calculated.

WRITING FOR PUBLICATION

Although different journals require their own individual variations in presentation, the format of a research report typically contains the following sections: introduction, aims, methods, results, discussion, and summary. The introduction should show how previous work leads up to the questions to be asked, which should be clearly stated in the second section: Description of the method should include the apparatus used, the experimental design and reasons for its choice, details of the subject population, and the procedures adopted. The results section is likely to contain tables, graphs, and diagrams as outlined above. It should also contain a verbal account of the main findings. The discussion should say whether the results support the experimental hypotheses, how the findings relate to other published work, and suggestions for future research. The summary should include why the work was done, how it was accomplished, what was found, and what the results suggest. Reports should be free of ambiguity, orderly in their presentation of ideas, and smooth in flow. Colloquial expressions and cliches should be avoided and jargon kept to a minimum. A good test of a paper's readability is whether it is comprehensible to an educated layman.

The title of the paper is important as it largely determines whether the paper is read. In selecting the most appropriate title an effort should be made to balance a high information content with a style that attracts the reader. Headings in the more reputable journals will provide useful models in this respect.

Short words are easier to comprehend than long ones but there are times when one long word expresses an idea better than several short words. Writing only in short simple sentences produces choppy prose but writing exclusively in long, involved sentences creates difficult, if not unreadable material. Varying sentence length gives writing relief and interest. Similar comments apply to the length of paragraphs.

Sudden shifts in tense should be avoided. Past tense is usually appropriate for a literature review or describing the experimental design and procedure inasmuch as it is a historical account. Present tense should be used to describe and discuss the results that are literally there before the reader. Future tense is rarely needed. Frequently an author uses synonyms or near-synonyms to avoid repetition of a term. Although this intention is laudable the result may seriously detract from the flow of the paper. When a synonym is used the reader cannot know if the intention is to convey the same meaning as the first term or if a subtle difference in meaning is intended. If monotony occurs it may be from repeating ideas as well as words.

The tradition of using the third person, passive voice, in scientific writing is gradually disappearing and most journals no longer insist on this style. The argument that it preserves objectivity is no longer accepted and some use of the first person, active voice, is generally encouraged.

Several strategies can contribute to producing a coherent paper such as recording it on tape and playing it back. Asking a colleague to criticize a paper often leads to valuable comments, particularly if the critic is from outside the specialist research area. Re-reading a paper several days or weeks after completing a first draft is a useful strategy for approaching the paper with a fresh perspective.

BIBLIOGRAPHY AND REFERENCES

American Psychological Association Publication Manual. 2nd edn. (1974). American Psychological Association

Armitage, P. (1974). *Statistical Methods in Medical Research*. Blackwells Scientific Publications

Bennett, A. E. and Ritchie, K. (1975). *Questionnaires in Medicine*. Oxford University Press.

Bolton, B. (1974). *Introduction to Rehabilitation Research*. Chas. C. Thomas.

Hayslett, M. S. (1967). *Statistics Made Simple*. W. H. Allen

Hersen, M. and Barlow, D. M. (1976). *Single Case Experimental Design: Strategies for Studying Behaviour Change*. Pergamon General Psychology Series

Maxwell, C. (1973). *Clinical Research for All*. Cambridge Medical Publications Ltd.

Morton, L. (1977). *Use of Medical Literature*. Butterworths

Nichols, P. J. R. (1975). 'Some psychosocial aspects of rehabilitation and their implications in research'. *Proc. Roy. Soc. Med.* 68, 537–544

Scientific Affairs Board. (1978). 'Ethical principles for research with human subjects'. *Bull. Brit. Psychol. Soc.* 31, 48–9

Thorne, C. (1970). *Better Medical Writing*. Pitman Medical and Scientific Co.

Index